Nursing Education and Quality Assurance in Nursing Colleges

Shyamala D Manivannan
RN RM MSc (N) PhD (N)
Professor and Director
Faculty of Nursing
Dr MGR Educational and Research Institute
Chennai, Tamil Nadu, India

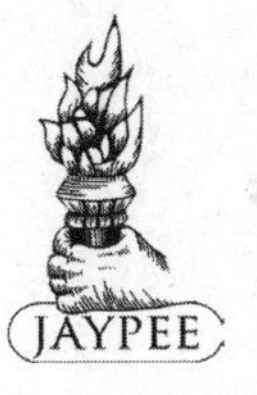

The Health Sciences Publisher
New Delhi | London | Panama | Philadelphia

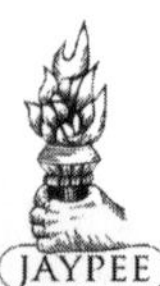

Jaypee Brothers Medical Publishers (P) Ltd

Headquarters

Jaypee Brothers Medical Publishers (P) Ltd.
4838/24, Ansari Road, Daryaganj
New Delhi 110 002, India
Phone: +91-11-43574357
Fax: +91-11-43574314
Email: jaypee@jaypeebrothers.com

Overseas Offices

J.P. Medical Ltd.
83, Victoria Street, London
SW1H 0HW (UK)
Phone: +44-20 3170 8910
Fax: +44-(0)20 3008 6180
Email: info@jpmedpub.com

JP Medical Inc.
325 Chestnut Street, Ste 412
Philadelphia, PA 19106
Phone: +1-267-519-9789
Email: support@jpmedus.com

Jaypee Brothers Medical Publishers (P) Ltd.
Bhotahity, Kathmandu, Nepal
Phone: +977-9741283608
Email: kathmandu@jaypeebrothers.com

Jaypee-Highlights Medical Publishers Inc.
City of Knowledge, Bld. 237, Clayton
Panama City, Panama
Phone: +1 507-301-0496
Fax: +1 507-301-0499
Email: cservice@jphmedical.com

Jaypee Brothers Medical Publishers (P) Ltd.
17/1-B, Babar Road, Block-B, Shaymali
Mohammadpur, Dhaka-1207, Bangladesh
Mobile: +08801912003485
Email: jaypeedhaka@gmail.com

Website: www.jaypeebrothers.com
Website: www.jaypeedigital.com

Nursing Education and Quality Assurance in Nursing Colleges

First Edition: **2016**

ISBN: 978-93-85999-13-0

Printed at Rajkamal Electric Press, Plot No. 2, Phase-IV, Kundli, Haryana.

Dedicated to

This book is dedicated to my parents, Late Sri A Padmanaba Iyer and Smt S Venkattammal, and my teachers, who introduced me to this noble profession.

Preface

A learner tries to do many tasks during the journey of his/her education. Learning is an ongoing task that requires people to be lifelong learners to get the complete taste of education. Sharing the knowledge is the significant task of our caring profession. Learning and teaching are the two inseparable activities which complement each other and perpetuate an individual's life. Providing education and assuring quality are the two responsible activities that promote the excellence in teaching and learning. Statutory bodies of general and nursing education expect the educational institutions to assure quality and excellence in nursing education. Statutory bodies provide guidelines and assess nursing institutions to assure quality education to provide good-quality nursing care to the society.

Nursing Education and Quality Assurance in Nursing Colleges is packed under four sections. First section talks about the philosophies of education and nursing image. Second section deals with the essentials of curriculum, which are discussed in detail and provide the basis for curriculum planning and development. Teaching and learning process occupies the third section. This section explains the teaching and learning process. Quality assurance section runs in four chapters under the fourth section. This explains in detail about the quality assurance process in the nursing colleges that are built keeping in mind the mission, vision and objectives of the nursing schools and colleges. In addition, research works related to certain chapters are highlighted for enhancing the students' knowledge in the field of application and integration of the current learning.

This book addresses various aspects and also the quality assurance in nursing education. It also deals with the essential elements of nursing education and covers the syllabus for the undergraduate and postgraduate nursing students. It would be useful to the undergraduate as well as the postgraduate nursing students and teachers, who are the major components of teaching, learning and the quality assurance process of nursing. Enhancing the readers' knowledge would assure quality nursing education that further leads to assuring quality care to the society.

Shyamala D Manivannan

Acknowledgments

The provision of opportunity, motivation, timely support, help and encouragement are the most essential factors that take a project to the desired point of destiny. I would like to submit my thanks to the Lord Almighty for providing me the necessary wisdom and strength to complete this project. I would like to extend my thanks to all my teachers (who are deeply seated in my heart), and friends and philosophers of various disciplines who molded me. I would like to extend my love and thanks to my husband, A Manivannan for his continuous moral support and encouragement to complete this work. My affectionate hugs and thanks to my son, Karthik, my daughter Sinduja, and my daughter-in-law, Abhilasha Karthik for providing me a supportive environment.

I cannot find enough words to express my gratitude to Jaypee Brothers Medical Publishers (P) Ltd, New Delhi, India for their acceptance in publishing the work, and their professionalism during the entire process. I am especially grateful to Shri Jitendar P Vij (Group Chairman), Mr Ankit Vij (Group President), Ms Chetna Malhotra Vohra (Associate Director), Ms Payal Bharti (Project Manager), Mr Samir Khan (Project Coordinator), Mr Harsh Pal Singh Rawat (Graphic Designer), and Mr Manas Yadav (Typesetter) for shaping up the book and making all the changes without any complaints.

INC Syllabus

MSc (Nursing)

Nursing Education

I. Introduction

Education: Definition, aims, concepts, philosophies and their educational implications, impact of social, economic, political and technological changes on education:

- Professional education
- Current trends and issues in education
- Educational reforms and National Educational Policy, various educational commissions-reports
- Trends in development of nursing education in India.

II. Teaching learning process

Concepts of teaching and learning: Definition, theories of teaching and learning, relationship between teaching and learning.

Educational aims and objectives; types, domains, levels, elements and writing of educational objectives.

Competency-based education (CBE) and outcome-based education (OBE).

Instructional design: Planning and designing the lesson.

Writing lesson plan: Meaning, need and importance, formats.

Instruction strategies: Lecture, discussion, demonstration, simulation, laboratory, seminar, panel, symposium, problem-solving, problem-based learning (PBL), workshop, project, role-play (socio-drama), clinical teaching methods, programmed instruction, self-directed learning (SDL), micro-teaching, computer-assisted instruction (CAI), computer-assisted learning (CAL).

III. Instructional media and methods

Key concepts in the selection and use of media in education.

Developing learning resource material using different media.

Instructional aids: Types, uses, selection, preparation, and utilization.

Teacher's role in procuring and managing instructional aids: Projected and nonprojected aids, multimedia, video-teleconferencing, etc.

IV. Measurement and evaluation

Concept and nature of measurement and evaluation, meaning, process, purposes, problems in evaluation and measurement.

Principles of assessment, formative and summative assessment, internal assessment, external examination, advantages and disadvantages.

Criterion and norm-referenced evaluation.

V. Standardized and nonstandardized tests

Meaning, characteristics, objectivity, validity, reliability, usability, norms, construction of tests.

Essay, short-answer questions and multiple-choice questions.

Rating scales, checklist, OSCE/OSPE (Objective structured clinical/practical examination).

Differential scales, and summated scales, sociometry, anecdotal record, attitude scale, critical incident technique.

Question bank: Preparation, validation, moderation by panel, utilization.

Developing a system for maintaining confidentiality.

VI. Administration, scoring and reporting

Administering a test; scoring, grading versus marks.

Objective tests, scoring essay test, methods of scoring, item analysis.

VII. Standardized tools

Tests of intelligence: Aptitude, interest, personality, achievement, socio-economic status scale, tests for special mental and physical abilities and disabilities.

VIII. Nursing educational programs

Perspectives of nursing education: Global and national.

Patterns of nursing education and training programmes in India. Non-university and university programs: ANM, GNM, Basic BSc Nursing, Post Certificate BSc Nursing, MSc (N) programs, MPhil and PhD) in Nursing, Post Basic Diploma programs, nurse practitioner programs.

IX. Continuing education in nursing

Concepts, definition, importance, need, scope, principles of adult learning, assessments of learning, needs, priorities, resources.

Program planning, implementation and evaluation of continuing education programs.

Research in continuing education.

Distance education in nursing.

X. Curriculum development

Definition, curriculum determinants, process and steps of curriculum development, curriculum models, types and framework.

Formulation of philosophy, objectives, selection and organization of learning experiences; master plan, course plan, unit plan.

Evaluation strategies, process of curriculum change, role of students, faculty, administrators, statutory bodies and other stakeholders.

Equivalency of courses: Transcripts, credit system.

XI. Teacher's preparation

Teacher: Roles and responsibilities, functions, characteristics, competencies, qualities.

Preparation of a professional teacher.

Organizing professional aspects of teacher preparation programs.

Evaluation: Self and peer.

Critical analysis of various programs of teacher's education in India.

XII. Guidance and counseling

Concept, principles, need, difference between guidance and counseling, trends and issues.

Guidance and counseling services: Diagnostic and remedial.

Coordination and organization of services.

Techniques of counseling: Interview, case work, characteristics of a counselor, problems in counseling.

Professional preparation and training for counseling.

XIII. Administration of nursing curriculum

Roles of a curriculum coordinator: Planning, implementation and evaluation.

Evaluation of educational programs in nursing: Course and program.

Factors influencing faculty staff relationship and techniques of working together.

Concept of faculty supervisor (dual) position.

Curriculum research in nursing.

Different models of collaboration between education and service

XIV. Management of nursing educational institutions

Planning, organizing, staffing, budgeting, recruitment, discipline, public relation, performance appraisal, welfare services, library services, hostel.

XV. Development and maintenance of standards and accreditation in nursing education programs

Role of Indian Nursing Council, State Registration Nursing Councils, Boards and University.

Role of professional associations and unions.

Contents

Section I

Education and Nursing Education

1. Education
2. General Branches of Philosophy and Its Elements
3. Idealism
4. Naturalism
5. Pragmatism
6. Modern Philosophies of Education
7. Nursing Image and Nursing Profession

1

Education

Chapter Highlights

- Origin and Meaning of Education
- Concept of Education and Emergence of Philosophers
- Definition of Education
- Nature of Education
- Aims of Education
- Special Features of Education
- Different Aims of Education

Learning Objectives

Upon completion of this chapter, the students will be able to:

- State the origin and meaning of education
- Define education
- List the aims of education
- Describe the special features of education
- State the origin and meaning of education
- Interpret the nature of education
- List the special features of education
- Classify the different aims of education

INTRODUCTION

A born baby does not speak any particular language. It does not know its language, religion, caste, creed and wealth for the matter anything of this world except the warmth and comfort and its hunger and pain. During second month of its life, the baby recognizes the mother tries to make cooing sound. Where does it learn this? Baby starts learning in a nonformal way. The environment takes the role to teach the baby. From the womb to tomb, the man repeatedly undergoes one or the other learning practice that enriches him to be a social being. All these are act of education. Education is not alone the content oriented paper pencil work in the formal venues like schools and colleges. During life, any self-learning practice or others to self that modify some behavior or inculcate some new behavior is education. Education enables us achieve our fullest potentials in all aspects of our life. Educated are addressed as cultured. Education helps man to climb in a ladder of social respect. Through education, he develops all round abilities and earns his lively bread. Educated are well behaved and able to disseminate the knowledge to the followers. Educated can become as the teacher, mentor and guide of their family, friends and society. Society opens the ears to educated, develops and accepts them as role models and leaders. Education can maintain, strengthen the health of the family, nation and ultimately the world. We do not deny the fact that comforting technology oriented life of today is the gift of education. Education does wonders in every individual and empowers the human brains to walk in the earth and communicate to the moon and Mars. Education is so important that it will continue even in eternity.

Education has been described as a process of waking up to life: Ancient Tamil poet Thiruvalluvar in his Thirukkural,

"Men who learning gain have eyes, men say;
Blockheads' faces pairs of sores display.
The deeper a sand-well is dug the freer is its flow of water.
Even so, the deeper a man's learning the greater is his wisdom.
The learned make each land their own, in every city find a home;
Who, till they die, learn naught, along what weary ways they roam!"

MEANING OF THE WORD 'EDUCATION'

In English the term 'Education' has been derived from two Latin words Educare (Educere) and Educatum. The educatum word itself is composed of two words, 'E' and 'Duco'. 'E' means a progress from inward to outward while 'duco' means developing or progressing. Therefore education means developing from inside to outside. 'Educare' means to train or mold. It again means to bring up or to lead out or to draw out, propulsion from inward to outward. The term 'Educatum' denotes the act of teaching. It throws light on the principles and practice of teaching. The term Educare or Educere mainly indicates development of the latent faculties of the child. However, child does not know these possibilities. It is the educator or the teacher who can know these and take appropriate methods to develop those powers.

In Hindi, the term 'Siksha' has come from the Sanskrit word 'Shash'. 'Shash' means to discipline, to control, to order, to direct, to rule, etc. Education in the traditional sense means controlling or disciplining the behavior of an individual. In Sanskrit 'Shiksha' is a particular branch of the Sutra literature, which has six branches –Shiksh, Chhanda, Byakarana, Nirukta, Jyotisha and Kalpa. The Sutra literature was designed to learn the Vedas. Siksha denotes rules of pronunciation. There is another term in Sanskrit, which throws light on the nature of education. It is 'Vidya' which means knowledge. The term 'Vidya' has originated from 'Bid' meaning knowledge.

CONCEPT OF EDUCATION AND EMERGENCE OF PHILOSOPHERS

Children are born illiterate and innumerate, and ignorant of the norms and cultural achievements of the community or society into which they have been thrust; but with the help of professional teachers and the dedicated amateurs in their families and immediate environs (educational resources made available through the media and nowadays the internet), within a few years they can read, write, calculate, and act in culturally-appropriate ways. Some are born in wealthy background others are not so; some learn these skills with more facility than others and so education also serves as a social-sorting mechanism and undoubtedly has enormous impact on the economic fate of the individual.

Education being an important social domain has attracted the attention of philosophers for thousands of years; especially the complex issues of education have attracted great philosophical thoughts. Dewey pointed out that the primary ineluctable facts of the birth and death of each one of the constituent members in a social group make education a necessity, for despite this biological inevitability —the life of the group goes on (Dewey, 3).

DEFINITIONS OF EDUCATION

Here are some of the definitions given by the great educators of the east and the west to have a clearer picture of the nature and meaning of the term education:

- Education is the manifestation of perfection already in man. Like fire in a piece of flint, knowledge exists in the mind. Suggestion is the friction; which brings it out. —*Swami Vivekananda*
- By education I mean an all-round drawing out of the best in child and man's body, mind and spirit. —*Mahatma Gandhi*
- The highest education is that which does not merely give us information but makes our life in harmony with all existence. —*Rabindranath Tagore*
- Education is something, which makes a man self-reliant and self-less. —*Rigveda*
- Education is that whose end product is salvation. —*Upanishada*
- Education according to Indian tradition is not merely a means of earning a living; nor it is only a nursery of thought or a school for citizenship. It is initiation into the life of spirit and training of human souls in the pursuit of truth and the practice of virtue. —*Radhakrishnan*
- Education develops in the body and soul of the pupil all the beauty and all the perfection he is capable of. —*Plato*
- Education is the creation of sound mind in a sound body. It develops man's faculty specially his mind so that he may be able to enjoy the contemplation of supreme truth, goodness and beauty. —*Aristotle*
- Education is the child's development from within. —*Rousseau*
- Education is enfoldment of what is already enfolded in the germ. It is the process through which the child makes the internal-external. —*Froebel*
- Education is the harmonious and progressive development of all the innate powers and faculties of man-physical, intellectual and moral. —*Pestalozzi*
- Education is the development of good moral character. —*J.F. Herbert*
- Education is not a preparation for life, rather it is the living. Education is the process of living through a continuous reconstruction of experiences. It is the development of all those capacities in the individual which will enable him to control his environment and fulfill his possibilities. —*John Dewey*
- Education is the complete development of the individuality of the child so that he can make an original contribution to human life according to the best of his capacity. —*T.P. Nunn*
- Education according to George Knight (1980) is a lifelong learning process that can take place in an infinite variety of circumstances and contexts.
- According to Kleining (1985), education is 'The range of activities both formal and informal whereby people are initiated into or realigned with the evolving traditions, structures, and social relations which are taken to constitute their education.'
- Peter (1975) wrote: 'Education consists in initiating others into activities, modes of conduct and thoughts which have standards written into them by references to which it is possible to act, think and feel with varying degrees of relevance and taste.'
- True education means more than the pursue of a certain course of study. It means more than a preparation for the life that now is. It has to do with the whole being and with the whole period of existence possible to man. It is the harmonious development of the physical, the mental, and the spiritual powers. It prepares the student for the joy of service in this world and for the higher joy of wider service in the world to come (White, 1903, p13).

Different educationists have defined education in various ways. It is hard to give a specific definition on education since it is very vast. Each definition differs from others except in few common aspects. Different philosophers have different perceptions and interpretations on concepts of education. Some educationists have defined only one aspect of education whereas the others emphasize its other phases. According to Idealists, the aim of life is spiritual development. As such, they regard education as a spiritual process, which aims at bringing together the soul and the creator leading to self-realization. Pragmatists think about education as a process of social progress. Actually, education is a sort of synthesis of all the above viewpoints.

NATURE OF EDUCATION

As the meaning of education, its nature too is very complex. The natures of education are:

- ***Education is life long process*** because every stage of life of an individual is important from educational point.
- ***Education is a systematic process:*** Refers to transact its activities through a systematic institution and regulation.
- ***Education is development of individual and the society:*** A force for social development, which brings improvement in every aspect in the society.
- ***Education is modification of behavior:*** Human behavior modified or improved through educational process.
- ***Education is a training:*** Human senses, mind, behavior, activities; skills are trained in a constructive and socially desirable way.
- ***Education is instruction and direction:*** It directs and instructs an individual to fulfill his desires and needs for exaltation of his whole personality.
- ***Education is life:*** Life without education is meaningless and like the life of a beast. Every aspect and incident needs education for its sound development.
- ***Education is continuous reconstruction of our experiences:*** As per the definition of John Dewey education reconstructs and remodels our experiences towards socially desirable way.
- ***Education is a power and treasure in human being*** through which he is entitled as the supreme master on the earth.

Therefore, the role of education is countless for a perfect man and society. It is necessary for every society and nation to bring holistic happiness and prosperity to its individuals.

NEED FOR AIMS OF EDUCATION

Education is a purposeful activity. By education, we intend to bring certain desirable changes in the students. Education is a conscious effort and, as such, it has definite aims and objectives. In the light of these aims, the curriculum is determined and the academic achievements of the student are measured. Education without aim is building without a foundation. Aims give direction to activity. Absence of an aim in education makes it a blind alley. Every stage of human development had some aim of life. The aims of life determine aims of education.

SPECIAL FEATURES OF EDUCATION

Education is both unilateral as well as bi-polar in nature.

- It is a continuous process.
- It is knowledge or experience.

- It is development of particular aspects of human personality or a harmonious integrated growth.
- It is conducive for the good of the individual or the welfare of the society.
- It is a liberal discipline or a vocational course.
- It is stabilizer of social order, conservator of culture, an instrument of change and social reconstruction.

Primary Aims of Education

Concerning Philosophical Principles the primary aim of education in the broadest sense is to 'form a man' or to help a child attain full formation or completeness as a man.

The other broader aims of education

- To convey the heritage of culture of a given area of civilization,
- To prepare for life in society and for good citizenship
- To secure mental equipment required for implementing a particular function in the social whole for performing family responsibilities, and for making a living.
- The above mentioned are corollaries and essential but secondary aims.

Parenthetically, education in the broad sense of the word continues during the entire lifetime of every one of us. The school system is only a partial and inchoative agency with respect to the task of education. Man learns through every moment of his life formally or informally. Each learning task, constantly prepares man to be a cultured person with certain moral and ethical values.

CLASSIFICATION OF DIFFERENT AIMS OF EDUCATION

The aims of education can be classified under various headings.

The vocational aim: The vocational aim is also known as 'the utilitarian aim or the bread and butter aim.' Education must help the child to earn his livelihood. Education, therefore, must prepare the child for some future profession or vocation or trade. The vocational aim is a narrow aim of education. Therefore, the vocational aim is not a complete aim by itself.

The knowledge or information aim: Knowledge is indispensable for all right action and it is the source of all power. It is knowledge which makes a realist a visionary successful in any profession. Knowledge makes a person wiser in nature. Information is the wealth of the individual.

The culture aim: Man has no culture when he is born. The cultural aim of education is recommended to supplement the narrow view of knowledge aim. The cultural aim of education is no doubt a nice aim as it produces men of culture. However, the cultural aim is ambiguous and has too many meanings. It cannot serve as the major aim of education. Nevertheless, any educational curriculum emerges out of cultural commitments and constraints.

The character formation aim or the moral aim: Character is the very basic of life and, as such, it should be the aim of education. Vivekananda and Gandhiji both emphasized character building in education. Character formation or moral education is concerned with the whole conduct of man. The Secondary Education Commission (1951–52) stated that the character education has to be visualized with reference to contemporary socioeconomic and political situation.

The spiritual aim: The idealist thinkers have opined that the spiritual development of an individual should be the supreme aim of education. Spirituality gives strength, wisdom and good direction for life and the adjustments. Mahatma Gandhi has attached great importance to spiritual values in education.

The adjustment aim: Adjustment is the basic for human life. He has to adjust to environment and other living and nonliving things of his environment. None can survive without adjustment. Life is a struggle for adjustment. In the words of Horney: Education should be man's adjustment to his nature, to his fellows and to the ultimate nature of the cosmos.

The leisure aim: Leisure equals the 'Free and unoccupied time' of an individual. This leisure time must be utilized in a creative way. During leisure we can pursue an activity for own sake and not for earning a living, which is dull and monotonous. During leisure, we can also regain our lost energy and enthusiasm. Leisure can make our life dynamic and charming. A person can work for his own choices in his leisure time. Person actually refreshes his mind during leisure time.

The citizenship training aim: Education should help children perform and discharge their various civic duties and responsibilities successfully. The Secondary Education Commission in India (1951–1952) has greatly emphasized citizenship training in schools. Such training includes the development of certain qualities to character such as clear thinking, clearness in speech and writing, art of community living, cooperation, toleration, and sense of patriotism and sense of world citizenship.

The complete living aim: Some educationists have insisted upon the need of an all-comprehensive aim of education. This viewpoint has led to the development of two aims—'the complete living aim' and the 'harmonious development aim.' According to Horney 'there is no one final aim, subordinating all lesser aims to itself… There is something in all these aims but not everything in anyone of them.'

The harmonious development aim: Educationists are of the opinion that all the powers and capacities inherited by a child should be developed harmoniously and simultaneously. Gandhi is a strong advocate of the harmonious development.

The social aim: Man is a social animal. No individual can live and grow without social context. Individual life became boring to man and that is why he formed society. Individual security and welfare depend on the society. Individual improvement is conditioned by social progress. Education should make each individual socially efficient. A socially efficient individual is able to earn his livelihood amidst of all the enjoyments as a complete man in the society.

Conclusion

Education concentrates on various aspects of mankind. Many philosophers were attracted to contribute to education because it is a social subject with complex issues. Literature reveals that the philosophers viewed few issues in common and as well they are repeated by the followers. Some of them are character building, man making, harmonious human development, preparation for adult life, -development of citizenship, utilization of leisure, training for civic life, training for international living, achieving social and national integration, scientific and technological development, education for all, equalizing educational opportunities, strengthening democratic political order and human source development. The ultimatum is developing a good human being.

2

General Branches of Philosophy and Its Elements

Chapter Highlights

- Meaning of Philosophy
- Scope of Philosophy of Education
- Metaphysics
- Importance of Metaphysics
- Elements of Metaphysics
- Metaphysics Sub-branches
- Axiology
- Importance of Ethics
- The Key Elements of Ethics
- Esthetics
- Importance of Esthetics
- Elements of Esthetics
- Politics
- Epistemology
- Typical Epistemological Questions
- Importance of Epistemology
- Elements of Epistemology

Learning Objectives

Upon completion of this chapter, the students will be able to:

- State the meaning of philosophy
- List the main branches of philosophy
- Describe the elements of metaphysics, axiology and epistemology
- Explain the scope of philosophy of education
- Describe the importance of metaphysics, axiology and epistemology

INTRODUCTION

Generally philosophy means the maturation of thoughts. Tacit thoughts and ideas gets molded with experience and comes in established form for open sharing. The ideas of Aristotle and Plato still serve today as models of clear and rational thinking about highly abstract and difficult questions. Philosophy makes real foundation for critical thinking and analytical abilities. No organization runs without philosophy and no curriculum building without the philosophical foundations.

MEANING OF PHILOSOPHY

Why Do We Learn Philosophy

Philosophy helps us learn about ourselves and the world. It teaches us how to grapple intelligently with basic questions such as:

- "Who am I?"
- "Does God exist?"
- "How should I live?"

- "Should I do what society tells me to do?"
- "Can I be sure of any of my beliefs?
- "Does my life have meaning?
- "Are values just a matter of opinion?"
- "What is the nature of mind, language, and thought?"

Philosophy means 'love of wisdom.' It is made-up of two Greek words, Philo, meaning love, and sophos, meaning wisdom. Philosophy helps teachers to reflect on key issues and concepts in education, usually through such questions as: What is being educated? What is the good life? What is the nature of learning? What is teaching? Philosophers think about the meaning of things and interpretation of that meaning.

SCOPE OF PHILOSOPHY OF EDUCATION

Different scholars view philosophy in using their own perceived ideas, opinions and experiences. There are some definitions given by some philosophers defining this as a method of experience and other few have stated that it is a comprehensive synthetic science.

Philosophy is a Critical Method of Approaching Experience

- Edgar S Brightman: 'Philosophy is essentially a spirit or method of approaching experience rather than a body of conclusions about experience'.
- Clifford Barrat: 'it is not the specific content or these conclusions, but the spirit and method by which they are reached, which entitles them to be described as philosophical.'
- CJ Ducasse: 'where I limited to one line for my answer to it, I should say that philosophy is general theory of criticism.'

Philosophy develops our ability to: Reason clearly
- Distinguish between good and bad arguments
- Think and write
- Clearly see the big picture Look at different views and opinions.

*Nurses need to definitely build the above abilities to function as a professional.

Philosophy is a comprehensive synthetic science.

- Joseph A Leighton: 'philosophy, like science, consists of theories of insight arrived at as a result of systematic reflection.'
- Herbert Spencer: 'philosophy is concerned with everything as a universal science'
- Roy Wood Sellers: 'our subject is a collection of sciences, such as theory of knowledge, logic cosmology, ethics and aesthetics as well as a unified survey'.

Philosophy of education is one of the areas of applied philosophy. This include the main branches of philosophy namely 'metaphysics, axiology and epistemology.

Metaphysics

It is the study of the ultimate nature of reality. This deals with issues of reality, God, freedom and the soul. Metaphysics is the branch of philosophy responsible for the study of existence. It is the foundation of a world view. It is concerned with explaining the fundamental nature of being and the world. *Metaphysics* is the study of the nature of things. Metaphysicians ask what kinds of things exist, and what they are like. They reason about such things as whether or not people have free will, in what sense abstract objects can be said to exist, and how it is that brains are able to generate minds.

Typical metaphysical questions: What is reality?
Does God exist, and if so, can we prove it?
Are human actions free, or are they determined by some forces outside of our control?
Do minds/souls exist, or are humans simply complex physical objects?
What is time? What is the meaning of life?

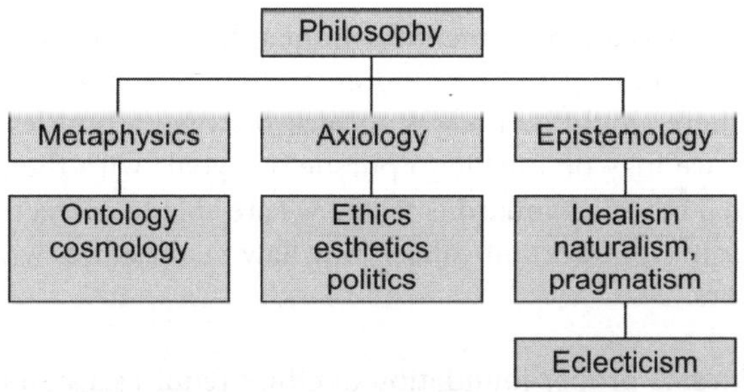

Fig. 2.1: Main branches of philosophy

Importance of metaphysics : Metaphysics is the foundation of philosophy. Without an explanation or an interpretation of the world around us, we would be helpless to deal with reality. We could not feed ourselves, or act to preserve our lives. The degree to which our metaphysical world view is correct is the degree to which we are able to comprehend the world, and act accordingly. Without this firm foundation, all knowledge becomes suspect. Any flaw in our view of reality will make it more difficult to live.

Elements of metaphysics: Reality is absolute. It has a specific nature independent of our thoughts or feelings. The world around us is real. It has a specific nature and it must be consistent to that nature. A proper metaphysical world view must aim to understand reality correctly.

The physical world exists, and every entity has a specific nature. It acts according to that nature. When different entities interact, they do so according to the nature of both. Every action has a cause and an effect. Causality is the means by which change occurs, but the change occurs via a specific nature.

Metaphysics sub-branches

Ontology: What issues are related to nature, existence, or being? Is child inherently evil or good? How might your view determine your classroom management?
Cosmology: What is the nature and origin of the cosmos or universe? Is the world and universe orderly or is it marked by chaos? What would one or the other mean for a classroom?

Axiology

Deals with issues of value in three areas: Ethics, social/political philosophy, and esthetics. *Ethics* The study of moral principles, attempts to establish rational grounds for good conduct. Ethics is the branch of study dealing with what is the proper course of action for man. It answers the question, 'What do I do?' It is the study of right and wrong in human endeavors. At a more fundamental level, it is a method to categorize our values and pursue them.

- Typical ethical questions:
- What is good/bad?
- What is right/wrong?
- What is the foundation of moral principles?
- Are moral principles universal?

Importance of ethics: Ethics is a requirement for human life. It is our means of deciding a course of action. Without it, our actions would be random and aimless. There would be no way to work towards a goal because there would be no way to pick between a limitless number of goals. Even with an ethical standard, we may be unable to pursue our goals with the possibility of success. To the degree which a rational ethical standard is taken, we are able to correctly organize our goals and actions to accomplish our most important values. Any flaw in our ethics will reduce our ability to be successful in our endeavors.

The key elements of ethics: A proper foundation of ethics requires a standard of value to which all goals and actions can be compared to. This standard is our own lives, and the happiness which makes them livable. This is our ultimate standard of value, the goal in which an ethical man must always aim. It is arrived at by an examination of man's nature, and recognizing his peculiar needs. A system of ethics must further consist of not only emergency situations, but the day to day choices we make constantly. It must include our relations to others, and recognize their importance not only to our physical survival, but to our well-being and happiness. It must recognize that our lives are an end in themselves, and that sacrifice is not only not necessary, but destructive.

Esthetics

Esthetics is the study of art. It includes what art consists of, as well as the purpose behind it. Does art consist of music, literature, and painting? Or does it include a good engineering solution, or a beautiful sunset? These are the questions that aimed at in esthetics. It also studies methods of evaluating art, and allows judgments of the art. Is art in the eye of the beholder? Does anything that appeals to you fit under the umbrella of art? Or does it have a specific nature? Does it accomplish a goal?

Importance of esthetics: Art has existed through all of recorded human history. It is unique to humans because of our unique form of thinking. Its importance is based on this nature, specifically, man's ability to abstract. Art is a little understood tool of man to bring meaning to abstract concept. Esthetics is important because it delves into the reason why art has always existed, the burning need of mankind through the ages to see the world in a different, clear way. It further evaluates art by the standard of human life, and whether it accomplishes the job of satisfying man's intellectual needs, or whether it tends to hurt or make worse those needs.

Elements of esthetics: Art is a selective recreation of reality. Its purpose is to concretize an abstraction to bring an idea or emotion within the grasp of the observer. It is a selective recreation, with the selection process depending on the value judgments of the creator. These value judgments can be observed and evaluated via the field of ethics.

Politics: Politics is ethics applied to a group of people. Politics tells you how a society must be set up and how one should act within a society. Except for hermits, this comes up a lot.

The requirement for a political system is that the individuals within that system are allowed to fully function according to their nature. If that's not the case, they will either rebel, as in Czarist Russia, or the system will eventually collapse, as in Communist Russia.

Reason is man's prime means of survival. A human being cannot survive in an environment where reason is ineffective, and will thrive or starve to a degree in proportion to the effectiveness of reason. This means that the prime goal of a political system must be the preservation and enabling of the faculty of reason.

Epistemology

Epistemology is the study of our method of acquiring knowledge. It answers the question, 'How do we know?' It encompasses the nature of concepts, the constructing of concepts, the validity of the senses, logical reasoning, as well as thoughts, ideas, memories, and all things mental. It is concerned with how our minds are related to reality, and whether these and whether these relationships are valid or invalid. It also forms one of the pillars of the new sciences of cognition, which developed from the information processing approach to psychology, and from artificial intelligence, as an attempt to develop computer programs that mimic a human's capacity to use knowledge in an intelligent way.

Typical epistemological questions

- What is knowledge and how does it differ from belief or opinion?
- What is truth, and how can we know if a statement is true?
- What are the sources of knowledge?
- Do absolutes exist, and if so, can we know them?
- What is the relationship between faith and reason?

Importance of epistemology : Epistemology is the explanation of how we think. It is required in order to be able to determine the true from the false, by determining a proper method of evaluation. It is needed in order to use and obtain knowledge of the world around us. Without epistemology, we could not think. More specifically, we would have no reason to believe our thinking was productive or correct, as opposed to random images flashing before our mind. With an incorrect epistemology we would not be able to distinguish truth from error. The consequences are obvious. The degree to which our epistemology is correct is the degree to which we could understand reality, and the degree to which we could use that knowledge to promote our lives and goals. Flaws in epistemology will make it harder to accomplish anything.

Elements of epistemology: Our senses are valid, and the only way to gain information about the world. Reason is our method of gaining knowledge, and acquiring understanding. Logic is our method of maintaining consistency within our set of knowledge. Objectivity is our means of associating knowledge with reality to determine its validity. Concepts are abstracts of specific details of reality, or of other abstractions.

Ways through which we happen to know or sources of knowing:

Scientific Inquiry, Senses and feelings, From authority or divinity, Empiricism (experience), Intuition, Reasoning or Logic.

What reasoning processes yield valid conclusions?

Deductive: Reasoning from the general to the particular *All children can learn. Bret is a fifth grader. He has a learning disability. Can Bret learn?*

Inductive: Reasoning from the specific to general. *After experimenting with plant growth under varied conditions, students conclude plants need water and light.*

Few major educational philosophies emerged within the epistemological frame that focuses on the nature of knowledge and how we come to know. These educational philosophical approaches are currently used in classrooms all over the world. These educational philosophies will be discussed in the subsequent sections of this chapter.

3

Idealism

Chapter Highlights

- Fundamental Principles of Idealism
- Aims of Education in Idealism
- The Idealist Teacher
- The Idealist's Curriculum
- Methods of Teaching Adopted in Idealism
- Strengths and Weaknesses of Idealism
- Contributions of Idealism to Education

Learning Objectives

Upon completion of this chapter, the students will be able to:

- List the fundamental principles of idealism
- State the aims of education in idealism
- Describe the idealist teacher
- Describe the idealist's curriculum
- Describe the methods of teaching adopted in idealism
- Enumerate the strengths and weaknesses
- List the contributions of Idealism to education

INTRODUCTION

Idealism is one of the oldest schools of thought, originating in human nature itself continuing from the primitive man to his present counterpart. The word idealism is derived from two distinct sources—the idea and the ideal. Idea means true and testified knowledge. The word ideal stands for the perfected form of an idea or ideas. An idealist does not have considerations for material values of life. Idealism considers 'Mind and Self'. Adams stated that idealism in one form or other permeates the whole of the history of philosophy. Idealism refused to believe that the world is a great machine. Idealism believed that the world has a meaning, a purpose, perhaps a goal.

Fundamental Principles of Idealism

- **Universe exists in spirit:** Idealism believes in spiritual world and material world, but gives more importance to spiritual world in comparison to the material world. According to Idealism the spirit is the fundamental constituent of the universe. They believe that spiritual world is real and the ultimate truth whereas the material world is transitory and moral. Every individual human mind is part of the universal mind outside which nothing exists. Therefore, the spiritual knowledge is the only true knowledge.

- **Ideas are more important than object:** According to Idealists, knowledge of mind and soul can be obtained through ideas only. Hence, they have given more importance to ideas over the objects and material or later. In the words of Plato 'Ideas are of the ultimate cosmic significance. They are rather the essences that give form to cosmos. These ideas are eternal and unchanging.'
- **Importance of man over nature:** To Idealists, man is more important than material nature. It is because man can think and experience about material objects and material phenomena. Hence, the thinker or the one who experiences is more important than the object or the phenomena experienced. Man is endowed with intelligence and a sense of discrimination. Thus, he is not a slave of the environment as animals are but the moulds and transforms the environment for his own good and welfare of the society. In short, he creates his own world of virtue and his creativity achieves higher and higher levels of art in many areas.
- **Faith in spiritual values:** According to Idealists, basic aim of life is to achieve spiritual values, truth, beauty and goodness. These spiritual values are permanent and never die. One can achieve realization of god through achieving these values. Using these absolute values man rises in the moral plane till he attains divinity. For the achievement of these spiritual values one has to develop his capacities of knowing, feeling and willing.
- **Importance of personality development:** Idealists insist on fullest development of the personality of an individual. According to them, the development of personality means achievement of 'perfection'. Plato rightly speaks that each individual has an ideal self. He tries to develop that ideal 'self' more and more. This self-realization is the true sense of the term. This self-realization can only be achieved in society. Hence, development of social qualities is very essential for self-realization. Idealism believes in the welfare of whole human community.
- **Full support to the principle of unity in diversity:** Idealists give full support to the principle of Unity in Diversity. They believe that is of spiritual nature. This may be called Universal Consciousness or Divinity. This underlying divine force maintains the existence and working of all entities. Idealists call this power as God, the Supreme Force which is omnipotent and omnipresent.

IDEALISM AND AIMS OF EDUCATION

Idealism prescribes certain fundamental aims of education which are directly influenced by the aims and principles of life. In this context Ross puts forth the view, 'The function of education is to help us in our exploration of the ultimate universal values so that truth of the universe may become our truth and give power to our life.' Some of the important aims of education as laid down by idealists are:

- **Self realization:** According to idealism man is the most beautiful creation of god. It lays great stress on the exaltation of human personality it is self-realization. The aim of education is to develop the self of the individuals higher till self-realization is achieved. It is in fact making actual or real the highest potentialities of the self.
- **Universal education.** Education according to idealism should be universal in nature. The universe is regarded as a thought process. Education should be based on the teaching of Universal truth from the stand-point of rationality of the Universe.
- **Spiritual development:** Idealists give greater importance to spiritual values in comparison with material attainments. According to Rusk, 'Education must enable Mankind through its culture to enter more and more fully into the spiritual realm, and also enter more and more fully into the spiritual realm, and also enlarge the boundaries of spiritual realm.'

- **Transmission and promotion of cultural heritage:** The aim of idealistic education is the preservation; enrichment and transmission of culture, Education must contribute to the development of culture. It should help in enlarging the boundaries of spiritual realm.
- **Cultivation of moral values:** According to idealism, man is essentially a moral being. Therefore, moral, intellectual and esthetic aspects of his personality should be promoted.
- **Preparation for a holy life:** Idealism prepares an individual for a holy life. Froebel says— 'The object of education is the realization of a faithful, pure, inviolable and hence holy life.'
- **Development of intelligence and rationality:** Idealism wishes that education should develop the mind fully. Only the highly developed mind can understand the all pervading force. The idealists believe that education must help in the full evolution of mind, the emancipation of spirit, self-realization and the realization of higher values of life and to train the whole man completely and fully for manhood and not some part of man.

IDEALISM AND CURRICULUM

While developing curriculum, idealists give more importance to thought, feelings, ideals and values than to the child and his activities. They firmly hold that curriculum should be concerned with the whole humanity and its experiences. The curriculum should give good mental experience of all types. So cognition (knowing) affecting (feeling) and conation (striving) should find due place.

Sciences and art should be taught as fully integrated. Since the main aim of education according to the philosophy of idealism is to preserve and advance the culture of human race, so subjects like Religion, Ethics, philosophy, History, Literature, etc. should be provided in the curriculum. Healthy mind is found in healthy baby only. So health, hygiene, games and sports should find an important place in the curriculum.

Idealism and Methods of Teaching

Idealism has not prescribed specific methods of teaching. According to idealism, classroom is a temple of spiritual learning, a meeting place of human minds—a place for self education. For this no particular method has been suggested. However, the following methods have been advocated by different idealists:

- Learning through reading
- Learning through lecturing
- Learning through discussion
- Learning through imitation
- Desecrates employed the device of simple to complex.

Idealism and Discipline

Idealism wants discipline the children. Idealists believe that there can be no spiritual development of the child without discipline. This leads to inner discipline. 'The discipline is not to be imposed on pupils. The teacher has only to help them to develop self discipline and through that self-knowledge.'

Self-insight and self-analysis are the main disciplinary factors. The main task of education is the cultivation of higher values of life through moral and religious education. It requires the teacher to present a good example and exercise lasting impact upon the pupil's mind. A teacher is an ideal person to play the role model of his pupil.

Idealism and Teacher

Idealism assigns a special role to the teacher. It considers teacher as a spiritual guide for the child. The teacher serves as a living model for the student. He sets the environment in which education takes place. He carries the child from darkness to light. He is to guide the student towards utmost possible perfection. Idealism regards the teacher as the priest of man's spiritual heritage. He is a co-worker with God in perfecting man. An idealist teacher is a philosopher, friend and guide. According to Gentle–A teacher is 'a spiritual symbol of right conduct.' He is thus, an indispensable necessity.

According to Froebel, the school is a garden, the teacher is a cautious gardener and the child is a tender plant. The plant can grow, no doubt, without help but the good gardener sees that the plant grows to the finest possible perfection. Through teacher's guidance the child can make his natural development into a process leading to perfection and beauty.

CONTRIBUTIONS OF IDEALISM TO EDUCATION

Idealistic philosophy in education emphasizes 'the exaltation of personality', which is the result of self-realization, achieved by spiritual knowledge, self-discipline and dignified teacher. Idealism assigns a very important place to the teacher who is respected as a guide, and philosopher. They emphasize the importance of moral and spiritual education and points out the values of humanities, social sciences, art and literature. It emphasizes man's perfection in various facets of life-physical, spiritual, intellectual, moral, esthetic and social.

Strengths of Idealism

- Idealistic education emphasizes the inculcation of highest values namely, Truth, Beauty and Goodness
- It aims at self–realization of all individuals by one's own efforts. Hence, it promotes universal education
- The teacher assigned a very important role. The teacher influences the child by his high ideals of life and by his sympathetic encouraging behavior
- Idealism emphasizes the principle of self-discipline
- Because of the Idealistic philosophy and education, the school has grown into an important social organization.

Weaknesses

- The common criticism regarding Idealism is that it is an abstract and vague
- It avoids the present realities and prepares the child for the next world
- It emphasizes upon the achievement of immortal values namely, Truth, Beauty and goodness
- Methods of teaching emphasize cramming and rote memory. In modern education, these methods are given little importance
- Humanities are given greater importance for the spiritual development of the child, while the present age of science lays great stress upon scientific subjects in the curriculum.

4

Naturalism

Chapter Highlights

- Basic Concept of 'Naturalism'
- Metaphysics and Naturalism
- Epistemology and Naturalism
- Axiology and Naturalism
- Naturalism in Education
- Aims and Objectives of Education
- The Concept of Student
- Naturalists' Curriculum
- Teaching Methodology
- Concept of Discipline
- Agencies of Education
- Strengths of Naturalistic Education
- Weaknesses of Naturalistic Education

Learning Objectives

Upon completion of this chapter, the students will be able to:

- Describe the basic concepts of naturalism
- Describe the aims and objectives of naturalists education
- Describe the curriculum and teaching methods adopted by naturalists
- Explain the concepts of education in naturalists education
- List the strengths and weaknesses of naturalists' education

INTRODUCTION

Naturalism wants the child to learn in the lap of the nature. Naturalism believes that laws of nature govern the whole universe and these laws are changeable. The senses works like real gateways of knowledge and exploration is the method that helps in studying nature. The naturalist philosopher derives the aims and ideals, the methods of teaching and the principles of curriculum and school management from the nature.

BASIC CONCEPT OF 'NATURALISM'

Naturalists are not dependent on schools and books but on manipulation of the actual life of educand. Naturalism rejects all spiritual and supernatural explanations of the world and holds that science is the sole basis of what can be known. All religious truth is derived from nature and natural causes, and not from revelation. Naturalism is the doctrine which separates nature from God, subordinates spirit to matter and sets up unchangeable laws as supreme.

Metaphysics and Naturalism

Concept of god: Naturalist God is within Nature. He is not all nature nor more than nature. He is that particular structure in nature, which is sufficiently limited to be described as making possible the realization of value and as the foundation of all values.

The concept of self: The self seems to be an organization of experience in each individual which is constantly developing and changing. The human self is seen by naturalism as an offshoot of Nature, and not as springing from beyond Nature.

Naturalists are not much interested in the concept of soul of man. According to them, man is the child of nature; in the evolutionary processes that have been at work in the universe so far, he is on the very crest of the wave.

Epistemology and Naturalism

In terms of theory of knowledge, naturalism highlight the value of scientific knowledge, through specific observation, accumulation and generalization. It also lays emphasis on the empirical and experimental knowledge. Naturalism stresses on sensory training as senses are the gateways to learning.

The logic of naturalism: Simple induction is the logic of naturalism. Simple induction involve careful observation of nature, accurate description of what is observed, and caution in formulating generalizations.

Axiology and naturalism: Naturalists believe that nature is versatile. Instincts, drives and impulses need to be expressed rather than repressed. According to them, there is no absolute good or evil in the world. Human needs create the values for life.

Ethical value: Ethics of naturalism is hedonistic. The highest good is the most highly refined and abiding pleasure.

Esthetic value: The principles enunciated above regarding the ethical values of naturalism hold also for esthetic values. They, too, are rooted in nature and do not depend on any source outside nature for their validation. Nature itself provides the criterion for beauty.

Religious value: The prime imperative of a naturalistic religion is that its adherents ally themselves with the value-realizing force in Nature and help to bring into existence values which are not actual in the present.

Social value: Rousseau's naturalism rooted man in nature rather than society. So much did he regard man as a child of Nature, as over against society, that he proposed in his Emile to keep Emile away from society until adolescences. Individual man, he contended, is not a man unless he is free; if he is in bondage, he is less than a man.

NATURALISM IN EDUCATION

We are born weak, we need strength; helpless, we need aid; foolish, we need reason. All that we lack at birth, all that we need when we come to man's estate, is the gift of education

—Jean Jacques Rousseau

Naturalism as a philosophy of education, developed in the 18th century.

Wholeness of reality: It is based on the assumption that nature represents the wholeness of reality. Nature, itself, is a total system that contains and explains all existence including human beings and human nature.

Conformity on readiness to do: Education must conform to the natural processes of growth and mental development. The make-up of the learner determines the character of the learning process, not the designs of teachers of the learner. Child needs to enjoy education, must learn in pleasurable environment. Children have a good time when they are doing things, which the present development of their physical and mental equipment makes them ready to do. This readiness for specific kinds of activity is evidenced by their interest.

The interest: Consequently, interest in a subject and interest in ways of doing things are guides to parents and teachers, both as to subjects of study and methods of teaching for which children have a natural readiness at any given stage of development.

Self activity: Education should engage the spontaneous self-activity of the child. The child educates himself in great pleasure, most of his knowledge is base on what he discovers in his own active relations with things and people. Adults are foolish, if they do not use this native self-activity as an ally in their teaching. Spencer advised, to teach the learner as little as possible and induce him to discover as much as possible.

AIMS AND OBJECTIVES OF EDUCATION

Naturalists represent a complete reversal of traditional purposes of the school, chiefly, perfecting of man's highest powers via study of literature, philosophy, and classics.

Education is for the body as well as the mind. Even if it were possible, there is no point in making a man mentally fit for life and neglecting his physical fitness. Mind and body must both be cared for and the whole being of the student unfolded as a unit. A child is bad because he is weak, make him strong and he will be good. The naturalist education proposes that the child be given opportunity to grow physically, mentally, socially, emotionally, esthetically, vocationally, under the auspices of the school.

The school's most important job as an educational agency is to see to it that the child learns how to preserve his own physical health and well-being.

'Complete living' is the general aim as this is not very explicit term, it may be made more understandable by a parallel attempt at generalization. This impression is borne out by the specific objectives, which are now to be discussed.

- *Self-preservation:* In order to live completely as man, first he has to live, then continue his own existence. While instinct is the chief guarantee of this objective, education may also help by acquainting the learner with the laws of health and enabling him to earn a living. The school's most important job as an educational agency is to see to it that the child learns how to preserve his own physical health and well-being.
- *Securing the necessities of life:* It is especially in the realm of developing economic efficiency that education helps in preserving life. Money is not life, but it is a necessity in maintaining life. Education should train directly for success in this important function.
- *Raising children:* Spencer stated that the most important function that most men and women have to perform is that of being parents. Therefore education should deal unashamedly both with the care of children in the nursery and the discipline of them as growing boys and girls.
- *Social and political relations:* Beyond the home in the far-reaching social structure, man must have some understanding and mastery of social and political processes if living is to be complete. He must be a wise citizen who is equipped for effective social and political action.

- *Enjoyment of leisure:* Life is not all serious struggles, keeping physically strong, earning a living, being a responsible parent and an earnest citizen. Complete living also includes freedom from struggle some of the time for 'gratification of the tastes and feelings.'

The concept of teacher: The teacher's role is to remain behind the scene and observe. The natural development of child should be stimulated since, nature, considered to be the best educator.

According to naturalists, the teacher is the observer and facilitator of the child's development rather than a giver of information, ideas, ideals and will power or a molder of character. In the words of Ross 'teacher in a naturalistic setup is only a setter of the stage, a supplier of materials and opportunities, a provider of an ideal environment, a creator of conditions under which natural development takes place. Teacher is only a non-interfering observer'.

For Rousseau, the teacher, first, is a person who is completely in tune with nature. He has a profound faith in the original goodness of human nature. He believes that human beings have their own timetable for learning. For each stage of development, the child, shows certain signs that he is ready to learn what are appropriate to that stage. Significantly, the teacher who is aware of human nature and its stages of growth and development, does not force student to learn but rather encourages learning, by insulating him to explore and to grow by his interactions with the environment.

Rousseau opines that teacher should not be in a hurry to make the child learn. Instead, he should be patient, permissive and non-intrusive. According to him the teacher is an invisible guide to learning. While ever-present, he is never a taskmaster. Naturalists are of the view that teacher should not be one who stresses books, recitations and massing information in literary form, 'rather he should give emphasis on activity, exploration, and learning by doing'.

Great emphasis was placed upon the study which teachers should make of the environmental background of each student, since unacceptable behavior was rooted there rather than in the pupil's ill will. Teachers were advised to learn of the racial, national, and religious backgrounds of their students if a pupil caused trouble or lacked initiative in school, the home conditions should be studied to see whether a home broken by divorce, death, or marital conflict is responsible for the child's difficulties. If a teacher were unable to manage a class, he was held responsible because he lacked insight into child nature.

The Concept of Student

Rousseau once commented that everything is good as it comes from the hands of the author of nature. Man meddles with them and they become evil. True, all God's creation was good, but man's own free acts had ushered in sin and evil. Everything is good as it comes from the hands of the author of Nature; but everything degenerates in the hands of man. He will leave nothing as nature made it, not even man. Like a saddle horse that must be trained for man's service, he must be made over according to his fancy, like tree in his garden.

The teachers must teach the pupil not subjects. This means the pupil need to be the focus. The pupil is to the teacher what man is to the philosopher. Therefore, the doctrine of the pupil is virtually the doctrine of man in the classroom.

'I hate books; they only teach us to talk about things we know nothing about.' —*Jean Jacques Rousseau*. Its curriculum is usually based on the needs, interests and abilities of the child in relation to its levels of development. So, a child-centered curriculum forms an amicable answer of the Naturalist. It helps in recognizes individual differences and experiences of the child should form the core element of the curriculum in like manner the curriculum of the naturalists might be classified as experience-centered.

Professional courses in child and educational psychology became the center of the educational program for teachers. 'Know the child and you will know what to teaches' became the slogan of the naturalists.

Naturalists' Curriculum

As a doctrine, naturalism does not favor in imposing any boundary on the children. So advocates of this theory have not framed any curriculum of education. A child will gather experience from nature according to his own demand. He is not to be forced to practice any fixed curriculum. This concept about curriculum existed till the time of Rousseau but it changed after wards. Later on naturalism was influenced by scientific development. So the thinkers think that to give natural pleasure to man, science should be utilized in life. Hence, their concept of curriculum also changed.

- Science dealing with nature will include Physics, Chemistry, Botany, etc. These branches of science will help children to be acquainted with nature.
- Mathematics and language will be included because these will help to acquire the subjects of science.
- History and Social Science: in order to acquire modern knowledge, one should practice the process of evolution. It will also help to realize the importance of those in their present life.
- Agriculture and Carpentry will offer opportunity to the children to act them in freedom and will increase their power of observation.
- Naturalists felt the importance of Physical Education and Health Training for self-protection. But they did not form any particular curriculum for this. They say that the children should be given opportunity for their free movement of bodies in natural environments. They will thus acquire techniques of self-protection from nature and expose themselves in nature.
- Naturalists have considered drawing as the main technique of self-expression.
- They have included drawing as compulsory in the curriculum.
- Health and physical education become an integral part of the curriculum because they contribute to 'self-preservation.'
- Household and industrial 'arts' take their place in the curriculum because they meet the legitimate demands of the students.
- Humanistic studies, considered recreational rather than essential. Advised these for leisure time learning. Modern languages replace classical ones because they are useful.

Naturalists have also commented about ethical and spiritual training in the curriculum. They were against spiritual training as according to them children should pick their own religion from experiences they acquire. They also said that ethical training should not be imposed on children. They will build their own ethical sense in natural order by receiving rewards and punishments.

Teaching Methodology

- Naturalism advises to teach as little as possible and encouraging student to discover as much as possible for himself.
- Difficult tasks are not to be excluded, however, be made pleasant.
- Naturalism show both a reaction against traditional educational methods and a proposal for substituting 'natural' methods in their place.
- The natural mode of self-expression is play and learning should be done through cheerful spontaneous creativity of play.

- The process of discovery is given importance. The activities like excursions, fieldtrips and practical experiments are recommended to enhance learning. According to Spencer the experience is the only teacher. Spencer, the scientific naturalist stated that the 'experimentation' as the only valid method of teaching.
- All teaching methods should include pupil activity involving direct or vicarious experience; the pupil must educate himself.
- Readiness of the organism for any given learning need to be confirmed. Negatively stated, this principle means that it is not the teacher or society that determines what the child should learn, but his own developmental. The pupil will learn about his physical environment when his interests and instincts lead him to such learning.
- Educational activities should be enjoyable to the child. The tasks assigned by traditionalist teachers were designed to discipline the student and therefore were considered unpleasant by the student, but the naturalist felt that any task that went 'against the grain' for the pupil should be avoided.
- Observe how quickly children learn and what they enjoy. Number games, word games, reading stories, studying plants or animals in their natural habitats, the skills of wood wording, household arts, drama constitute real enjoyment for the learner.
- Any teaching-learning methods, which make the material distasteful to the pupils, should be avoided. Spencer attaches great importance to sense training as he believes senses are the gate ways of knowledge.

Concept of Discipline

- Punishment should be constituted by natural consequences of wrong deeds; should be certain, but tempered with sympathy. Naturalism emerged at a time when education was confined within the rigid rules of discipline by the influence of Idealism. Naturalism aims at making education free from the bondage of rigid discipline under which children were tortured. Naturalism, as a philosophy of education advocates maximum freedom for the child and further stresses in freeing the child from the tyranny of rigidity, interference and strict discipline. The freedom of child disciplines him and he is naturally controlled by his own learning and experiences. There is stress given to discipline by natural consequences.
- The situation will provide a form of innate discipline that should replace the teacher. To illustrate, a child learns to avoid hot objects because he has experienced the discomfort and pain which follow his touching them the pupil learn to cooperate with other pupil when he finds himself ostracized by his class mates.
- There are no harsh words, no snapping and snarling. Nature quickly teaches the normal child the dangers of fire, and exemplifies for parents and teachers what is desirable in corrective relations with children.
- If a child is slow in dressing, for a walk, leave him at home. If he breaks a window, let him sit in the cold. If he overeats, let him be sick. In fact, let him suffer the consequences for which he is responsible himself for going against nature.
- It is easier for parent or teacher to hold a firm position with the child and yet not lose rapport with him completely. Even the disobedient child should feel that he has not lost all the sympathy of his guardians. But in the common snapping and snarling of parents, the emotional break between parent and child is too sharp and may do more damage than the punishment does good

AGENCIES OF EDUCATION

If naturalism is true, then it may follow that mothers and/or fathers are the natural teachers, and there is no firm basis for adding to institutions, Rousseau, proposes that formal schooling is both unnecessary and harmful to education 'according to nature.' Even the tutor's role must be subordinated to that of the home and nature. His function is a negative one: to keep the child and youth from the evil influence of corrupt institutions and society. The foundations of good physical and mental health are laid during infancy. Other naturalists believed that although the parents' role is very important in the child's education, one should have formalized institutions whose very existence is rooted in nature. They acknowledge the important function that secondary educational agencies serve. Mass communication media such as radio, television, movies, newspapers, all play important parts in the modern child's education.

Strengths of Naturalistic Education

- Child centered education: Naturalists gave importance to both mind and body.
- Freedom to child: 'learning is naturally pleasurable.'
- Conformity on child's readiness to learn.
- Learning by doing: The naturalist reminds all educators to utilize direct experience whenever possible to insure meaningful and lasting learning.
- Naturalists recognized the failure of traditional education in regard to this rather obvious fact and offered both theoretical and practical means for adapting content and method to individual differences.
- No punishment or autocracy from the tutor
- Parents considered to be the learning base
- Family the institution is given more importance.

Weaknesses of Naturalistic Education

- Has no permanent goal for education. Without specific aims of education can easily become a haphazard.
- By designating experience as the sole source of knowledge naturalism limits itself to one methodology and to a narrow curriculum
- Any appeal to sources outsider nature for improvement of the educative process is miseducative since it violates the very foundations upon which education should be built.

RESEARCH LINK

Hussey. T. (2011) Naturalistic nursing. Nurs Philos 12 (1): 45–52.

Where nurse education aims to provide an overarching intellectual framework, this paper argues that it should be the framework of naturalism. After an exposition of the chief features of naturalism and its relationship to science and morality, the paper describes naturalistic nursing, contrasting it with some other perspectives. There follows a defense of naturalism and naturalistic nursing against several objections, including those concerning spirituality, religion, meaning, morality, and alternative sources of knowledge. The paper ends with some of the advantages of the naturalistic approach.

5

Pragmatism

Chapter Highlights

- Principles of Pragmatism
- Pragmatic Principles of Curriculum Development
- Educational Implications of Pragmatism
- Teaching Methods Followed in Pragmatism
- Process of Discipline in Pragmatism

Learning Objectives

Upon completion of this chapter, the students will be able to:

- Explain the principles of pragmatism
- Describe the pragmatic principles of curriculum
- State the educational implications of pragmatism development
- Describe the methods of teaching followed in pragmatism
- Explain the process of discipline in pragmatism

INTRODUCTION

Pragmatism emerged at the end of the nineteenth century as the most original contribution of American thought to the enterprise of philosophy (Stumpf, 1966). The term pragmatism derives its origin from a Greek word meaning to do, to make, to accomplish. So the use of words likes 'action' or 'practice' or 'activity'. Action gets priority over thought. Experience is at the center of the universe. According to pragmatism values are instrumental only. There are no final or fixed values. They are evolved and are not true for all times and for all situations.

PRINCIPLES OF PRAGMATISM

- *Pluralism:* Philosophically, the pragmatists are pluralists. According to them there are as many words as human beings. The ultimate reality is not one but many. Everyone searches truth and aim of life according to his experiences.
- *Emphasis on change:* The pragmatists emphasizes change. The world is a process, a constant flux. Truth is always in the making. The world is ever progressing and evolving. Therefore, everything here is changing.
- *Utilitarianism:* Pragmatists are utility is the test of all truth and reality. A useful principle is true. Utility means fulfilment of human purposes. The results decide the good and evil of anything, idea, beliefs and acts. Utility means satisfaction of human needs.

- *Changing aim and values:* The aim and values of life change in different times and climes. The old aims and values, therefore, cannot be accepted as they are. Human life and the world is a laboratory in which the aims and values are developed.
- *Individualism:* Pragmatists are individualists. They put maximum premium upon freedom in human life. Liberty goes with equality and fraternity. Everyone should adjust to his environment.
- Emphasis on social aspects—Since man is a social animal therefore, he develops in social circumstances. His success is success in society. The aim of education is to make him successful by developing his social personality.
- *Experimentalism:* Pragmatists are experimentalists. They give more importance to action than ideas. Activity is the means to attain the end of knowledge. Therefore, one should learn by doing constant experimentation, which is required in every field of life.

Pragmatism and Educative Process

Pragmatism approaches the problems of education from the 'progressivits' view point 'progress implies change. Change further implies novelty', so education cannot be conceived of as acquired once for all. Problem-solving is at the core of all education. The educative process thus becomes empirical, experimental, and piecemeal: in a word pragmatic.

Educational Implications

- *Education as life:* Pragmatists firmly believe that old and traditional education is dead and lifeless. Education is a continuous re-organizing, reconstructing and integrating the experience and activities of race. They want to conserve the worthwhile culture of the past, think out the solutions to meet the new situations and then integrate the two. Real knowledge can be gained only be activity, experiments and real life experiences.
- *Education as growth:* Thus education will be useful if it brings about the growth and development of the individual as well as the society in which he lives. Education is meant for the child and child is not meant for education and child is not empty bottle to be filled up by outside knowledge. Each child is born with inherent capacities, tendencies and aptitudes, which are drawn out and developed by education. One of the aims of education is to develop all the inherent capacities of the child to the fullest extent.
- *Education as a social process:* To pragmatism, man is a social being. He gains more and more knowledge through personal experiences than he gets from books. According to pragmatism, the education of the child should be through the medium of society so that develops in him socially desirable qualities which promote his welfare and happiness. John Dewey rightly speaks out—Education is the social continuity of life.
- *Education a continuous restructuring of experience:* Education is a process of development. Knowledge is gained by experiences and experiments, conducted by the learner himself. One exercise leads to another and so on and the area of knowledge is widened by the child. The process of reconstruction of experience goes on and leads to adjustment and development of personality. For pragmatists educational process has no end beyond itself. In addition to the individual, it is continuous reorganizing restructuring and integrating the experience and activities of the race.
- *Education the responsibility of state:* Education is the birth right of each individual and may not be within the right of the individual, so the state should shoulder the responsibility. The refusal of the state to do so may not lead the nation to suffering. It is for the state to make the child capable and confident to meet the problems and challenges of life successfully.

Aims and Pragmatism

Pragmatists do not believe in any preconceived aims of education. Human experience is prone to change. Therefore, the need to reshape our aims to meet the needs of such a dynamic environment as ours has become where the invention of every machine means a new social revolution. So it has been said that education has no aims.

Pragmatism and Curriculum

Principles of curriculum development in pragmatism.

- *Principle of utility:* According to this principle, only those subjects, activities and experiences should be included in the curriculum which are useful to the present needs of the child and also meet the future expectations of adult life as well. As such Language, physical well-being, physical training, Geography, History, Science, Agriculture and Home science for girls should be included in the curriculum.
- *Principle of interest:* According to this principle, only those activities and experiences wherein the child takes interest should be included in the curriculum. According to John Dewey these interests are of four varieties namely: (1) interest in conversation, (2) interest in investigation, (3) interest in construction and (4) interest in creative expression. Keeping these varieties of interests in view, at the primary stage, the curriculum should included Reading, Writing, Counting, Art, Craft-work, Natural science and other practical work of simple nature.
- *Principle of experience:* The third principle of pragmatic curriculum is the child's activity, vocation and experience. All these three should be closely integrated. The curriculum should consist of such varieties of learning experiences which promote original thinking and freedom to develop social and purposeful attitudes.
- *Principle of integration:* Pragmatic curriculum deals with the integration of subjects and activities. According to pragmatism knowledge is one unit. Pragmatists want to construct flexible, dynamic and integrated curriculum which aids the developing child and the changing society more and more as the needs, demands and situation require.

Pragmatism and methods of teaching

The whole emphasis of method of teaching in pragmatism is on child, not the book, or the teacher or the subject. The dominant interest of the child is 'to do and to make'. The method should be flexible and dynamic. It must be adaptable and modifiable to suit the nature of the subject matter and potentiality of the students. The whole emphasis of method of teaching in pragmatism is on child, not the book, or the teacher or the subject. The dominant interest of the child is 'to do and to make'.

Project method is a contribution of pragmatist philosophy in education. The child learns by doing says John Dewey. All learning must come as a product of action. Learning by doing makes a person creative, confident and cooperative. They believe in discovery and enquiry methods. Problem-solving, play methods and experiments in laboratory were emphasized.

Teacher

Pragmatism regards teacher as a helper, guide and philosopher. The chief function of pragmatic teacher is to suggest problems to his pupils and to stimulate them to find by themselves, the solutions, which will work. The teacher must provide opportunities for the natural development of innate qualities of children. His main task is to suggest problems to his pupils and to guide them to find out solutions.

Pragmatic Discipline

To utilize the interest of the pupil is the basis of discipline here. The teacher and pupils attack a problem jointly. Teacher's role is that of a guide and a director; it is the pupil who acts, learning this becomes a cooperative venture—a joint enterprise. Pursuit of common purposes enforces it own order. Education becomes a social process of sharing between the members of the various groups and all are equal partners in the process. That is no rewards also there are no placing for the martinet so any punishments. The discipline proceeds from the life of the school as a whole.

6

Modern Philosophies of Education

Chapter Highlights

- Modern Philosophies of Education
- Meaning of Perennialism
- Curriculum in Perennialism
- Curriculum Process in Essentialism
- Focus of Teachers in Essentialists' Curriculum
- Curriculum as Per Reconstructionist's Philosophy of Education
- Salient Features of Existentialism

Learning Objectives

Upon completion of this chapter, the students will be able to:

- List the modern philosophies of education
- Interpret the meaning of perennialism as an educational philosophy
- Describe the process of curriculum in perennialism
- Describe the curriculum process in essentialism
- Explain the focus of teachers in essentialists' curriculum
- Explain the curriculum as per reconstructionists' philosophy of education
- Describe the salient features of existentialism
- State the role curriculum, teacher and student in existentialism

INTRODUCTION

Two thousand years ago Greek philosopher Aristotle wrote: 'In modern times there were opposing views about the practice of education. There is no general agreement about what the young should learn either in relation to virtue or in relation to the best life; nor is it clear whether their education ought to be directed more towards the intellect than towards the character of the soul. And it is not certain whether training should be directed at things useful in life, or at those conducive to virtue, or at non-essentials and there is no agreement as to what in fact does tend towards virtue. Men do not all prize most highly the same virtue. So naturally they differ also about the proper training for it.'

Through the centuries, many philosophies of education have emerged, each with their own beliefs about education. In this chapter, we will discuss four philosophies, namely; perennialism, essentialism, progressivism and reconstructionism proposed by Western philosophers. Also, discussed are the viewpoints of three Eastern philosophers; namely, al-Farabi, Tagore and Confucius.

Meaning of Perennialism

Perennial means 'everlasting', like a perennial flower that blooms year after year.

Perennialism, the oldest and most conservative educational philosophy has its roots in the philosophy of Plato and Aristotle. Two modern day proponents of perennialism are Robert Hutchins and Mortimer Adler. The perennialists believed that humans are rational and the aim of education is 'to improve man as man' (Hutchins, 1953). The answers to all educational questions derive from the answer to one question: What is human nature? According to them, human nature is constant and humans have the ability to understand the universal truths of nature. Thus, the aim of education is to develop the rational person and to uncover universal truths by training the intellect. Towards developing one's moral and spiritual being, character education should be emphasized.

Perennialism is based on the belief that some ideas have lasted over centuries and are as relevant today as when they were first conceived. These ideas should be studied in school. Perennialism is a teacher-centered educational philosophy that focuses on everlasting ideas and universal truths learned from art, history, and literature. The curriculum of perennialism stems from the 'Great Books', a collection of literature deemed in Western culture to be foundational, significant, and relevant, regardless of the time period. These books include the works of Socrates, Aristotle, Homer, Plato, Geoffrey Chaucer, and William Shakespeare.

Perennialists' Curriculum

The study of philosophy is a crucial part of the perennialist curriculum. This was because they wanted students to discover those ideas that are most insightful and timeless in understanding the human condition.

Perennialism is similar to essentialism in that teachers guide the educational process. It is also closely associated with the Socratic method of teaching, which promotes an open dialogue between teacher and student. Perennialism in the classroom involves students gaining cultural literacy through the Great Books and proving their understanding through tests, writing, and behavior. A perennialism teacher has a duty to help students to become cultural citizens and to understand the principles of human knowledge.

Curriculum

Hutchins sought to open up the dialogue between teachers and students, and to foster an environment of debate that could help students relate to these ancient values. 'The purpose of the university is nothing less than to procure a moral, intellectual, and spiritual revolution throughout the world,' he said. Perennialists were not keen on allowing students to take electives (except second languages) such as vocational and life-adjustment subjects. They argued that these subjects denied students the opportunity to fully develop their rational powers.

The perennialists, criticized the vast amount of disjointed factual information that educators have required students to absorb. They urge that teachers should spend more time teaching concepts and explaining how these concepts are meaningful to students.

The perennialists advise that students should not be taught information that may soon be obsolete or found to be incorrect because of future scientific and technological findings.

At the secondary and university level, perennialists were against reliance on textbooks and lectures in communicating ideas. Emphasis should be on teacher-guided seminars, where students and teachers engage in dialogue; and mutual inquiry sessions to enhance understanding of the great ideas and concepts that have stood the test to time. Student should learns to learn, and not to be evaluated. Universities should not only prepare students for specific careers but to pursue knowledge for its own sake.

Teaching reasoning using the 'Great Books' of Western writers is advocated using the Socratic method to discipline the minds of students. Emphasis should be on scientific reasoning rather than mere acquisition of facts. Teach science but not technology, great ideas rather than vocational topics.

School should teach religious values or ethics. The difference between right and wrong should be emphasized so that students will have definite rules that they must follow.

ESSENTIALISM

The term essentialism as an educational philosophy was originally popularized in the 1930s by William Bagley and later in the 1950s by Arthur Bestor and Admiral Rickover. Essentialism comes from the word 'essential' which means the main things or the basics. As an educational philosophy, it advocates instilling in students with the 'essentials' or 'basics' of academic knowledge and character development.

William Bagley was considered the founding philosopher of the Essentialist movement. Bagley's philosophy of education argued that students should learn 'something' in addition to the process of thinking. The philosophy also asserted that other philosophies over-emphasized the process of learning instead of content knowledge in the curriculum (Null, 2003).

Essentialists Philosophy of Education

Schools should transmit traditional moral values and intellectual knowledge that students need to become model citizens. Teachers should instill traditional virtues such as respect for authority, fidelity to duty, consideration for others and practicality.

Essentialism stresses on science and understanding the world through scientific experimentation. To convey important knowledge about the world, essentialist educators emphasized instruction in natural science rather than nonscientific disciplines such as philosophy or comparative religion.

The Essentialists' Curriculum

Based on the beliefs of essentialism, the curriculum proposed has the following characteristics: The 'basics' of the essentialist curriculum are mathematics, natural science, history, foreign language, and literature. Essentialists disapprove of vocational, life-adjustment, or other courses with 'watered down' academic content.

Elementary students receive instruction in skills such as writing, reading, and measurement. Even while learning art and music (subjects most often associated with the development of creativity) students are required to master a body of information and basic techniques, gradually moving from less to more complex skills and detailed knowledge.

Only by mastering the required material for their grade level are students promoted to the next higher grade.

Essentialist programs are academically rigorous, for both slow and fast learners. Subjects are common for all students regardless of abilities and interests. Nevertheless, how much is to be learned is adjusted according to student ability. It advocates a longer school day, a longer academic year, and textbooks that are more challenging.

Essentialist Teachers

Essentialists maintain that classrooms should be oriented around the teacher, who serves as the intellectual and moral role model for students. Teachers need to be mature and well educated, who know their subjects well and can transmit their knowledge to students.

Teaching is teacher-centered and teachers decide what is most important for students to learn with little emphasis on student interests because it will divert time and attention from learning the academic subjects. Essentialist teachers focus heavily on achievement test scores as a means of evaluating progress.

In an essentialist classroom, students are taught to be 'culturally literate,' that is, to possess a working knowledge about the people, events, ideas, and institutions that have shaped society. Essentialists hope that when students leave school, they will possess not only basic skills and extensive knowledge, but also disciplined and practical minds, capable of applying their knowledge in real world settings.

Discipline is necessary for systematic learning in a school situation. Students learn to respect authority in both school and society.

RECONSTRUCTIONISM

Reconstructionism is a philosophy that believes in the rebuilding of social and cultural infrastructures. Students are to study social problems and think of ways to improve society. Reconstructionism was largely the brain child of Theodore Brameld from Columbia Teachers College. He began as a communist, but shifted to reconstructionism. Reconstructionists favor reform and argue that students must be taught to bring about change.

The Reconstructionist Curriculum

- In the reconstructionist curriculum, it was not enough for students to just analyze interpret and evaluate social problems. They had to be committed to the issues discussed and encouraged to take action to bring about constructive change.
- The curriculum is to be based on social and economic issues as well as social service. The curriculum should engage students in critical analysis of the local, national and international community. Examples of issues are poverty, environment degradation, unemployment, crime, war, political oppression, hunger, etc.
- There are many injustices in society and inequalities in terms of race, gender, and socioeconomic status. Schools are obliged to educate children towards resolution of these injustices and students should not be afraid to examine controversial issues. Students should learn to come to a consensus on issues and so group work was encouraged.
- The curriculum should be constantly changing to meet the changes in society. Students be aware of global issues and the interdependence between nations. Enhancing mutual understanding and global cooperation should be the focus of the curriculum.
- Teachers are considered the prime agents of social change, cultural renewal and internationalism. They are encouraged to challenge outdated structures and entrusted with the task of bringing about a new social order which may be utopian in nature.
- In general, the curriculum emphasized the social sciences (such as history, political science, economics, sociology, religion, ethics, poetry, and philosophy), rather than the sciences.

EXISTENTIALISM

The seeds of existentialism may be traced back to an earlier period of the history of philosophy. During the 18th century reason and nature were given more importance, objectivity was very much emphasized, leading to industrial and technological developments and science was given utmost importance. From the scientific viewpoint, man was also regarded as an object. Man became a slave to machines in developing industrial society. Against this situation existentialism emerged as a protest against the society and asserted the supremacy of individuality of man. The existentialist philosophy is not a creation of any single philosopher. In American education, such people as Maxine Greene, George Kneeler, and Van Cleve Morris, are well-known existentialists who stress individualism and personal self-fulfillment.

Soren Kierkegaard (1813–1855) is regarded as the father of modern existentialism and is the first European Philosopher who bears the existentialist label.

Importance to Subjectivity

Existentialism is a philosophical movement that is generally considered a study that pursues meaning in existence and seeks value for the existing individual. It, unlike other fields of philosophy, does not treat the individual as a concept, and values individual subjectivity over objectivity. For the existentialist man is never just part of the cosmos but always stands to it in a relationship of tension with possibilities for tragic conflict.

Salient Features of Existentialism

The aim of education: Existentialists believe that the most important kind of knowledge is about the human condition and the choices that each person has to make; education is a process of developing consciousness about the freedom to choose and the meaning of responsibility for one's choices. Hence, the notion of group norms, authority, and established order like social, political, philosophical, religious, and so on are rejected.

All round development: The existentialists have aimed at total development of personality through education. Education should aim at the whole man. It should aim at character formation and self-realization. In the existentialist classroom, subject matter takes second place to helping the students understand and appreciate themselves as unique individuals who accept complete responsibility for their thoughts, feelings, and actions.

Subjective knowledge: The advancement of science has made too much of objective knowledge, so much so, that the term has come to mean unreal, non-sense, ignorant and irrelevant. The existentialists point out that subjective knowledge is even more important than objective knowledge. They believe that truth is subjectivity; it is a human value and values are not facts. Therefore, along with the teaching of science and mathematics, the humanities, art, literature should be also be given suitable place in curriculum at every stage of education.

Importance of environment: The present industrial, economic, political and social environment is valueless. The existentialists seek to provide an environment proper to self-development and self-consciousness.

Child centered education: Existentialist education is child centered. It gives full freedom to the child. The teacher should help the child to know himself and recognize his being. Education should be according to the individual's needs and abilities of the child.

Curriculum: Learners to choose what to study and also determine what is true and by what criteria to determine these truths. The curriculum would avoid systematic knowledge or structured disciplines, and the students would be free to select from many available learning situations. They are explored as a means of providing students with vicarious experiences that will help unleash their own creativity and self-expression. Existentialist's approach to education is almost an inversion of the realist approach. The classroom would be rich in materials that lend themselves to self-expression, and the school would be a place in which the teacher and students could pursue dialogue and discussion about their lives and choices.

Existentialist Teacher and Student

Existentialist methods focus on the individual. Learning is self-paced, self-directed, and includes a great deal of individual contact with the teacher, who relates to each student openly and honestly. The student should feel completely free for realizing his self. Under the guidance of the teacher, the student should try to realize his self through introversion. The student accepts the discipline prescribed by the teacher and does not become irresponsible. The purpose of freedom given to him should be to enable him to effect the full development of his individuality.

Existentialists lay emphasis upon religion and moral education. Religion allows a person to develop himself. Religious education gives him an understanding of his existence in the cosmos. It shows the religious path of self-realization.

7

Nursing Image and Nursing Profession

Chapter Highlights

- Nursing Image
- Concepts of Profession
- Use of Different Approaches to Determine Profession
- Pavalko's Eight Dimensions of Profession
- Hallmarks of the Professional Nursing Practice and Environment

Learning Objectives

Upon completion of this chapter, the students will be able to:

- Identify and interpret the societal perceptions on nursing image
- Infer the specific concepts of profession
- Describe the different approaches to determine profession
- Demonstrate skills in applying these approaches in recognizing the profession
- Explain the hallmarks of professional nursing practice and environment

INTRODUCTION

Florence Nightingale, founder of modern nursing used her wisdom, knowledge and her untiring efforts to initiate her service to humankind. She wanted the nurses to get trained in formal institutions, nursing schools. Florence Nightingale laid foundation for the professional nursing education in well-defined schools. This gave the guidance and support to nurses climbing further on the education and practice ladder. During the Victorian age, nursing was perceived as women's work all the altruistic qualities were observed and valued in nurses. In 1800s, the males only could be physicians and only females could be nurses. The characteristics demanded from nurses were altruism, sacrifice and submission.

Nursing Image

To debate or discuss on the question 'Is Nursing a profession?' We need to know about perceptions of the society. Kalisch and Kalisch identified six periods during which distinct corresponding images of the nursing profession were seen:

Period 1: Angel of Mercy (1854–1919): There were two prominent images of nurses. One image, in novel by Charles Dickens, was Sairy Gamp who worked in primitive conditions, the poorly educated alcoholic nurse who performed domestic duties. Second one, Florence nightingale, the original ***'Angel of Mercy.'*** In early 1900s, nurses were viewed as honorable, moral, spiritual, self-sacrificing and ritualistic. From 1916–1918 nursing profession received the greatest attention. The nurse was portrayed as an autonomous and intelligent health care provider.

Period 2: Girl Friday (1920–1929): Nursing students were exploited as cheap labor, literally staffing entire hospitals. Nurses were described as faithful, dependent, cooperative, long suffering and subservient. Nurses were shown as remedies for the emotional turmoil that active soldiers suffered and endured.

Period 3: Heroine (1930–1945): Nursing was acknowledged as a worthy profession. Nurses were identified for their education and abilities. Seven films on nursing profession were released in 1930s. These stressed the education and work of professional nurses. The film White Parade nominated for the 1934 academy award for best picture showed in it the heroine rejected a millionaire's offer of marriage to continue her career as a nurse.

Period 4: Mother (1946–1965): Nurses were chronicled as maternal, compassionate, unassertive, submissive and domestic. Mainly they considered for raising the children. Nevertheless, they were portrayed as intelligent and altruistic.

Period 5: Sex Object (1966–1982): After 1966, the mother image changed to the sex object image. Nurses were increasingly depicted as being sexually promiscuous, self-indulgent, superficial and unreliable. Dickson noted, media images are important because they have an impact on clients and their families.

Period 6: Careerist (from 1983): During this period nurses were portrayed as intelligent, logical, progressive, sophisticated, empathetic and assertive. Men and women of nursing were dedicated and provided high standards of care to the society.

Having known the nursing image has emerged out of societal perceptions and public opinions as portrayed in the television, cinema and magazines. Therefore, it is important for nurses to keep up the honesty and dignity of the professional discipline to pronounce and maintain 'nursing as a profession.

Concepts of Profession

There is always confusion exists in using the terms 'Job', 'occupation' and 'profession'. While using these terms, no attention is being paid to assess the inner meaning of it. Is nursing a profession is not the question of today. It has been attempted by many professionals to address our 'nursing' as a profession. To get idea about the profession let us view the following definitions:

Job: A group of positions those are similar in nature and level of skill that can be carried out by one or more individuals.

Occupation: A group of jobs that are similar in type of work and that are usually found throughout an industry or work environment.

Profession: Profession is a type of occupation that meets certain criteria that raise it to a level above that of an occupation.

Use of Different Approaches to Determine Profession

For decades many experts were trying to find the proper approach through which they determine the profession but they had only a minimal success. Three common models are the process approach, the power approach, and, most widely accepted, the trait approach.

Process Approach

The process approach views all occupations as points of development into a profession along a continuum ranging from position to profession.

Strengths of this approach: This approach gives very explanatory consumer oriented criteria for differentiating an occupation from profession.

Weaknesses of this approach: The major difficulty with this approach is that it lacks **criteria** on which to ***base*** judgments. There is no objectivity to measure and say where exactly we are:

The status of an occupation or profession depends almost completely on public perception of the activities of that occupation. As we know, nursing has always had a poor public image when it comes to being viewed as a profession.

Continuum of Professional Development:

Position ⟵⟶ Profession

Power Approach

The power approach uses two criteria to define a profession:

a. How much independence of practice does this occupation have?
b. How much power does this occupation control?

The concept of power refers to political power and the amount of money that the person in that occupation earns. Using this determinant, occupations such as medicine, law, and **politics** would clearly be considered professions. The members of these occupations earn high incomes, practice their skills with a great deal of independence. Nursing, of course, with its relatively poor salaries, low membership in organizations, and perceived lack of political power, would clearly not meet the power criteria for a profession.

Trait Approach

Many researchers and theorists who have attempted to identify the traits that define a profession, Flexner, Bixler, and Pavalko are most widely accepted as the leaders in the field. These three social scientists have determined that the following common characteristics are important:

- High intellectual level
- High level of individual responsibility and accountability
- Specialized body of knowledge
- Knowledge that can be learned in institutions of higher education
- Public service and altruistic activities
- Public service valued over financial gain
- Relatively high degree of autonomy and independence of practice
- Need for a well-organized and strong organization representing the members of the profession and controlling the quality of practice
- A **code of ethics** that guides the members of the profession in their practice
- Strong professional identity and commitment to the development of the profession. Demonstration of professional competency and possession of a legally recognized license.
- According to Catalano, Joseph T. 2006) the profession of nursing meets most of the criteria but falls short in a few areas.

Pavalko's Eight Dimensions Profession are:

- A profession has relevance to social value.
- A profession has a training or educational period.
- Elements of self motivation address the way in which the profession serves the client or family and larger social system.
- A profession has a code of ethics
- A professional has a commitment to life-long work
- Members control their profession
- A profession has a theoretical framework on which professional practice is based
- Members of a profession have a common identity and distinctive subculture.

According to Catalano, Joseph T. (2006) the profession of nursing meets most of the criteria but falls short in a few areas. Though many scholars claim that nursing is a profession and possesses all the characteristics of profession, some scholars deny saying that it has to strive hard and must perform and prove in the areas of deficit to achieve and maintain the status of professional excellence.

An editorial appeared in the New York Medical Journal in 1914 claiming that nursing is not a profession: Nursing is not, strictly speaking, a profession.

As a response to above MARY A. MESSER, (1914) claimed that nursing is a profession (in the year 1914 in American journal of nursing) in her writings: With all due respect to the New York Medical Journal, nursing today does require, not only skill and intelligence but education. It is true that there are many mechanical duties in a nurse's life, which require only skill, but to be an efficient nurse, demands also special knowledge and attainments. It took more courage to train for nurses in the early days than at present, for since only ignorant women of a low standard of morality had attended the sick, people could not understand why young unmarried women were willing to spend two or three years in a hospital that they might become trained helpers at the bedside. However, since courage and persistence will conquer untold obstacles, the work went steadily on. Institutions for instruction in nursing were established, good, earnest women were called into the work, until now it would seem that we could just claim the right to the term 'professional nurse.'

Her respectful words would have definitely alerted and warned the concerned party to think many times to speak or degrade any profession. Even after 100 years of journey from this date of issue, we are standing courageously to say that we are professionals of nursing profession. Still we are debating and pulling the evidences to speak on our behalf.

There are nursing theorists who had contributed theoretical base to nursing knowledge from the period of Florence Nightingale, the founder of modern nursing. The nursing domain had borrowed considerable amount of theoretical base from other sciences like sociology, psychology. In this advancing world of knowledge, it is observable and acceptable using knowledge from interdisciplinary sciences. At same time, professionals need to strive hard to involve themselves in evidence-based practice. The nursing scholars, academicians, and practitioners need to get involved more and more in seeking empirical evidence to have its own knowledge. From bottom level to top level, need to show their commitment and loyalty to the profession. Professional organizations and regulatory authorities should be continuously monitoring and contributing to the growth of the profession. Nursing administrators and leaders who are the guides for the nursing schools and colleges should set themselves as the living examples of the profession.

Profession in general needs to be meeting the needs of its stakeholders with honest methods and appreciable identities, this will serve as the revelation to improve public image. An excellent nursing college that meets all the set standards of the statutory body is on its way to achieve its professional excellence. Nursing education is taking its broader and deeper steps to produce the qualified nurses, academicians and practitioners who would serve the humankind as ***nursing professionals***, uplift and maintain the ***nursing profession*** at its highest levels by providing ***excellent nursing education***.

HALLMARKS OF THE PROFESSIONAL NURSING PRACTICE AND ENVIRONMENT

Hallmarks are characteristics of the practice setting that best support professional nursing practice and allow baccalaureate and higher degree nurses to practice to their full potential. These Hallmarks are present in health care systems, hospitals, organizations, or practice environments that:

- **Manifest a philosophy of clinical care emphasizing quality, safety, interdisciplinary collaboration, continuity of care, and professional accountability, for example:**
  - The organization has a philosophy and mission statement that reflects these criteria
  - Nursing staff have meaningful input into policy development and operational management of issues related to clinical quality, safety, and clinical outcomes evaluation
  - Nurse staffing patterns have an adequate number of qualified nurses to meet patients' needs, including consideration of the complexity of patient care
  - Nursing is represented on the organization's staff committees that govern policy and operations
  - The organization has a formal program of performance improvement that includes a focus on nursing practice, safety, continuity of care, and outcomes
  - Nursing staff assume responsibility and accountability for their own nursing practice.
- **Recognize contributions of nurses' knowledge and expertise to clinical care quality and patient outcomes, for example:**
  - The organization differentiates the practice roles of nurses based on educational preparation, certification, and advanced preparation
  - The organization has a compensation and reward system that recognizes role distinctions among staff nurses and other expert nurses, e.g. based on clinical expertise, reflective of nursing practice, education, or advanced credentialing
  - The organization's performance improvement program has criteria to evaluate whether nursing care practices are based on the most current research evidence
  - Professional and educational credentials of all disciplines, including nurses, are recognized by title on nametags and reports
  - Nurses and other disciplines participate in media events, public relations announcements, marketing of clinical services, and strategic planning
  - Nurses are encouraged to be mentors to less experienced colleagues and to share their enthusiasm about professional nursing within the organization and the community and
  - Advanced nursing roles, including clinical nurse specialists, nurse practitioners, scientists, educators, and other advanced practice roles, are utilized in the organization to support and enhance nursing care.
- **Promote executive level nursing leadership, for example:**
  - Nurse executive participates on the governing body
  - Nurse executive reports to highest level operations or corporate officer

- Nurse executive has the authority and accountability for all nursing or patient care delivery, financial resources, and personnel
- Nurse executive is supported by adequate managerial and support staff.

- **Empower nurses' participation in clinical decision-making and organization of clinical care systems, for example:**
  - Decentralized, unit-based program or team organizational structure for decision-making
  - Organization or system-wide committee and communication structures include nurses
  - Demonstrated leadership role for nurses in performance improvement of clinical care and the organization of clinical care systems
  - Utilization review system for nursing analysis and correction of clinical care errors and patient safety concerns
  - Staff nurses have the authority to develop and execute nursing care orders and actions and to control their practice.
- **Maintain clinical advancement programs based on education, certification, and advanced preparation, for example:**
  - Financial rewards available for clinical advancement and education
  - Opportunities for promotion and longevity related to education, clinical expertise and professional contributions
  - Peer review, patient, collegial, and managerial input available for performance evaluation on annual or routine basis
  - Individuals in nursing leadership/management positions have appropriate education and credentials aligned with their role and responsibilities.
- **Demonstrate professional development support for nurses, for example:**
  - Professional continuing education opportunities available and supported
  - Resource support for advanced education in nursing, including RN-to-BSN completion programs and graduate degree programs
  - Preceptorships, organized orientation programs, re-tooling or refresher programs, residency programs, internships, or other educational programs available and encouraged
  - Incentive programs for registered nursing education for interested licensed practical nurses and non-nurse health care personnel
  - Long-term career support program targeted to specific populations of nurses, such as older individuals, home care or operating room nurses, or nurses from diverse ethnic backgrounds
  - Specialty certification and advanced credentials are encouraged, promoted, and recognized
  - APNs, nurse researchers, and nurse educators are employed and utilized in leadership roles to support clinical nursing practice
  - Linkages are developed between health care institutions and baccalaureate/graduate schools of nursing to provide support for continuing education, collaborative research, and clinical educational affiliations.
- **Create collaborative relationships among members of the health care provider team, for example:**
  - Professional nurses, physicians, and other health care professionals practice collaboratively and participate in standing organizational committees, bioethics committees, the governing structure, and the institutional review processes

  - Professional nurses have appropriate oversight and supervisory authority of unlicensed members of the nursing care team
  - Interdisciplinary team peer review process is used, especially in the review of patient care errors.
- **Utilize technological advances in clinical care and information systems, for example**:
  - Documentation is supported through appropriate application of technology to the patient care process
  - Appropriate equipment, supplies, and technology is available to optimize the efficient delivery of quality nursing care
  - Resource requirements are quantified and monitored to ensure appropriate resource allocation.

Section II

Curriculum Essentials

8

The Curriculum

Chapter Highlights

- Introduction to Curriculum
- Concepts Related to Curriculum
- Definitions of Curriculum
- Intellectual Development as a Purpose of the Curriculum
- Approaches of Curriculum Development Process
- The Reasons for Adopting Common National Curriculum:
- Different Thoughts and Opinions on Curriculum Construction
- Curriculum is the Orbit of any Educational Program
- Curriculum and the Novice Nurses of Today

Learning Objectives

Upon completion of this chapter, the students will be able to:

- Define different terms fall under the concepts of curriculum
- Interpret curriculum definitions of various edcationalists
- Identify the reasons for adopting national curriculum in nursing
- Explains different perspectives on curriculum construction
- Recognize the curriculum as orbit of the educational program

INTRODUCTION TO CURRICULUM

A curriculum originates from certain values, beliefs and philosophical orientations in coordination with the conceptions of learning and the demands of society. In simple words, the structural base and molding process adopted, the kind of environment, period of time and discipline selected with a due consideration to societal demands, vision, mission and values of the organization to teach and develop an individual or group of learners as worthy players of the field. Curriculum word is strictly followed mostly in 'formal educational' settings where the government or the private organizations offering a program for the specified groups of the concerned discipline. It is a difficult task to give a standard definition for the word curriculum. There are many scholars defined 'curriculum' based on their perceptions and philosophy of education. Nursing schools, colleges pull out the meaning of curriculum as a related concept, which reflect the educational philosophy, beliefs, values of the school, learners and society as the core with the standards of the concerned regulatory bodies of the state and nation as the base. The task of defining the concept of curriculum is the most difficult, for the term *curriculum* has been used with quite different meanings ever since the field established.

The term curriculum refers the existing contract between society, the state and educational professionals with regard to the educational experiences that learners should undergo during a certain phase of their lives. For the majority of authors and experts, the curriculum defines: 1. why; 2. what; 3. when; 4. where; 5. how; and 6. with whom to learn.

The curriculum, in the context of education, the basic foundations of educational contents, their sequencing, continuity and integration in order to educate and bring about the set behavioral modifications based on the learning objectives with the extensive use of learning resources that include effective and efficient teachers who facilitate learning to provide various learning experiences. After the work of Stenhauser and some researchers, major part of the academic community consider curriculum to have political, technical or professional dimensions.

Originally, the curriculum considered as the product of a technical process: Depending on the state of the art of disciplinary and pedagogical knowledge, curriculum experts prepare the document. There is a long chain of factors involved in curriculum development like the school, teacher, learner, society, the program content, the philosophy, values and beliefs of the organization and the standards and regulations of the statutory bodies. As a planner and nursing administrator, we need to consider money (financial support without which any drawn curriculum cannot be implemented); manpower (curriculum experts, many faculty brains to contribute on teaching resources as well plan and deliver the content). Material (nursing curriculum is delivered in formal buildings of schools and colleges that possess the needed facilities as per the norms) and time (to plan and execute all the mentioned sequences we need to have adequate time).

Since the school is a social institution, it is obligated to consider all the aspects of the learning, further consider the student as an individual his own background. All these provide us the base to note that curriculum is not an isolated phenomenon of single object; it is a system with inputs seeking to provide quality products. Curriculum is a continuous process seeks its ongoing assessment and review to get the feedback on its performance. Since, curriculum occurs as a outcome of fed input and the processed throughput we could confidently agree the statement that it is a process.

CONCEPTS RELATED TO CURRICULUM

The word **curriculum** derives from the Latin word *currere* meaning 'to run'. This implies that one of the functions of a curriculum is to provide a template or design, which enables learning to take place. Curricula usually define the learning, expected to take place during a **course** or **program of study** in terms of knowledge, cognitive skills, interpersonal skills and numerical skills, information technology skills and psychomotor skills. Curriculum should specify the teaching, learning and assessment methods and indicate the learning resources required to support the effective delivery of the course. This also would include faculty members and their qualification required for teaching in the program. Many of us use the words curriculum and syllabus synonymously, but those are not the same. A curriculum is more than a syllabus. A **syllabus** describes the content of a program and seen as one part of a curriculum. The curriculum, written and published, for example as course documentation, is the ***official*** or ***formal*** curriculum. Most times, official curriculum becomes as ***functional*** and implemented. A curriculum is developed with certain beliefs and orientations, conceptions of learning and the demands of society.

The official curriculum is different from the **hidden, unofficial** or **counter curriculum.** The hidden curriculum describes those aspects of the educational environment and student learning (such as values and expectations that students acquire, as a result of going through an educational process) which are not formally or explicitly stated but relate to the culture and ethos of an organization. This highlights that the **process** of learning is as important as its product and as teachers, we need to be aware of both the formal and informal factors, which influence learning.

Definitions of Curriculum

- John Dewey (1902): Curriculum is a continuous reconstruction, moving from the child's present experience out into that represented by the organized bodies of truth that we call studies...the various studies...are themselves experience—they are that of the race.
- Franklin Bobbitt (1918): Curriculum is the entire range of experiences, both directed and undirected, concerned in unfolding the abilities of the individual.
- Herald O. Rugh (1927): The curriculum is a succession of experiences and enterprises having a maximum lifelikeness for the learner...giving the learner that development most helpful in meeting and controlling life situations.
- Hollis Cawell (1935): The curriculum is composed of all the experiences children have under the guidance of teachers.... Thus, curriculum considered as a field of study represents no strictly limited body of content, but rather a process or procedure.
- Ralph Tyler (1957): The curriculum is all the learning experiences planned and directed by the school to attain its educational goals.
- Robert Gagne (1967): Curriculum is a sequence of content units arranged in such a way that the learning of each unit may be accomplished as a single act, provided the capabilities described by specified prior units (in the sequence) have already been mastered by the learner.
- James Propham and Eva Baker (1970): Curriculum is all planned learning outcomes for which the school is responsible.... Curriculum refers to the desired consequences of instruction.
- JLMC Brien and R. Brandt (1997): Curriculum refers to a written plan outlining what students will be taught (a course of study). Curriculum may refer to all the courses offered at a given school, or all the courses offered at a school in a particular area of study.
- Indiana Department of Education (2010): Curriculum means the planned interaction of pupils with instructional content, materials, resources, and processes for evaluating the attainment of educational objectives.
- Definition 8: Curriculum is all the experiences that learners have in the course of living. (Marsh, 2003)
- A systematic arrangement of the sum total of the learning experiences planned by a school for a desired group of students to attain the aims of a particular educational program (Florence Nightingale International Foundation Basic Education).
- A composite of entire range of experiences the learner undergoes under the guidance of the school (Lambertson, Eleaner, Education for Nursing Leadership).
- The planned opportunities subject matter (body of knowledge, skills, values and attitudes) and learning activities that the faculty plan and implement in all settings (class room, laboratory, hospital, community health agency, etc.) for a particular group of students for a specified time period (Heidgerkhen, Teaching and Learning in Schools of Nursing).

Whatever way we define the curriculum, the main goal is to nourishing the minds of the students with knowledge and skills that would aid them function as an effective professional in the society; in addition, that gives him a means and way to earn and live in this world.

INTELLECTUAL DEVELOPMENT AS A PURPOSE OF THE CURRICULUM

Fox in 1961 identified five positions regarding the meaning of intellectual development as a purpose of the curriculum (Cited by Loretta E Heidgerken in 1992):

- Intellectual development is conceived as a mastery of subject matter achieved primarily through teacher exposition, drills, tests, etc. The primary purpose is to build a storehouse of information, skills and values, which may be useful to the individual in his future life. The traditional subject-matter curriculum is an example of this concept. The early nursing curricula were essentially of this type. The so-called formal classes doctors lecturers and nurses classes constituted the nursing curriculum.
- Intellectual development is conceived as being directed toward the development of the process itself, i.e. problem-solving, creative thinking, etc. Mastery of subject matter in and of itself is secondary; it serves as resource with primary emphasis on problem solving. Curricula developed between 1920's and 1930's were of this nature, nursing too advocates to use problem solving approach in teaching.
- Intellectual development of an individual is related to and dependent on the development of all aspects of personality, growth of the learner is interrelated—emotional health, personal and social adjustment, skill in-group interaction, physical health, all contribute and are essential to intellectual effectiveness. Therefore, the curriculum must give consideration not only to class and related activities but also to those activities commonly referred to as co-curricular activities, such as student government, social clubs and dormitory living. India's national leader Mahatma Gandhiji stressed on all round development of the students and he believed in eclectic thoughts.
- Intellectual development is important, but development for effective functioning in all areas of living is important in and of itself; therefore, the school has a responsibility to provide for the students' development for citizenship, parenthood, religious development, etc.

Approaches of Curriculum Development Process

Literature reveals that there are two types of curriculum development process.

'Bottom-up' curriculum development process: Proceeds from the bottom upwards. In this case, as well, four different phases identified:

- What the society want
- Responses provided by teachers in the schools
- The collection of these responses and the effort to identify some common aspects
- The development of common standards and their evaluation. The majority of decentralized countries follow this type of curriculum development process.

'Top-down' process curriculum development process: Proceeds from the top downwards. The most usual term to indicate this type of process is the English expression 'top-down'. In this case, curriculum development processes occur through four phases:

- The curriculum presented to teachers
- The curriculum adopted by teachers
- The curriculum assimilated by learners and
- The evaluated curriculum.

The majority of centralized countries follow this type of curriculum development process.

Regulatory bodies for nursing or for higher education develop a national curriculum for nursing programs (Indian nursing council controls the nursing education through release of syllabus for each nursing program delivered in India, e.g. Bachelor of Science in Nursing, Master of Science in Nursing, etc. The basic aim of Indian nursing council is to establish a uniform standard of training for nurses, midwives and health visitors. Most countries are interested in national curriculum to maintain uniform standards and meet the societal needs considering cultural patterns of the country.

Reasons for Adopting Common National Curriculum

- The minimum standards of nursing education should be nationally determined to ensure safe care for the population.
- National guidelines ensure good quality of education for learners.
- Uniformity in curriculum allows the nurses and midwives to take up job in any part of the country without extra preparations since the curriculum taught and the statutory requirements are the same all over the country.
- This also helps us focus on national priorities in nursing education.
- National curriculum reviews can also contribute to improving quality on a national basis. Curriculum specialists and leaders should develop this national curriculum, since such development may require major reorientation in nursing education.

Different Thoughts and Opinions on Curriculum Construction

The two foundational works on curriculum, one by Ralph Tyler (1949) and the other by Jerome Bruner (1960) provided a good beginning since the ideas of them perceived as the most rationalized ones. Bruner wrote, Learning should not only take us somewhere; it should allow us later to go further more easily... The more fundamental or basic is the idea, the greater will be its breadth of applicability to new problems'. Bruner advocated that these fundamental ideas should be constantly revisited, and re-examined so that understanding deepens over time. This notion of revisiting and re-examining fundamental ideas over time is what has become known as a 'spiral curriculum.' Students return repeatedly to the basic concepts, building on them, making them more complex, and understanding them more fully.

This short monograph by Tyler, 'The basic principles of curriculum instruction' help educational institutions engage in curriculum building. The four steps include defining goals, establishing corresponding learning experiences, organizing learning experiences to have a cumulative effect, and evaluating outcome into practice, everywhere. Tyler's principles were the accepted approach to curriculum development for almost 30 years. People add their newer ideas to modify Tyler's work but foundation principles remain the same.

In response to the curriculum approach advocated by Tyler, often called the *product approach*, appeared the *process approach*. Wiggins and Mc Tighe's (1998, 2005) authored the book '*Understanding by Design*'. The authors call their approach 'backward design' and, sure enough, they cite Ralph Tyler's (1949) model as providing the logic behind their 'new' idea. It starts from the end, the desired results, first, and then works backward to a curriculum based on acceptable evidence of learning.

Curriculum is the Orbit of any Educational Program

Curriculum is the orbit and the educational program revolves around this. Curriculum regulates certain principles and uniformity in the offered course or a program. Educational organizations are bound to meet the educational and teaching obligations mentioned in the curriculum. The curriculum becomes as a guiding star for the faculty leaders (Deans, principals), faculty, students ultimately the organizations: government or private. Any problem in the program plan or delivery ultimately ends up with curriculum review and plan to bring a change. It is not that easy to demolish the foundation (curriculum) of all the time. We can strengthen the curriculum, modify the curriculum; but planning to change the entire curriculum in a short notice is a daydream. The ongoing evaluation strengthens the curriculum to keeping current. Adapting changes through analyzing the societal needs by paying due consideration to present generation, culture, technology and trends happening in the profession all over the world would help us move our profession with innovations, modern thoughts and ideas.

Curriculum and Novice Nurses of Today

Present day's curriculum designers need to consider generation gap and preferences, advancement in professional field and technology, innovative teachers and teaching strategies and appropriate clinical placements for hands on experiences in addition to the regular curriculum needs. As nursing is moving more towards commercial side, careful approach is essential to avoid the factors diluting the process of curriculum construction and need to assure quality in every aspect of the process. Curriculum need to consider the teacher as the facilitators. Curriculum should provide firsthand experience. Especially, the nursing graduates to be prepared as critical thinkers and skillful professionals. Accordingly, the curriculum planners of nursing have to consider various dimensions to plan a curriculum for the nursing graduates of today and tomorrow. Simultaneously the curriculum needs to perpetuate faculty of today for tomorrow.

9

Concepts Related to Curriculum Planning

Chapter Highlights

- Terminologies Used as Base in the Process of Curriculum Planning and Development
- Ten Axioms of Curriculum Planning
- Man Power Planning, Human Dimensions in Curriculum Planning
- Curriculum at National Level
- Curriculum at Institutional Level
- The Major Stakeholders to be included in Curriculum Planning
- Curriculum Planning at Different Levels

Learning Objectives

Upon completion of this chapter, the students will be able to:

- Define the terminologies used in the process of curriculum planning and development
- List down ten axioms of curriculum planning
- Interpret curriculum planning in human institutional level
- Explain curriculum planning at national and dimensions

Curriculum is not static; it is an ever-changing phenomenon, sensitive to the needs of the society and happenings in the world. Nursing is a discipline and nursing education is also sensitive to world happenings and the societal needs. Education is considered as one of the institutions activated by the curriculum that is sensitive to the forces affecting the education.

TERMINOLOGIES USED AS BASE IN THE PROCESS OF CURRICULUM PLANNING AND DEVELOPMENT

The *curriculum* is perceived as a plan for the learning experiences that young people encounter under the direction of the school. The preliminary phase, when the curriculum workers make decisions and take actions to establish the plans that teachers and students will carry out, is known as ***curriculum planning***. The process of keeping the curriculum running smoothly is commonly known as ***curriculum development***. The translation of plans into action is ***Curriculum implementation***. The intermediate and final phase of development in which results assessed and successes of both the learners and the programs are determined is known as ***curriculum evaluation. Curriculum revision*** is used to refer to the process for making changes in an existing curriculum or to the changes themselves and is substituted for *curriculum development* or *curriculum improvement*.

Nursing teachers and specialists who participate in efforts to improve the curriculum should consider some general principles of curriculum development. Prior to planning the planners must give due considerations and respect to the time, money and intellectual investments of the previous curriculum planners even though they possess new ideas and strategies that would infuse new ideals and identities for the profession. Novel ideas come up while addressing the work of previous planners.

Ten Axioms of Curriculum Planning

The following are the axioms of curriculum planning according to Peter F. Oliva William R. Gordon:

- Change is both inevitable and necessary, for it is through change that life forms grow and develop.
- A school curriculum not only reflects but also is a product of its time.
- Curriculum changes made at an earlier period of time can exist concurrently with newer curriculum changes at a later period of time.
- Curriculum change results from changes in people.
- Curriculum change is effected as a result of cooperative endeavor on the part of groups.
- Curriculum development is basically a decision-making process.
- Curriculum development is a never-ending process.
- Curriculum development is a comprehensive process.
- Systematic curriculum development is more effective than trial and error.
- The curriculum planner starts from where the curriculum is, just as the teacher starts from where the students are.

Man Power Planning, Human Dimensions in Curriculum Planning

Curriculum development is a 'people' process, a human endeavor. The curriculum planning means the work of continuous chain of people. The human players accept and carry out mutually reinforcing roles in a curriculum process. This human touch will be obvious at any part of the speaking curriculum of nursing.

Curriculum at National Level

Curriculum committee, in nursing colleges, function within its scope and limitations of the country's 'curriculum planning approach': 'top to bottom' or 'bottom to top'. Curriculum developers mainly concentrate on the phases of planning, implementation and evaluation. Regulatory bodies for nursing or for higher education often develop a national curriculum for specific nursing program. Indian nursing council, the statutory body that functions at central level to prescribe, control and coordinate the curriculum of all the nursing programs in India.

The people who develop the national curriculum or national curriculum guidelines are also responsible for making sure that local educational institutions have the resources to implement the guidelines. If the essential resources are not available, guidelines are unrealistic such curriculum cannot be authentically implemented.

Curriculum at Institutional Level

The institutional level curriculum planning is equally important. The institutional curriculum is built upon the national curriculum, each institution interprets the national curriculum through their own teaching and learning philosophy, beliefs and values that builds and molds the students who join the institutions. The teaching/learning philosophy of the local institution, the characteristics of local students and many other factors make such local interpretation essential (Walker, 2003). A formally elected curriculum committee works on the institutional curriculum. On which all major stakeholders are represented.

The Major Stakeholders to be Included in Curriculum Planning (Young, 1998)

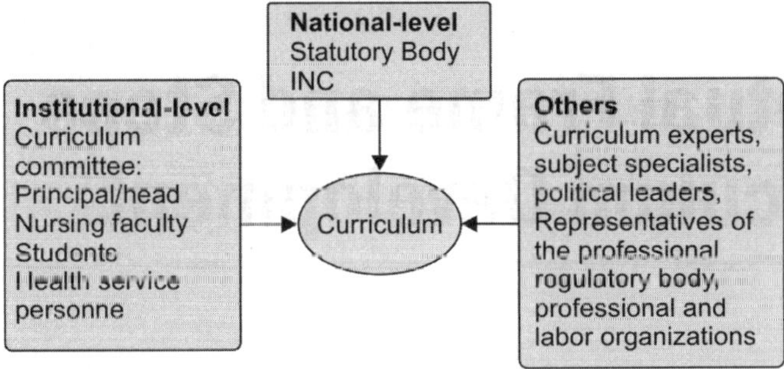

- Nursing faculty members at all levels of the nursing schools and colleges, to ensure deep understanding of the context of the teaching/learning and the curriculum, and to support implementation.
- Current and past students, to ensure that their experience of the current teaching/learning is taken into account, and to obtain their support for implementation.
- Health service personnel, to get the input from the practice site of students and graduates, and to improve understanding of vision and goals.
- Community members, to ensure that the needs of the community are addressed, and their support for change obtained. Usually the curriculum committee members are chosen from these stakeholders.

Many others, such as curriculum experts, subject specialists, political leaders, representatives of the professional regulatory body, professional and labor organizations could also be included from time to time.

Curriculum Planning at Different Levels

People who are not well oriented to the word, 'curriculum' usually associate the word 'curriculum' with a course, textbook, or syllabus. The term curriculum is broad and refers to the whole learning experience of students. For example, it can include a formal plan, global objectives, and the methods of educational delivery. Usually academicians of nursing field view the word, 'curriculum' in a more worldly sense. Curriculum is a comprehensive plan for learning. This plan is a vision and structural frame that is converted into learning experiences for the student of a particular program of the educational institution. Curriculum development is a process that organizes that considers and bases itself on the values of the community, school, and educator. The value preferences are the most important phenomenal influence for forming the philosophical base for the curriculum development. Curriculum planning should begin with a series of questions that reveal the value preferences and the answers serves as the basis of planning efforts and program evaluation. The value preferences as revealed by the answers are referred to as the educational philosophies.

A good curriculum development process includes:

- The analysis of purpose
- The arrangement of a program
- Putting into action related learning events an
- The evaluation of the program and feedback.

The following chapters will deal with the steps and other details of the curriculum development.

10

Conceptual Frame and Steps in Curriculum Development

Chapter Highlights

- Stages of Curriculum Development
- Conceptual Frame for Steps in Curriculum Development
- Establishment of the Purposes
- Philosophy and Curriculum Planning
- Goals
- Objectives
- Focusing on Needs and Selection of Learning Experiences
- Selection of Learning Experiences
- The Organization of Learning Experiences
- Grouping Learning Experiences Under Subject Headings
- Placement

Learning Objectives

Upon completion of this chapter, the students will be able to:

- List down the stages of curriculum development
- Interpret the conceptual frame of curriculum development
- Define philosophy, goals and objectives
- State the features of philosophy that correspond the curriculum views of curriculum developer
- Demonstrate skill in selecting and organizing the learning experiences

CURRICULUM DEVELOPMENT: INTRODUCTION

Curriculum development is not an 'easy one shot work'. Curriculum development is a complex process need intellectual planning that include many stages. From the 1920s, a technical approach to creating curricula was in practice, reaching an apex in nursing with the influential models developed by Tyler (1950) and Taba (1962). Steps in the technical approach to **curriculum development** include:

- Define the goals; purposes, or objectives
- Define experiences or activities related to the goals
- Organize the experiences and activities
- Evaluate the goals.

'Curriculum development is a deliberate process, not an event, which takes concentrated time, effort and faculty commitment' (Dillard and Laidig, 1998, p. 78). The process consists of a series of systematic, logical, dynamic, spiraled, and progressive stages (Torres and Stanton, 1982) that can be time-consuming and labor-intensive (Hull, St. Romain, Alexander, Schaff, and Jones, 2001).

In 1998, Wiggins and Mc Tighe changed the order of the stages to what has been called a backward design. The steps in this design include:

- Identify the desired results
- Determine the acceptable evidence

- Plan teaching experiences and instruction based on standards, as opposed to a curriculum based on activities. In a study designed to compare results from a backward designed curriculum with those from a traditional curriculum, students from the backward designed curriculum outperformed traditional students in meeting outcome goals (Kelting-Gibson, 2005).

Stages of Curriculum Development

- Identify the characteristics desired of the graduate of the program. Review of the recent literature, discussion with service leaders and other members of the community, and consultation are several strategies that can be useful.
- Concurrently, review the 5 to 10 year trends in the internal and external environment that might affect the characteristics desired of the graduate. An example of such a trend is the changing characteristics of potential students.
- Revise and refine desired characteristics of the graduate accordingly.
- Identify philosophical beliefs and values of the faculty that are relevant to the curriculum, taking into consideration the mission and goals of the parent institution. Clearly identify characteristics and needs of potential students.
- Clarify the main concepts identified in the philosophy. Clearly define each concept based on faculty beliefs. This statement will be the basis for all subsequent curriculum work.
- Link the concepts into coherent propositions that form a conceptual **framework** for the curriculum. This might be eclectic or based on an extant framework for nursing (e.g. Orem, Roy, Neuman, Leddy).
- Identify a structure for the curriculum that will accommodate general education, supporting (e.g. anatomy and physiology, general psychology), and nursing courses. Also reconsider the existing organization of the faculty, which should be consistent with the philosophy (e.g. a developmental organization, such as infants/children, adolescents, adults, elderly; or a health/illness continuum, such as health, chronic/long-term, acute).
- Using the philosophy and program outcomes as guides, identify the vertical and horizontal strands of the evolving curriculum. Develop a **matrix** of these strands. For example, if leadership is one of the horizontal strands, an increasing complexity of leadership skills should be demonstrated as the student progresses vertically through the program.
- Using the curriculum framework and the strand matrix as guides, determine names, placement, and objectives of courses.
- Flesh out the course sequence with content, teaching/learning and evaluation activities. Ensure that all matrix strands are appropriately represented.
- Identify an evaluation plan for the entire curriculum.

Before detailing each of these steps, it is important to note that much of the success or failure of curriculum development is determined by the group communication processes of the faculty.

Role of Faculty Members in Curriculum Planning

'The greater the amount of participation of the faculty, the greater the degree of success' (Torres and Stanton, 1982, p. 7).

- There should be clear delegation of assignments to various committees. One person should make final decisions about the role and functions of committees.
- There need to be realistic goals and adequate support and resources for the work of the committees.
- A timetable for the total curriculum process should be developed at the start of the process.

- Faculty need to be proactive, active, involved, and enthusiastic. Creativity is essential, so faculty members need to brainstorm and promote a free flow of ideas and information.
- To the extent possible, faculty should listen and not argue. Seek first to understand and then to be understood.
- Think win-win. Curriculum revision should not be a power play but a mutual and noncompetitive process.
- Avoid **negative synergy** because it is debilitating. It includes talking about other people dishonestly, politicking, rivalry, masterminding, and second-guessing outcomes for self-gain. Negative synergy can be contagious if not confronted, and can ultimately derail the process. Instead, celebrate accomplishments, no matter how small.
- Take care of yourself. The curriculum process is time-consuming and may be associated with increased stress and uncertainty. Try to remain calm and peaceful, and stay up-to-date on information about the revision.
- Try to provide a documented rationale to support the changes that you think should be made. This will help to avoid emotional defense of the status quo.
- Group process among the faculty may need development through strategies such as small group work with a consultant, critical incidents/role play, or storyboarding.
- Recognize and respect each person's unique contribution

Curriculum Development Requires:

Goldenberg, Andrusyszyn, and Iwasiw (2004) suggest that curriculum development requires:

- **Commitment** of time, energy, and resources.
- **Compatibility,** which is the ability of the group to harmonize and function as a whole. This requires a focus on common ground and the curriculum as a whole rather than as individual courses.
- **Communication.** Consider having a facilitator to keep faculty on task and to referee conflicts. A gatekeeper can regulate communication and allow each person to be heard, set up the agenda, and summarize accomplishments. A harmonizer promotes group cohesion and diffuses tension (e.g. rejection, defensiveness), and a housekeeper can record minutes, secure and prepare meeting rooms, and serve as timekeeper. These roles should be rotated among the faculty members.
- **Contribution**. Curriculum development work requires consensus, which is derived from communication, compromise, and negotiation.

CONCEPTUAL FRAME FOR STEPS IN CURRICULUM DEVELOPMENT

The construction of the nursing curriculum is the responsibility of the schools/colleges of nursing, and just as the philosophy, resources and other conditions will vary from one school to another, so will the curriculum. What will be common to all the curricula in one state or country will be the requirements, which are prescribed by the statutory body (in this case Indian Nursing Council) in the form of a syllabus. The syllabus is however the minimum required by the law, and in constructing their own curricula, schools can add whatever required to meet their own particular objectives. The curriculum therefore includes all the subject matter and experiences which a particular school of nursing plan for its own students and which is developed by the members of its own curriculum committee. Curriculum development is an ongoing activity.

Purpose ⇒ Goals ⇒ Objectives ⇒ Needs Focusing ⇒ Curriculum Alignment ⇒ Instruction

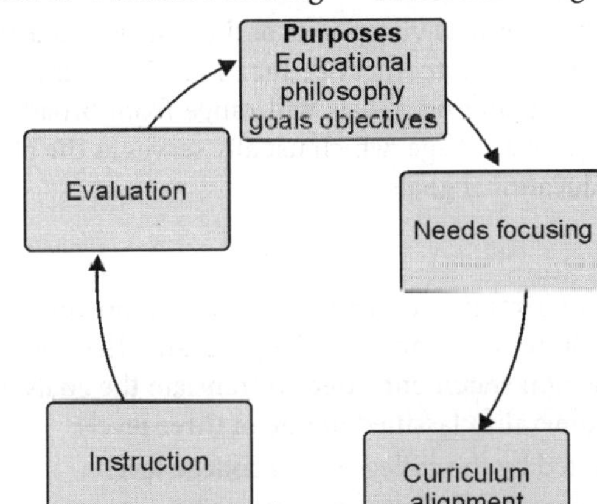

I. Establishment of the Purposes

The clarification of purpose involves identifying a philosophy (refer to one of the philosophies). The philosophy serves as the basis for clarifying the values and beliefs about the purpose, goals, and objectives of a program. Only by developing a philosophy, can curriculum-planning progress. A popular method of creating a philosophic statement is to have the individuals involved in the curriculum process develop their own belief statements. The statements will reflect the various beliefs about the purpose of education and values. The philosophic statement that is created will most likely show that the program exists to meet the needs and interests of students.

II. Philosophy and Curriculum Planning

'The purpose of the curriculum philosophy is to guide the educational process of the learner' (Torres and Stanton, 1982, p. 30). 'A curriculum **philosophy** is a speculative and analytical examination of beliefs which are logically conceptualized. However, beliefs are accepted opinions or convictions of the truth that are not necessarily supported by scientific knowledge…The purpose of the curriculum philosophy is to guide the educational process of the learner' (Torres and Stanton, 1982, p. 30). Educational philosophy is the core of curriculum development that aids in answering the value-laden questions and making curricular choices. The philosophy is the most essential component that gives meaning and base to any curriculum development work. Formulation educational philosophy, always demand the curriculum planners consider their values as pertaining to education.

A philosophy that accurately reflects the beliefs and values of the curriculum developer can accomplish the following:

- Provide the intent and purpose of the existence of the program
- Define the roles of the persons directly associated with the program and school/college
- Clarify the objectives of the program
- Clarify the learning activities in the program
- Direct the selection of learning strategies and tactic to be used in the classroom

Goals

Goals are derived from the philosophical viewpoints of the college, department and community. The goals are statements pertaining to the outcomes of education. Goals, like the statement of philosophy, are a foundation of curriculum planning. Goals will range from broad statements to specific. For example, the mission statement of a college, which usually serves as the philosophical statement, will be supported by the broad educational goals.

Objectives

Objectives also guide the long-range curriculum planning process. They are the operational statements that describe the desired outcomes of the program. The objectives are derived from the goal statements and are the action statements used to translate the goals into a working educational program. Objectives can be generally classified in one of three levels:

Level 1: Broad objectives created by the college at the college level

Level 2: General statements, but more specific, created at the department or program level

Level 3: Behaviorally stated objectives created by program instructor or instructors

III. Focusing Needs and Selection of Learning Experiences

People feel happy when needs of them are met, same way pupils too. Any organization exists for serving and meeting the needs of its client or the stakeholders and educational organizations holds responsibility of supplying good products by giving a great emphasis on molding its students. Until unless the organization know the needs of its stakeholders (students, hospital, nursing colleges, schools, public and wherever the students going to work after completing their programs.)

Needs focusing is an assessment of the needs of the learner and represents an investigation into how outside factors such as local population characteristics affect the program. This inquiry can result in an adjustment of the curriculum goals, objectives, instructional techniques, and student expectations.

The first step of needs assessment is to decide what data is needed to help in decision making and the second step is developing a strategy for gathering the data.

Selection of Learning Experiences

A learning experience is something in which the student actively participates and which result in change of behavior. There are desirable and undesirable learning experiences. In an education program, a desirable experience is one, which results in the change of behavior (in terms of knowledge, skills and attitude) outlined in the objectives of the program. The teacher should select only experiences, which will result in desirable outcomes in both the hospital and community. The use of the term 'learning experience' instead of curriculum content is however, preferable as it implies the involvement of the student. The kind of learning experience, which the student will require, will depend on the objectives of the curriculum.

In his classic text on curriculum, Tyler defined the term learning experiences as follows:

The term 'learning experience' is not the same as the content with which a course deals nor the activities performed by the teacher. The term 'learning experience' refers to the interaction between the learner and the external conditions in the environment to which he/she can react. Learning takes place through the active behavior of the student. (p. 63)

Five general principles in selecting learning experiences

Tyler stated five general principles in selection of learning experiences

- The learning experience must give students the opportunity to practice the desired behavior. If the objective is to develop problem-solving skills, the students should have ample opportunity to solve problems. For example, if the objective is to help the student acquire demonstrate skills in immunization of infant, the learning would be acquired by experience in immunization clinics, rather than in a pediatric ward.
- The learning experience must give the students satisfaction. Students need satisfying experiences to develop and maintain interest in learning; unsatisfying experiences hinder their learning.
- The learning experience must 'fit' the students' needs and abilities. This infers that the teacher must begin where the student is ability-wise and that prior knowledge is the starting point for new knowledge.
- Multiple learning experiences can achieve the same objective. There are many ways of learning the same thing. A wide range of experiences is more effective for learning than a limited range.
- The learning experience should accomplish several learning outcomes. While students are acquiring knowledge of one subject or concept, they are able to integrate that knowledge in several related fields and satisfy more than one objective (Tyler, 1949).

IV. The Organization of Learning Experiences

To develop a reasonable set of topics, Davis (1993) recommends creating a list of all the content areas you *could* cover that are relevant to the subject of the course, and then 'severely' paring down the topics you have listed, distinguishing what you consider absolutely essential from the rest (p. 5). Build your course around these essential topics, choosing materials (books, articles, films, speakers, etc.) that will speak to these topics and help you accomplish your learning goals.

'Coverage is the enemy'. —Herb Simon, Carnegie Mellon University Professor and winner of the Nobel Prize for Economics

Organization and Sequencing

There are many—often equally effective ways to organize a course to accomplish a particular set of objectives. For example, a course could be arranged in any one of the following ways: chronologically, from concrete to abstract (or vice versa), from theory to application (or vice versa), around a set of questions, around a set of practical problems or case studies, according to disciplinary classifications and categories, etc. However we choose to organize the course, the goal should be to create a structure that supports the learning objectives we have identified.

In general, courses should build towards greater complexity, starting with component pieces and working towards synthesis and integration. As Fink (2003) puts it: 'The goal is to sequence the topics so that they build on one another in a way that allows students to integrate each new idea, topic, or theme with the preceding ones as the course proceeds' (p. 128).

Selecting a Teaching Strategy

Fink distinguishes overall teaching strategies from particular instructional strategies or techniques. A teaching strategy involves combining and sequencing a number of different instructional activities to help students accomplish the learning goals of the class. To determine an effective teaching strategy, think about what you want students to be able to *do* when they leave the course (e.g. apply certain formulas? Create an interactive animation? Debate the merits of particular policies? Create a stage design that reflects a critical reading of an historical play?).

Having identified the broad learning objectives, work backwards, asking yourself: What particular skills and knowledge will students need in order to accomplish these objectives? Then address the following questions:

- What kinds of activities will students need to engage in to acquire the necessary skills and knowledge?
- How can you organize these activities to provide sufficient practice?
- How can you sequence them so that skills build upon one another?

Ordering or Construction of Knowledge

Wiles and Bondi (2011) describe five patterns of constructing knowledge in a curriculum. All can be identified within nursing curricula.

Branching design is the variation of the building blocks design. The end points of learning are known in advance. The curriculum starts with foundational knowledge and then there is some choice within prescribed areas beyond the common experience.

Spiral design, the same knowledge areas are repeatedly revisited at higher levels of complexity. There can be some flexibility, but this likely limited as curriculum designers decide what knowledge needs to be re-examined and when.

Specific task or skills design, specific knowledge and experience are intended to assist students to achieve predetermined competencies. There can be flexibility in the content and ordering of content.

Process design there is a fluid organization of knowledge. The emphasis is on the process to be learned and content is the medium through which specified processes are addressed.

The spiral curriculum is predicated on cognitive theory advanced by Jerome Bruner (1960), who wrote, 'We begin with the hypothesis that any subject can be taught in some intellectually honest form to any child at any stage of development'. In other words, even the most complex material, if properly structured and presented, can be understood by very young children.

Based on the chosen pattern the institutions/curriculum committee/apex statutory bodies organize the selected learning experiences.

Grouping Learning Experiences Under Subject Headings

When all the learning experience have been selected, the next step is to organize them in such a way that the student will receive the maximum benefit. There are many theories regarding the most effective method of organizing the curriculum and it rests with the individual school of nursing to make their own choice. In the past the syllabus prescribed by Indian Nursing Council consisted of a list of subjects, which included anatomy and physiology, nutrition, microbiology, principles and practices of nursing, medical surgical nursing, midwifery and subjects specially included to promote professional understanding. More recently the subject headings have been expanded to include more of the physical, biological and social sciences, maternal and child health, psychiatric nursing, community health nursing, research methodology and subsequent organization and expansion of learning experiences have taken place.

There are several other ways of organizing learning experiences which can be explored and tried out by individual schools, but this practice of grouping them under subject headings is a method of organization which is extensively used for the subject and the clinical experience related to the subject together provide the desired learning experience for the subject.

Placement

When the broad plan for the organization of learning experiences has been decided upon, the next step is their placement in the total curriculum. They have to be distributed throughout the period of course in such a way that the principles of sequence and integration are observed.

Sequence entails the placement of content so that there is gradual progression from simple to complex and from normal to abnormal. For example, the teaching of the basic principles of psychology early in curriculum will help the student in her first year to understand the normal relations of any patient admitted to hospital. Teaching of more complex subject matter in relation to psychiatric nursing will be based on her previous learning of normal human behavior and in turn, prepare her to understand the abnormal behavior of the mentally ill. Similarly the development of an ability to accept responsibility of her own health by maintaining her own health record, then progressing to being responsible for the elementary nursing care of one or two patients during the early months of her training, the responsible for the total nursing care of several patients, until by her final year, she is introduced to responsibilities of ward management.

Integration requires that subjects and experiences which relate or contribute to the learning of one another should be so placed (horizontally) in the curriculum that possible for the students to put together all she learns into a unified, meaningful whole. For example 'food chemistry', 'the functions of digestive system', 'principles of nutrition' and 'pharmacology related to digestive system' complement one another and should be taught at the same time.

General Plan of the Curriculum

The actual mechanics of carrying out this organization may be simplified by preparing a general plan, which will show at a glance the placement of subject matter and clinical experience. Certain blocks of clinical experience statutory requirements; it may be found easier to arrange these first in an educationally sound sequence and then fill in such other clinical experiences as are required to meet the objectives of school. The subject matter teaching necessary for each of the clinical experience can then be charted with each experience. To this general plan may be added the number of hours to be spent in planned instruction and in clinical experience per week per month. The number and distribution of hours will depend on time required for an effective achievement the objectives outlined in the curriculum. These will be affected by the minimum hours required by the Indian Nursing Council.

Sample of a general plan of the curriculum and the rotation plan is illustrated in chart 3 which gives a broad picture of the total program. The following are some of its main features.

- It shows the relationship between classroom teaching and clinical experience.
- Each area of clinical experience is indicated by a code, to which a guide is attached.
- The period of clinical experience vary in length each year, but the total duration of such experience is same for all the students.
- Students of a same class are divided into small groups, and rotated through the same clinical areas.
- As it is not possible to repeat lectures before clinical placements to each group, provision is made for teaching towards the end of first academic year and end of second academic year the subjects for which clinical experience is given in the beginning of the second and third year. Specific theory related to specific placement can be given at the time of placement.

Correlation Chart

From the general plan the various subject with more detailed outlines prepared by respective tutors can be set out in a correlation chart, indicating what will be taught each week (or month) of each year and as far as possible correlating one subject with another as they are developed. Complete correlation is not always possible but if every effort is made to achieve it while planning the curriculum, the teaching staff will be in position to know what the students have or have not been taught in other classes and can adapt their teaching accordingly.

Organization of Clinical Experience

The plan for clinical experience, which is illustrated in the general plan, shows how one class can be divided into a number of groups, depending on the size of the class and the number of students the clinical area can accommodate at one time. The following principles are following in carrying out a rotation plan.

- Each block of clinical experience being used in the rotation should be of the same duration
- Each student must rotate through each block. Students can miss no block as the blocks have been planned to provide altogether the experience required to meet the objectives of curriculum.
- All students should enter and leave the block at the scheduled times so that the rotation plan can operate efficiently and the teaching within blocks carried out.
- Each block of experience is subdivided so that students can be rotated through a series of related experiences within the block.
- A block may consist of two or three unrelated experiences which have been fitted into makeup the requisite length of the block to facilitate the rotation. For example one week each in ENT ward, Casualty, Ophthalmology ward, Communicable disease ward and skin and VD department in a five week block.

Teaching Systems

One of the factors which influence the organization of the curriculum is the teaching system which is adopted. There are three methods commonly used in India, each of which has its own particular advantages.

- Teaching block
- The study day system
- Daily classes

Teaching Block: The teaching blocks are part of the total block system of training. It may be scheduled during a block of clinical experience to provide the instruction related to those experiences or may be strategically placed at intervals throughout the curriculum so that instruction relates to current clinical experience and to new blocks of clinical experience for which the students are due to be posted. It may also be used for review and evaluation. The advantages of this system are as follows:

- The students are freed from ward responsibilities while having a concentrated period of instruction.
- Classes can conveniently be given to the whole group.
- Curriculum planning is facilitated and planning of correlated teaching made easier.
- Students can have uninterrupted periods of clinical experience.
- Ward administration is made easier when students do not have to leave the ward daily to attend classes.

- Attention is drawn to the educational status of the student, although she does not necessarily spend any less time in the wards.
- When block system of teaching is used it is desirable that the school maintain contact with the students when they are not in the teaching block, by means of holding weekly or biweekly classes.

Partial Block System: This is the modification of the block system which can be used instead of block throughout the course or can replace the full block at particular times. In this system the students may be in the partial block system.

This is the modification of the block system which can be used instead of block throughout the course or can replace the full block at particular times. In this system the students may be in the teaching block each morning for two to three weeks and in the clinical area each afternoon. When the partial block system is used, more daily lecturers will be required to cover the course.

Study Day System: The study day system is literally a complete day spent by the student each week studying in the school instead of having one class each day. A different day of the week is assigned to each group of students except for those who are affiliated outside, who will have any required instruction at the institutions to which they are affiliated.

Daily Classes: If none of the above system is used, the fourth possibility is holding single classes, daily or several times per week. During the first year and second year frequent scheduling of classes will be required to cover the curriculum but sometimes, problems arise when a number of students have to be relieved on time from different wards. However, when the schedules are planned with view to service needs and normal ward routine, it is possible to arrange timings, which are reasonably convenient to the ward, school and the student. Daily classes will still be necessary now and then during course, even when the other two systems are operating, but will not be required frequently.

V. Implementation

Careful attention must be paid to issues of implementation. The curriculum developer must ensure that sufficient resources, political and financial support, and administrative strategies developed to implement the curriculum successfully.

VI. Evaluation and Feedback

This is the stage that takes the last place in the stages of curriculum development process but lays foundation for further planning.

Evaluation is a phase in the curriculum development model as well as a specific step. Two types of evaluation, formative and summative, are used during curriculum development. Formative evaluations are used during the needs assessment, product development, and in testing steps. Summative evaluations are undertaken to measure and report on the outcomes of the curriculum. This step reviews evaluation strategies and suggests simple procedures to produce valid and reliable information. A series of questions are posed to guide the summative evaluation process.

11

Curriculum Models

Chapter Highlights

- Assumptions of Curriculum Planning (Saylor and Alexander, 1966)
- Peter Oliva's Ten General Axioms of Curriculum Development
- Broader Classification of Curriculum Models
- The Tyler Model
- The Taba Model
- The Oliva Model
- The Leyton Soto Model
- Eisner: Systemic-Aesthetic Model
- Weinstein and Fantini: Humanistic Model

Learning Objectives

Upon completion of this chapter, the students will be able to:

- State the assumptions of curriculum planning
- List the ten axioms of curriculum planning by Oliva Peter
- List the broader classifications of curriculum model
- Describe Tyler's curriculum model
- Describe Taba's curriculum model
- Describe Oliva, Leyton Soto, Eisner and Weinstein's curriculum models

The programs of individual schools, classrooms and of individual students usually mirror distinctly the nature and extent of the planning and development of these programs by teacher and students (Saylor and Alexander, 1966). Curriculum development is a complex undertaking. Its complexity and difficulty are perhaps heightened by the usual absence of a set of clear ideas or models and planning and the how and theory of curriculum planning and development (Beauchamp, 1961). Models can assist curriculum developers to conceptualize the development process by pinpointing certain principles and procedures.

ASSUMPTIONS OF CURRICULUM PLANNING (SAYLOR AND ALEXANDER, 1966)

- Quality in educational program has priority in educational goals.
- The curriculum itself must be dynamic and ever changing as new developments and needs in our society arise.
- The process of curriculum planning must be continuous, not limited and must be dynamic.
- No master curriculum plans will serve all schools.
- Many individuals participate in curriculum planning.

Procedures of curriculum planning vary from system to system, from school to school, and from classroom to classroom, but they must be logical, consistent and identifiable in each situation.

By examining models for curriculum development, we can analyze the phases the originators or authors conceived as essential to the process of curriculum development. A model must show phases or components, not people. The specification of curriculum goals must chart a progression of steps from departmental committee to school faculty curriculum committee or extended school committee, to principal, to district curriculum committee, to superintendent and to school board (Oliva, 1982).

Peter Oliva's Ten General Axioms of Curriculum Development

- **Curriculum change is inevitable, necessary, and desirable.**
  Schools and school systems grow and develop in proportion to their ability to respond to change and adapt to changing conditions. Society and its institutions continuously encounter problems to which they must respond.
- **Curriculum both reflects and is a product of its time.**
  The curriculum responds to, and is changed by, factors such as social forces, philosophical positions, psychological principles, accumulating knowledge, and educational leadership at its moment in history.
- **Curriculum changes made at an earlier period of time can exist concurrently with newer curriculum changes.**
  Curriculum revision rarely starts and ends abruptly. Changes can coexist and overlap for long periods of time. Usually curriculum is phased in and phased out on a gradual basis.
- **Curriculum change depends on people to implement the change.**
  People who will implement the curriculum should be involved in its development. When individuals internalize and own the changes in curriculum, the changes will be effective and long-lasting.
- **Curriculum development is a cooperative group activity.**
  Significant and fundamental changes in curriculum are brought about as a result of group decisions. Any significant change in the curriculum should involve a broad range of stakeholders to gain their understanding, support, and input.
- **Curriculum development is a decision-making process in which choices are made from a set of alternatives.**
  Examples of decisions curriculum developers must make include what to teach, what philosophy or point of view to support, how to differentiate for special populations, what methods or strategies to use to deliver the curriculum, and what type of school organization best supports the curriculum.
- **Curriculum development is an ongoing process.**
  Continuous monitoring, examination, evaluation, and improvement of curricula are needed. No curriculum meets the needs of everyone. As the needs of learners change, as society changes, and as new knowledge and technology appear, the curriculum must change.
- **Curriculum development is more effective if it is a comprehensive process, rather than a 'piecemeal' process.**
  Curriculum development should not be a hit or miss proposition, but should involve careful planning and be supported by adequate resources, needed time, and sufficient personnel.

- **Curriculum development is more effective when it follows a systematic process.** A set of procedures, or models, for curriculum should be established in advance, and be known and accepted by all who are involved in the process. The model should outline the sequence of steps to be followed for the development of the curriculum.
- **Curriculum development starts from where the curriculum is.** Most curriculum planners begin with existing curriculum. Oliva advises planners to 'hold fast to that which is good.'

Research Link: Aspects of curriculum and eclecticism in curriculum design

FEALY G.M. (2002) Aspects of curriculum policy in preregistration nursing education in the Republic of Ireland: issues and reflections. Journal of Advanced Nursing 37(6), 558–565

This article speaks about the aspects of curriculum, core principles and advises that the curriculum planner must be careful while using eclecticism and at the same time one can adopt eclecticism by concentrating on various aspects.

The Nursing Education Forum's recommendations related to curriculum regulation and design included a number of 'core principles', which the Forum asserted, should guide curriculum development and design. These were the principles of ***flexibility, eclecticism, transferability, progression, utility, evidence-based and shared learning.*** **'Flexibility'** referred to the need to have a curriculum that is responsive to local needs, while **'eclecticism'** referred to the need to have a curriculum that reflects diverse sources of knowledge and a variety of teaching/learning strategies. **'Transferability and progression'** indicated the need for parity of curricular experiences across programs in order to permit the transfer of students between programs. The principle of **'utility'** referred to the educational imperative of ensuring that the knowledge obtained is relevant to the discipline of nursing, while the principle of 'evidence base referred to the need to have' … educationally and clinically sound content' (p. 5). The final principle, that of **'shared learning'**, referred to the importance of encouraging nursing students to learn with and from other healthcare professionals. On the basis that it is especially germane to any consideration of policy decisions related to curriculum design and the content of instruction, the principle of eclecticism will be considered with reference to curriculum philosophy, nursing epistemology and pedagogical practice.

The selection of knowledge from 'diverse sources' and 'selecting the best elements' necessarily involves making value judgments about the intrinsic and, more especially, the extrinsic worth of that knowledge. It involves making choices about which sources of knowledge to turn to and, if it involves selecting knowledge, then it necessarily involves rejecting knowledge. The forum offers no indication as to the criteria that might apply in making such choices. Nor does it qualify what is meant by 'best'. Content may be 'best', in terms of its immediate contribution to nursing science, or it may be 'best' in terms of its capacity to contribute to the learner's intellectual skills, such as critical thinking.

Without clear guidance, eclecticism risks the inclusion of any aspect of content that would appear to be vaguely relevant and, in so doing, it can lead to a lack of deep understanding or critical reflection on the part of the learner (Mulholland 1997). By the same token, it risks the omission of areas of content that could constitute important elements of nursing science.

Curriculum development starts from where the curriculum is.

Most curriculum planners begin with existing curriculum. Oliva advises planners to 'hold fast to that which is good'.

BROADER CLASSIFICATION OF CURRICULUM MODELS

- Traditional deductive models, which are linear and prescriptive.
- Modern inductive models, which are nonlinear, and descriptive.

There are different models used by the curriculum planners for developing the curriculum. A deductive model proceeds from the general (examining the needs of society, for example) to the specific (specifying instructional objectives, for example). An inductive model starts with the development of curriculum materials and leads to generalization.

The Tyler Model

The Tyler Model is one of the best-known models for curriculum development. It is known for the special attention it gives to the planning phases. It is deductive for it proceeds from the general (examining the needs of society, for example) to the specific (specifying instructional objectives).

The First Part of this Model

This talks about the selection of objectives. Tyler recommended that curriculum planners identify general objectives by gathering data from the learners, contemporary life outside the school, and the subject matter. The numerous general objectives are refined by filtering them through two screens:

- Educational and social philosophy of the school and
- The psychology of learning and become specific instructional objectives.

Sources of Educational Goals in Tyler Model

The general objectives that successfully pass through the two screens (philosophical and psychological screen) become what are now popularly known as instructional objectives.

In describing general objectives Tyler referred them as 'goals', 'educational objectives', and 'educational purposes'. These are educational, social, occupational, physical, psychological and recreational. He recommended observations by teachers, interviews with students, interviews with parents, questionnaires and tests as techniques for collecting data about students. By examining these needs, the curriculum developer identifies a set of potential objectives.

Analysis of Contemporary Life

From the needs of society flow many potential educational objectives. For the source the curriculum planner turns to the subject matter, the disciplines themselves. From the three aforementioned sources, curriculum planners derive a multiplicity of general or broad objectives. Once this array of possible objectives is determined, a screening process is necessary to eliminate unnecessary and unimportant and contradictory objectives.

Four Democratic Goals of Tyler

- The recognition of every individual as a human being regardless of his race, national, social and economic status
- Opportunity for wide participation in all phases of activities in the social groups in the society
- Encouragement of variability rather than demanding a single type of personality
- Faith and intelligence as a method of dealing with important problems rather than depending upon the authority of an autocratic or aristocratic group.

In the Psychological Screen

The teachers must clarify the principles of learning that they believed to be sound. 'A psychology of learning as emphasized by Tyler not only includes specific and definite findings but it unified formulation of theory of learning which helps to outline the nature of the learning process, how it takes place, under what conditions, what sort of mechanism operate and the like'.

Significance of the Psychological Screen as per Tyler

- Knowledge in the psychology of learning enables us to distinguish changes in human beings that can be expected to result from a learning process from those that can not.
- A knowledge in the psychology of learning enables us to distinguish goals that are feasible from those that are likely to take a very long time or are almost impossible of attainment at the age level contemplated.
- Psychology of learning gives us some idea of the length of time required to attain an objective and the age levels at which the effort is most efficiently employed.

Tyler describes the next steps as the selection, organization, and evaluation of learning experiences. He defined learning experiences as 'the interaction between the learner and the external conditions in the environment to which he can react'. And teachers must give attention to learning experiences in order to:

- Develop skill in thinking
- Helpful in acquiring information
- Helpful in developing social attitude
- Helpful in developing interest

The Tyler Model

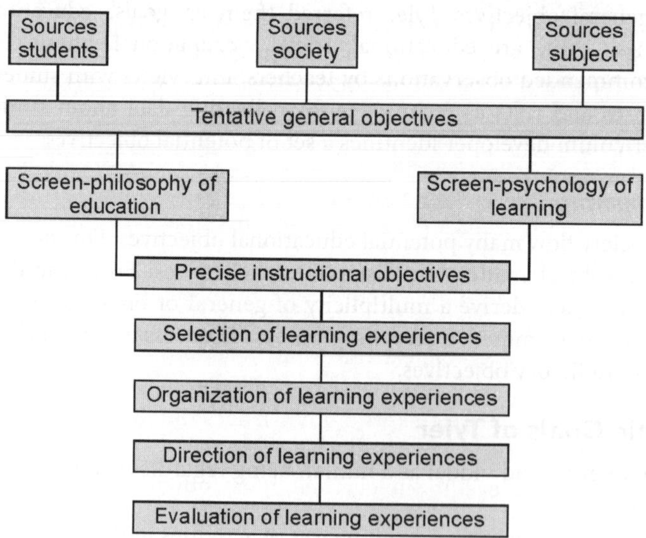

The Taba Model

Taba's Curriculum Designing Principles

- Hilda Taba believed in curriculum designed by the teachers rather than handed down by higher authority. She felt that teachers should begin the process by creating specific teaching-learning units for their students in their schools rather than by engaging initially in creating a general curriculum design.
- Taba advocated an inductive approach to curriculum development. In the inductive approach, curriculum workers start with the specifics and build up to a general design as opposed to the more traditional deductive approach of starting with the general design and working down to the specifics.

Elements of Taba's Curriculum

The model includes an organization of, and relationships among, five mutually interactive elements—objectives, content, learning experiences, teaching strategies, and evaluative measures—so that a system of teaching and learning is represented.

Taba's model contains within it a number of innovative aspects:

- Specificity in determining objectives and content
- Learning experiences selected and organized in accordance with specified criteria
- Teaching strategies that specify a variety of methods and technology
- Evaluative procedures and measures.

Factors external to the model that may affect its internal components:

Such factors include (a) the nature of the community in which the school is located—its pressures, values, and resources; (b) the policies of the school district; (c) the nature of a particular school—its goals, resources, and administrative strategies; (d) the personal style and characteristics of the teachers involved; and (e) the nature of the student population.

Objectives help to provide a consistent focus for the curriculum, to establish criteria for the selection of content and learning experiences, and to guide and direct evaluation of learning outcomes. At the same time that objectives, content, and learning experiences are being selected and organized, teaching strategies must also be planned and developed.

The process of determining objectives begins with the development of overall goals, originating from a variety of sources (for example, the demands of society, the needs of students, and the social science disciplines); is broken down into behavioral statements, classified in terms of the kinds of student outcomes expected (for example, the development of thinking skills, the acquisition, understanding and use of important elements of knowledge, and the like); and justified on the basis of a clearly thought out rationale.

The content for each grade level in the curriculum is contained within a number of teaching-learning units, all emphasizing to some degree a yearly theme. Each unit consists of three kinds of knowledge: key concepts (for example, interdependence, cooperation, cultural change, and social control), main ideas (that is, generalizations derived from key concepts), and specific facts (that is, content samples chosen to illustrate, explain, and develop the main ideas).

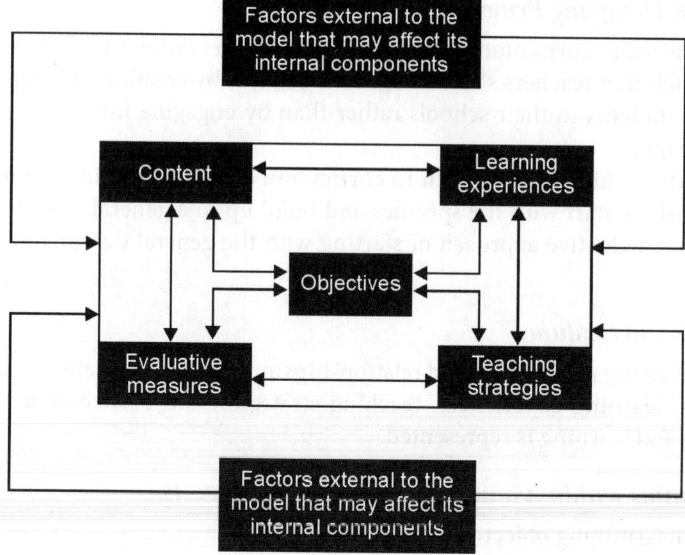

Fig. 11.1: Taba's instructional strategies model

The content contained in the units within a year's work is incorporated into learning experiences selected and organized in accordance with clearly specified criteria (for example, justifiability, transferability, variety of function, open mindedness, etc.). Care is taken to ensure that the learning experiences develop multiple objectives: thinking, attitudes, knowledge, and skills.

Especially designed teaching strategies that identify specific procedures that teachers may use are included within the curriculum. (This makes Taba's model unique.) Some have been designed to encourage students to examine their individual attitudes and values. Particularly innovative are certain strategies that promote the development of children's cognitive skills, such as comparing and contrasting, conceptualizing, generalizing, and applying previously learned relationships to new and different situations.

A variety of objective format devices have been prepared to measure the effectiveness of the curriculum in helping students to explain or recognize causal relationships, apply in new settings important generalizations developed in the curriculum, and to interpret social science data. Several open-ended devices have been designed to measure the quality of students' generalizations, the flexibility and variety of students' conceptualizations, and the variety and nature of the content that students use in response to open-ended questions. A coding scheme has been developed and used to analyze teacher-student discussions as to the levels of thinking that they exhibit, similar to Bloom and others' taxonomies (Durkin, 1993).

Taba's five steps sequence for accomplishing curriculum change

1. Production by teachers of pilot teaching-learning units representative of the grade level or subject area:
    a. Diagnosis of needs
    b. Formulation of objectives

   c. Selection of content
   d. Organization of content
   e. Selection of learning experiences
   f. Organization of learning experiences
   g. Determination of what to evaluate and the ways and means of doing it.
   h. Checking for balance and sequence
2. Testing experimental units
3. Revising and consolidating
4. Developing a framework
5. Installing and disseminating new units.

The Oliva Model

The Oliva Model is a deductive model that offers a faculty a process for the complete development of a school's curriculum. Oliva recognized the needs of students in particular communities are not always the same as the general needs of students throughout our society. According to Oliva, a model curriculum should be simple, comprehensive and systematic.

It is a comprehensive; step by step process that takes the curriculum planner from the sources of curriculum to evaluation.

The model shown represents the most essential components that can be readily expanded into extended model that provides additional detail and simplified process.

Flow Chart: A model for curriculum development (Oliva, 1976)

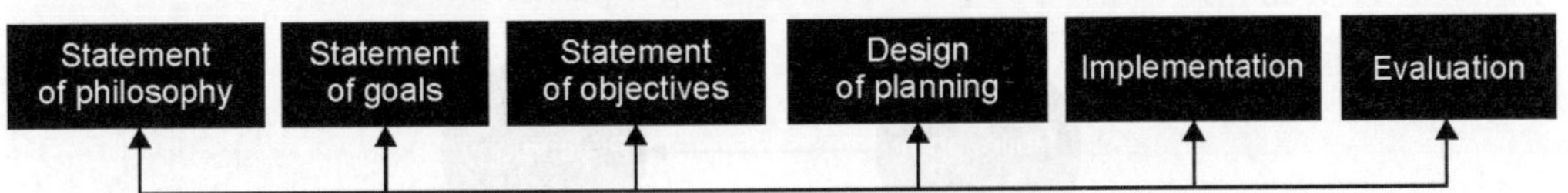

Another Oliva's model is a comprehensive step by step process that takes the curriculum planner from the sources of curriculum to evaluation. It has twelve components. The square represents planning phases and the circles, operational phases.

In Component I, it states the aim of education and their philosophical and psychological principles. These aims are beliefs that are derived from the needs of the individual and society, which incorporate concept similar to Tyler's 'screen'.

Components II requires an analysis of the needs of the community in which the schools are located as well as the needs of the students and the exigencies of the subject matter that will be taught in school.

Components III and IV call for specifying curricular objectives based on Components I and II.

The tasks of Component V are to organize and implement the curriculum, to formulate and establish the structure by which the curriculum will be organized.

In Components VI and VII an increasing level of specification is sought. Instructional goals and objectives are stated for each level of the subject. At this point it distinguish how the goals and objectives differ.

Component VIII shows how the curriculum worker chooses instructional strategies for use with students in the classroom. Simultaneously, the curriculum worker initiates Phase A of Component IX, preliminary selection of evaluation technique. At this stage, the planner thinks ahead and begins to consider ways she will asses students' achievement. The implementation of instructional strategies follows-component X.

Component XI is the stage when evaluation of instruction is carried out. Component XII completes the cycle with evaluation not of the student or of the teacher but rather of the curricular program.

The important features of the model are the feedback lines that cycle back from the evaluation of the curriculum to the curriculum goals and from the evaluation of instruction to the instructional goals. These lines indicate the necessity of continuous revision of the components of the respective subcycles.

THE LEYTON SOTO MODEL

Leyton Soto observed the linear nature of the Tyler model and the separation of the three sources of objectives. He eliminated some of the objectives to the Tyler model and added some of his refinements and clarifications. He charted three basic elements: philosophy, psychology and sources; three basic processes: selection, organization, and evaluation; and three fundamental concepts: objectives, activities, and experiences. Significantly he showed clearly the interrelationship among the various components of the model. He distinguished between learning experiences and learning activities. He defined objectives as the combination of experiences that the learner tries to achieve. Furthermore these experiences are the behaviors that are written into the objectives and activities are selected and organized, but only experiences, i.e. the terminal behaviors, are evaluated. Thus, the Leyton model presented an integrated or comprehensive model for curriculum development from the point of selecting objectives to the point of evaluating experiences.

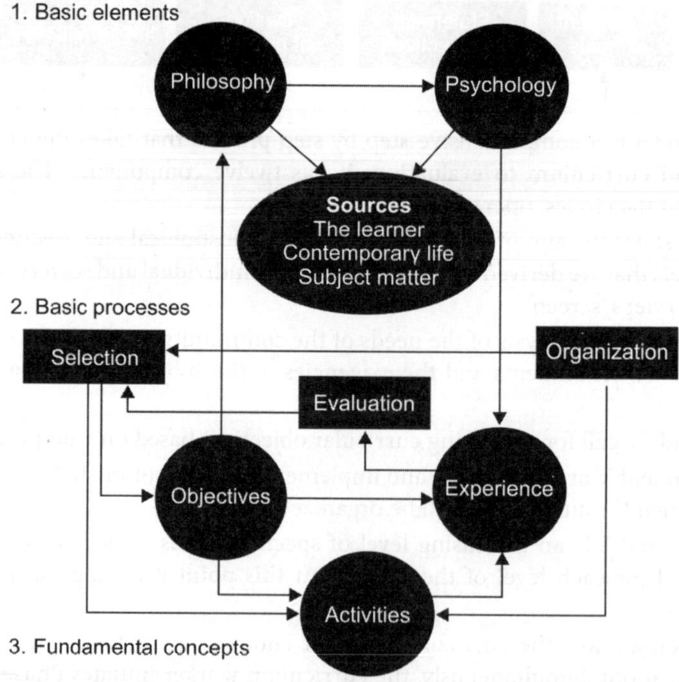

Eisner: Systemic-Aesthetic Model

Elliott Eisner (1991) offers a systemic and dimensional view of curriculum that combines behavioral principles with aesthetic components to form a curriculum planning model. Eisner indicated that if America is going to have the kind of schools it needs, it will need to pursue five dimensions:

- Intentional
- Structural
- Curriculum
- Pedagogical
- Evaluative
- **The intentional:** This refers to the serious, studied examination of what really matters in schools. To realize our intentions, we will need to address the characteristics of our curriculum, the features of our teaching, the forms of our evaluative practices, and the nature of our workplace.
- **The structural:** This dimension refers to how schools are structured, how roles are defined, and how time is allocated. All are important in facilitating and constraining educational opportunities. According to Eisner, the structural organization of schools has not changed much in the past one hundred years. We start school in September and end in June; school lasts twelve years with a prescribed curriculum for everyone; thirty students per class are taught by a single teacher; grades are given several times a year; and students are promoted to the next grade. Such a structure is restrictive.

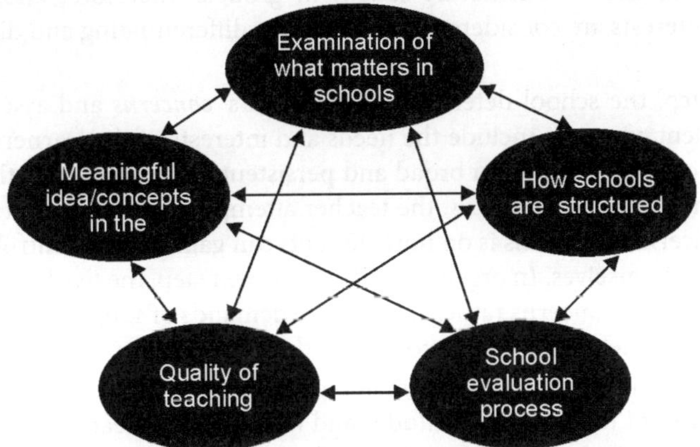

- **The curriculum:** The significance of ideas in a curriculum is of great importance. We need to think about those ideas more deeply and about the means through which students will engage them. The design of curriculum includes attention to ideas that matter, skills that count, and the means through which students and programs interact.
- **The pedagogical:** Whatever the virtues of a school's curriculum, the quality of teaching ought to be a primary concern of school improvement. To treat teaching as an art requires a level of scrutiny, assistance, and support that any performing art deserves. Schools need to be places that serve teachers so that they can serve students.
- **The evaluative:** School evaluation practices operationally define what really matters for students and teachers. Schools need to approach evaluation not simply as a way of scoring students, but as a way in which to find out how well we and our students are doing in order to better do what we do.

WEINSTEIN AND FANTINI: HUMANISTIC MODEL

Gerald Weinstein and Mario Fantini (1970) link socio psychological factors with cognition so learners can deal with their problems and concerns. For this reason, these authors consider their model a 'curriculum of affect'. In viewing the model, some readers might consider it part of the behavioral, managerial, or administrative approach, but the model shifts from a deductive organization of curriculum to an inductive orientation from traditional content to relevant content.

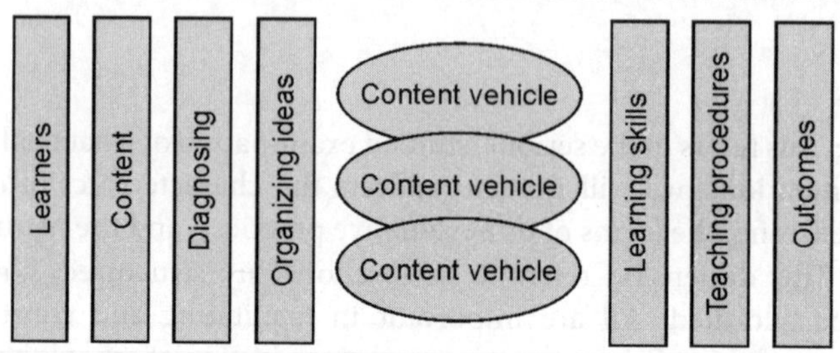

Fig. 11.2: Designing the curriculum a humanistic model

The first step, shown in Figure is to identify the *learners*, their age, grade level, and common cultural and ethnic characteristics. Weinstein and Fantini are concerned with the group, as opposed to individuals, because most students are taught in groups. Therefore, knowledge of common characteristics and interests are considered prerequisite to differentiating and diagnosing individual problems.

In the second step, the school determines the learners' *concerns* and assesses the reasons for these concerns. Student concerns include the needs and interests of the learners, self-concepts, and self-image. Because concerns center on broad and persistent issues, they give the curriculum some consistency over time. Through *diagnosis,* the teacher attempts to develop strategies for instruction to meet learners' concerns. Emphasis is on how students can gain greater control over their lives and feel more at ease with themselves. In *organizing ideas,* the next step, the teacher should select themes and topics around learners' concerns rather than on the demands of subject matter. The concepts and skills to be taught should help the learners cope with their concerns.

The *content* is organized around three major principles, or what Weinstein and Fantini call *vehicles*: life experiences of the learners, attitudes and feelings of the learners, and the social context in which they live. These three types of content influence the concepts, skills, and values that are taught in the classroom, and they form the basis for the 'curriculum of affect'.

According to the authors, *learning skills* include the basic skill of learning how to learn which in turn increases learners' coping activity and power over their environment. Learning skills also help students deal with the content vehicles and problem solving in different subject areas. Self-awareness skills and personal skills are recommended, too, to help students deal with their own feelings and how they relate to other people.

Teaching procedures are developed for learning skills, content vehicles, and organizing ideas. Teaching procedures should match the learning styles on their common characteristics and concerns (the first two steps). In the last step, the teacher evaluates the *outcomes* of the curriculum: cognitive and affective objectives. This evaluation component is similar to the evaluation components of deductive models of Tyler (1949), Beauchamp (1981), and Saylor et al. (1981), companion article; however, there is more emphasis on the needs, interests, and self-concept of learners—that is, affective outcomes.

Research Link

Carole Paulson, The experiences of Faculty Teaching in an Innovative Clinical Immersion Nursing Curriculum. Nursing Education Perspectives: November 2011, Vol. 32, No. 6, pp. 395–399.

The clinical immersion curriculum: The clinical immersion label pertains to the sequestering of clinical rotations to the senior year with field experiences, an open simulation laboratory, and work experience all part of the first three years of the program. Humanities are completed mainly in the freshman and sophomore years, and basic nursing concepts are integrated as soon as students are admitted to the major. In the sophomore year, general science courses, paired with pharmacology and pathophysiology, form the foundation for specialized nursing course work in the junior year. Sophomores and juniors participate in several observation or field experiences in a variety of community and acute care settings, such as rehabilitation and labor and delivery units.

Students are vicariously introduced to clinical settings and nursing competencies by way of the simulation laboratory. Here, using sophisticated technology under the direction of full-time laboratory personnel, students learn, through practice, the psychomotor skills needed for the senior immersion year. Students are referred back to the laboratory any time their actual clinical performance warrants the need.

Following completion of theory components, seniors are immersed in requisite medical-surgical, maternal-child, psychosocial, and community health clinical rotations that run three days per week over four weeks, comprising a total of six clinical courses. All clinical courses are pass/fail and supported with clear standards and competencies to which students are held accountable (Diefenbeck et al., 2006)

Every model has its own goals and objectives based from the needs of individuals, community and the society as a whole. The implementation process lies on the teachers as disseminators of learning and education.

According to Oliva, (1986) he pointed that before choosing a model or designing a curriculum, curriculum planners should attempt to outline the criteria they would look for in a model for curriculum improvement. A model must show the following component:

- Major components of the process
- Customary, but not inflexible, 'beginning and ending' points
- The relationship between curriculum and instruction
- Distinction between curricular and instructional goals
- Reciprocal relationship between components
- A cyclical rather than a linear pattern
- Feedback lines
- The possibility of entry at any point of the cycle
- An internal consistency and logic
- Enough simplicity to be intelligible
- Components in the form of a diagram or chart.

Of course Oliva's outline criteria will be very much helpful in understanding and laying foundation for developing new curriculum model. Whichever model is being chosen, curriculum planners need to consider the various dimensions of the curriculum before stepping in to the curriculum planning.

12

Curriculum Evaluation

Chapter Highlights

- Evaluating the Curriculum
- Four Parts of Evaluation in General
- Kirkpatrick's Four Levels of Evaluation in Training
- Nevo's 10 Major Issues in Curriculum Evaluation
- Curriculum Evaluation is a Part of Quality Assurance to Assure Quality in Education
- Evidence for Assuring Quality
- Steps in Curriculum Change Process
- Minor and Major Curriculum Changes

Learning Objectives

Upon completion of this chapter, the students will be able to:

- List the four parts of evaluation considered By evaluation models
- Describe nevo's 10 major issues in curriculum evaluation
- List some of the evidences to assure quality
- Identify the major and minor curriculum changes
- Identify kirkpatrick's four levels of evaluation in training
- Identify curriculum evaluation as a part of quality assurance in education
- Identify the steps in curriculum change process

EVALUATING THE CURRICULUM

The term 'evaluation' generally applies to the process of making a value judgment. In education, the term 'evaluation' is used in reference to operations associated with curricula, programs, interventions, methods of teaching and organizational factors. Curriculum evaluation aims to examine the impact of implemented curriculum on student (learning) achievement so that the official curriculum can be revised if necessary and to review teaching and learning processes in the classroom. Curriculum evaluation, is an essential phase of curriculum development. Through evaluation a faculty discovers whether a curriculum is fulfilling its purpose and whether students are actually learning. Anything and everything needs a check-point and curriculum is no exception. Curriculum needs to be periodically reviewed to meet the educational trends and challenges and societal needs. Many universities have a curriculum revision policy with a fixed time (once in 3 or 5 years) for curriculum revisions. But if necessity arises, they go for changing the curriculum, provided they have a curriculum change policy in place.

'The process of evaluation is essentially the process of determining to what extent the educational objectives are actually being realized by the program of curriculum and instruction. However, since

educational objectives are essentially changed in human beings, that is, the objectives aimed at are to produce certain desirable changes in the behavior patterns of the student, then evaluation is the process of determining the degree to which these changes in behavior are actually taking place'. Tyler's (1949) Basic Principles of Curriculum and Instruction Chicago: University of Chicago (pp. 105-106)

Evaluation is the process of conceiving, obtaining and communicating information for the guidance of educational decision-making with regard to a specified program (MacDonald, 1975)

It is the insistence on the expliciteness about criteria which distinguishes evaluation... from the 'everyday' use of the term. (Harlen)

Many models are used for evaluating the curriculum. Mostly they look at the strengths and weaknesses of something; the efficiency and effectiveness of how it is undertaken and the value to those who are involved. This evidence can be quantitative.

Strengths

- What were the good things about it—how can they be used in the future?
- What worked well? Why?—can this be applied to other lessons?
- What were the good results?—can they be replicated in the future?

Weaknesses

- What were the weak things about it?—how can they be overcome in the future?
- What did not work well? Why?—how could they be developed for the future?
- What were the poor results?—how can they be improved?

Efficiency

Efficiency is concerned with competence; the ability to do something well or achieve a desired result without wasting energy or effort, or the degree to which this ability is used.

- What things showed that the lesson was efficient, e.g. (reusable learning resources, recap of previous work to ensure all learners were ready to start, etc.). How can this efficiency be applied to other situations?
- What things suggested that the lesson was not efficient?—how can this be improved?

Effectiveness

Effectiveness is concerned with producing or causing a result; especially the desired or intended result. To be truly effective, the result should be striking especially in producing a strong or favorable impression on people.

- What things showed that the lesson was effective? (e.g. learners were involved and appeared to be learning; appropriate learning resources, recap of work at the end of the session which showed learners had learnt)—what lessons can I learn for my teaching?
- What things suggested that the lesson was not effective?

The value to those involved (value added)

- Sometimes social/personal things like teaching cannot be easily evaluated in terms of efficiency and effectiveness or based on qualitative or quantitative data. The extent to which the lesson (or more probably whole program of study) has contributed to the growth of the learner, although this may not appear in examination results, is very important. ***This is sometimes called 'value added'.***

For each of the issues considered in some models, it is important to establish a success criteria based on previous years, or national benchmark figures or on what the course team feels is appropriate. It is important to state how the success criteria has been reached.

- Success criteria should be observable and measurable
- Success criteria should be based on what the objective reasonably and legitimately requires
- Success criteria should be attainable—they should be designed to attain success rather than prevent it.

A useful model for teaching program evaluation is the Context-Input-Process-Product (CIPP) model (Daniel Stufflebeam 1966, 1967, 1971, 1972, 2000) which proposes a four-part evaluation for any program and suggests a number of questions which should be asked within those headings.

Four Parts of an Evaluation in General

- What needs to be done? (Context)
- How should it be done? (Input)
- Is it being done? (Process)
- Did it succeed? (Product)

Context: The setting of the course or subject, i.e. the aims. This can be seen in terms of the validity of what is being taught. External factors which impinge on the program and which may affect its outcomes might be considered here.

Input: The input element relates to the factors which contribute to the course, i.e. the tutor(s), the students, the resources, the environment.

Process: The process element concerns the appropriateness of what happens on the course, how the input elements are used to achieve the aims and objectives.

Product: The product concerns the outcomes—what has been gained (i.e. value added) and what has been achieved (i.e. qualifications).

Product element—subdivisions.

More recently the 'Did it succeed?' or product evaluation part itself is divided into:

Impact: Were the right beneficiaries reached? Was there a possible audience who were not reached—if so, why?

Effectiveness: Were their needs met? Was there an ineffective prioritization of one aspect of the curriculum over another. Could the program have been delivered in a more cost-efficient way with equal effectiveness? Do the results of the effectiveness evaluation suggest that changes should be made in specific areas?

Sustainability: Were the gains for the beneficiaries sustained? Was there a short-term improvement which was not evidenced some time after the program. Possible interview of past course members to ascertain the long-term program value.

Transportability: Did the processes that produced the gains prove transportable and adaptable for effective use in other settings? How will early adopters be reached? How will the more reticent early and late adopters be persuaded? Thus, the model can be remembered by the acronym CIPPIEST (C-Content, I-Input, P-Process, P-Product, I-Impact, E-Effectiveness, S-Sustainability, T-Transportability).

Kirkpatrick's Four Levels of Evaluation in Training

In Kirkpatrick's (1998) four-level model, each successive evaluation level is built on information provided by the lower level. According to this model, evaluation should always begin with level one, and then, as time and budget allow, should move sequentially through levels two, three, and four. Information from each prior level serves as a base for the next level's evaluation. Thus, each successive level represents a more precise measure of the effectiveness of the training program, but, at the same time, requires a more rigorous and time-consuming analysis.

Level 1: Evaluation—Reactions

Evaluation at this level measures how participants in a training program react to it. It attempts to answer questions regarding the participants' perceptions—Did they like it? Was the material relevant to their work? This type of evaluation is often called a 'smilesheet.' According to Kirkpatrick, every program should at least be evaluated at this level to provide for the improvement of a training program. In addition, the participants' reactions have important consequences for learning (level two). Although a positive reaction does not guarantee learning, a negative reaction almost certainly reduces its possibility.

Level 2: Evaluation—Learning

To assess the amount of learning that has occurred due to a training program, level two evaluations often use tests conducted before training (pretest) and after training (post-test).

Assessing at this level moves the evaluation beyond learner satisfaction and attempts to assess the extent students have advanced in skills, knowledge, or attitude. Measurement at this level is more difficult and laborious than level one. Methods range from formal to informal testing to team assessment and self-assessment. If possible, participants take the test or assessment before the training (pretest) and after training (post-test) to determine the amount of learning that has occurred.

Level 3: Evaluation—Transfer

This level measures the transfer that has occurred in learners' behavior due to the training program. Evaluating at this level attempts to answer the question—Are the newly acquired skills, knowledge, or attitude being used in the everyday environment of the learner? For many trainers, this level represents the truest assessment of a program's effectiveness. However, measuring at this level is difficult as it is often impossible to predict when the change in behavior will occur, and thus requires important decisions in terms of when to evaluate, how often to evaluate, and how to evaluate.

Level 4: Evaluation—Results

Level four evaluation attempts to assess training in terms of business results. In this case, sales transactions improved steadily after training for sales staff occurred in April 1997.

Frequently thought of as the bottom line, this level measures the success of the program in terms that managers and executives can understand—increased production, improved quality, decreased costs, reduced frequency of accidents, increased sales, and even higher profits or return on investment. From a business and organizational perspective, this is the overall reason for a training program, yet level four results are not typically addressed.

Methods for long-term evaluation include:

- Send post-training surveys
- Offer ongoing, sequenced training and coaching over a period of time
- Conduct follow-up needs assessment
- Check metrics (e.g. scrap, rework, errors, etc.) to measure if participants achieved training objectives
- Interview trainees and their managers, or their customer groups (e.g. patients, other departmental staff).

Nevo's 10 Major Issues in Curriculum Evaluation

David Nevo (1986) has attempted to clarify the meaning of evaluation by identifying 10 questions that represent the *'major issues addressed by the most prominent evaluation approaches in education'*

1. How is evaluation defined?

Educational evaluation is a systematic description of educational objects and/or an assessment of their merit or worth.

2. What are the functions of evaluation?

Educational evaluation can serve four different functions:

- formative (for improvement);
- summative (for selection and accountability);
- political (to motivate and gain public support); and
- administrative (to exercise authority).

3. What are the objects of evaluation?

Any entity can be an evaluation object. Typical evaluation objects in education are students, educational and administrative personnel, curriculum, instructional materials, programs, projects, and institutions.

4. What kinds of information should be collected regarding each object?

Four groups of variables should be considered regarding each object. They focus on:

- the goals of the object;
- its strategies and plans;
- its process of implementation; and
- its outcomes and impacts.

5. What criteria should be used to judge the merit of an object?

The following criteria should be considered in judging the merit or worth of an educational object:

- responding to identified needs of actual and potential clients;
- achieving national goals, ideals, or social values;
- meeting agreed-upon standards and norms;
- outdoing alternative objects; and
- achieving important stated goals of the objects.

Multiple criteria should be used for any object.

6. Who should be served by an evaluation?

Evaluation should serve the information needs of all actual and potential parties interested in the evaluation object (stakeholders). It is the responsibility of the evaluator(s) to delineate the stakeholders of an evaluation and to identify or project their information needs.

7. What is the process of doing an evaluation?

Regardless of its method of enquiry, an evaluation process should include the following three activities:

- focusing the evaluation problem;
- collecting and analyzing empirical data; and
- communicating findings to evaluation audiences.

There is more than one appropriate sequence for implementing these activities, and any such sequence can (and sometimes should) be repeated several times during the lifespan of an evaluation study.

8. What methods of enquiry should be used in evaluation?

Being a complex task, evaluation needs to mobilize many alternative methods of enquiry from the behavioral sciences and related fields of study and utilize them according to the nature of a specific evaluation problem. At the present state of the art, an *a priori* preference for any specific method of enquiry is not warranted.

9. Who should do evaluation?

Evaluation should be conducted by individuals or teams possessing:

- extensive competencies in research methodology and other data analysis techniques;
- understanding of the social context and the unique substance of the evaluation object;
- the ability to maintain correct human relations and to develop rapport with individuals and groups involved in the evaluation; and
- a conceptual framework to integrate the above-mentioned capabilities.

10. By what standards should evaluation be judged?

Evaluation should strike for an optimal balance in meeting standards of:

- utility (to be useful and practical);
- accuracy (to be technically adequate);
- feasibility (to be realistic and prudent); and
- propriety (to be conducted legally and ethically).

Institutions must have their own policies and regulations to evaluate the curriculum. In some countries, curriculum is evaluated by the apex level statutory body and curriculum changes are announced and adopted time to time. In some countries, the concerned nursing college and the curriculum committee takes the active role in changing or bringing in a new curriculum.

Curriculum Evaluation is a Part of Quality Assurance to Assure Quality in Education

Context (The setting of the course or subject)

Meeting Needs

- Are the aims consistent with the needs of the learner, industry or society?
- Does the curriculum develop links with the world of work?
- Does the curriculum meet current Government initiative, e.g. basic skills/key skills?

Proposed Course Structure

- Is the course structure the best way of achieving the desired outcomes?
- Are the aims updated regularly/has the course been updated in the light of national developments (e.g. basic skills/key skills, vocational developments)?

Encouraging Progression

- Do the aims encourage progression in further or higher education, or transferability to other programs?

Input (The input factors which contribute to the course)

Students

- Do the students possess the entry ability required by the course content?
- Did the students originally wish to do this course?

Tutors

- Are tutors/lecturers/professors appropriately qualified (an area of current interest in post compulsory education)?
- Are the faculty competent in the subject, in current teaching methods and, where necessary, in current industrial requirements?
- Are there adequate tutors for all aspects?
- Do tutors have adequate time for all the requirements of the course, e.g. IV/double marking/ tutorials?

Delivery

- Is there an appropriate amount of time in line with awarding body specifications?
- Are resources appropriate, adequate and available?
- Is the environment conducive to learning and appropriate to the world of work?

Process (The appropriateness of what happens on the course)

Students

- Do students have a 'voice' (e.g. staff/student forums)
- Are there appropriate course group support and interactivity facilities?
- Is there an effective student guidance/counseling system?

Tutors

- Do tutors receive/access, understand and use all available documents related to the curriculum, i.e. information from examining bodies regarding syllabus and assessment requirements?
- Are there regular and useful course team meetings?
- Do team members have access to necessary professional development?

Delivery

- Are teaching strategies appropriate?
- Are appropriate teaching aids and learning resources used?
- Is there appropriate/adequate general access to information technology?

- Is there appropriate/adequate general access to library and academic support?
- Are course accommodation and timetabling facilities maintained (e.g. no constant room or timetable changes)?

Monitoring and Assessment

- Is the monitoring/tutoring/support system appropriate and adequate?
- Is the assessment system valid and reliable?
- Is there an effective system of feedback to learners?

Product what has been gained (i.e. value-added) and achieved

Students

Attendance rate (and possible comparison to achievement)

- What is the staying-on rate as a trend (this year compared to the last 2 or 3 years)?
- What is the qualification achievement rate as a percentage of starters?
- Has the course contributed to the student's ability to meeting the needs of work, e.g. presentation skills?
- What is the progression rate to further industry?
- What was the student's response to the course–e.g. results of student perception questionnaires

Faculty and teaching staff

- What staff development was identified and satisfied at individual and course team level?
- Are tutors motivated by their involvement in the course?

Delivery

- To what extent has the course been modified in the light on on-going feedback?
- If appropriate, what do employers feel about the course?
- Is there an effective system for evaluating and gaining feedback about the program?

Evidence for Assuring Quality

Quantitative evidence

- Enrolments and patterns of enrolments (gender, ethnicity, widening participation, etc.)
- Attendance and partial attendance
- Course completion and retention
- Achievements and public outcomes
- Evidence of progression to further courses
- Evidence of progression to employment
- Three-year trends for any of the above
- Institutional comparisons for any of the above (e.g. attendance)
- National benchmarks with other institutional sectors

We should hunt for evidence, otherwise frame a system and start collecting the evidence.

Qualitative/quantitative evidence

Evidence from human sources can be turned into quantities.

- Evidence from the learners themselves
- Evidence from employers
- Evidence from parents

- Evidence from assessors [markers, examination boards, accreditation bodies]
- Evidence from moderators, internal and external verifiers
- Evidence from observers of teaching: formal teaching observations [including those by inspectors, consultants and 'critical friends'] and more informal peer observations and team-teaching
- Evidence from the course team and the teachers themselves

We also must consider how many of these would be useful to us in our course evaluations.

All these evidences will provide us build again to improve our quality of education what we provide.

Curriculum change processes

Ewell (1997) suggests that most curriculum changes are implemented piecemeal, and, in fact, 'without a deep understanding about what collegiate learning really means and the specific circumstances and strategies that are likely to promote it.'

Ideally, according to Lachiver and Tardif (2002), curriculum change is managed in a logical five-step process:

- an analysis of the current offerings and context;
- the expression of key program aims in a mission statement;
- a prioritization of resources and development strategies;
- the implementation of the targeted curricula change; and
- the establishment of monitoring tools and processes.

Factors influencing the decisions about curriculum change

- Influential or outspoken individuals.
- Financial pressures, including resource availability.
- Staff availability or workload.
- Employer or industry viewpoints.
- Current or prospective student viewpoints.
- Student abilities or limitations, or intake considerations.
- Pedagogical argument, or academic merit.
- University or government requirement or regulation.
- Professional accreditation needs, or syllabi set by professional bodies.
- Academic 'fashion', including the desire to remain in step with other institution.

Curriculum Change

This always takes definition and description from the apex bodies (Statutory bodies that have the control on the curriculum. It varies country to country like the nursing councils, higher education ministries, universities, individual institutions, etc. Whatever is the case, the technical advice is provided by the concerned discipline.

Curriculum changes can be classified as major and minor. This again gets the shape from the policies and procedures of the curriculum authorities.

The curriculum changes considered under 'major changes' are:

- Course creation
- Course deletion

- Changes in the academic units
- Revision of an existing program
- Increasing the physical facilities for running the program
- Raising the qualification requirements of the teachers required for teaching the subjects
- Raising the requirements of eligibility criteria
- Introducing the novel and highly technical content that require the teachers who meet the caliber and physical facilities.
- Increasing or decreasing the duration of the period of the program.

Minor Changes

- Prerequisites
- Corequisites
- Exemptions for certain categories
- Changes in unit objectives
- Changes in the title without changing the meaning
- Changes in assignments
- Changes in expected projects
- Adding new attributes to graduate
- Shifting the blocks in the master plans
- Choosing different hospitals that meet the set criteria
- Tutorial sessions (out of curriculum hours)
- Teaching learning strategies with a rationale after piloting
- Distribution of grades for internal and external examination
- Assessment strategies (Percentage allocation on quizzes, tests, viva voce, care plans, etc.)

Who would initiate the curriculum change?

Initiation for curriculum change may come from any related individuals, like the student, faculty, head of the department or even from the general public. But this always takes a series of hierarchy to reach the person of authority or the commission of authority to scrutinize and recommend the change to the statutory body for recognition and approval. Always submit the proposals as per the time mentioned by the regulatory authorities. This would help them initiate the change process on time if the curriculum change is accepted.

Section III

Teaching and Learning

13. Teacher Qualities and Teacher
14. Interdependence of Teaching and Learning
15. Learning Theories
16. Adult as a Learner
17. Learning Domains and Taxonomy of Education
18. Learning to Care: Nursing and Clinical Teaching
19. Teaching Methods
20. Audiovisual Aids
21. Measurement and Evaluation
22. Guidance and Counseling

13

Teacher Qualities and Teacher

Chapter Highlights

- Good Qualities of the Nurse Teacher
- Teaching Principles
- Characteristics of Teaching Models
- Twelve Qualities of a Teacher as a Mentor
- Teacher Development
- Standards for Effective Teacher Educators
- Functions of Teacher Educators

Learning Objectives

Upon completion of this chapter, the students will be able to:

- Describe the good qualities of the nurse teacher
- List down the characteristics of a teaching model
- Describe the process of teacher development
- List the functions of teacher educator
- Describe the principles of teaching
- List twelve qualities of a teacher as a mentor
- List down the standards for effective teacher educator

To be a good teacher/nursing lecturer is a great task to adapt, here you are going to train the hands and brain to care of the individuals who too have hands and brain in addition they are sick too. Here the responsibility on the teacher cannot be explained with mere words; because any 'wrong' in teaching ends up in 'wrong learning' and again 'the wrong learning' leads to another wrong. Ultimately, the 'wrong chain' rightly plays with the life of a human being leading to death. Nurse teachers being the molders of 'future nurses', need to possess good qualities to bring about quality nurses. The following are some of the good qualities of the nurse teacher.

GOOD QUALITIES OF THE NURSE TEACHER

- **Patience:** Patience is one of those obvious traits that is often surprisingly under-cultivated in teachers. Having patience both with students and yourself will create a more disciplined, more rational you. Patience can overcome anxiety, fear, discouragement and failure, which you can apply both to your own teaching style, but also impart to your students. How to get this coveted quality? Be patient in answering to students; progress by taking a few deep breaths and taking an extra 30 seconds to answer a student's question, make a diagnosis, or reply to an irate patient. Remind yourself that all things take time.
- **Emotional intelligence:** Part of a teacher's job is to help a student get through the course with success. Sometimes this means recognizing that specific students need extra help, and sometimes it means giving freer reign to a student who is doing especially well. Research tracking over 160

high performing individuals in a variety of industries and job levels revealed that emotional intelligence was two times more important in contributing to excellence than intellect and expertise alone. Emotional intelligence can help you discern what your students need, but it can also be a valuable tool to help you decide how to react in stressful teaching situations, navigate academic politics, and bond with students to give everyone a richer and more meaningful experience.

- **Dedication:** To be a nurse, a person needs endless dedication and a real belief that they are changing the world. To see dedication in a teacher inspires the students and shows them that even through many years of nursing, that the instructor has not lost their spark. In some ways, teaching a future nurse the art of determination is even more important than teaching those basic nursing skills. By being an example of dedication, the instructor is able to teach a valuable lesson that will help students break into their chosen profession and stay there.
- **Adaptability:** Adaptability is a key skill for a nurse educator because no two subjects (and indeed, no two students) are alike. It is impossible to apply the same template to every type of situation with which you are presented. It is worth noting, however, that being adaptable does not mean being a pushover! The nurse educators have a strict set of ethics and practices that demand hard work from their students, but these rules must be balanced by the recognition that you can always adjust things as you go along.
- **Social skills**: Basic social skills are important as a teacher, because you are a role model to your students. Emotionally, we learn to manage strong feelings, such as anger and show empathy for others, which can be helpful when managing difficult students. Ethically, we develop the ability to sincerely care for others and engage in socially responsible actions, which is of utmost importance when shaping the minds of future nurses. Behaviorally, we learn specific communication skills such as sharing and turn taking, which help as a core means of achieving our objectives in the hospital; we can well imagine a hospital without these skills, and you begin to realize how important they are.
- **Positive attitude:** Positive thinking can bring happiness and levity and helps a person cope with the setbacks of everyday life. Especially, when nurse educators find themselves dealing with the tedious minutia of academic life, filled with endless bureaucracy and regulations, a positive attitude can overcome even the worst day. Practice your own positive attitude by laughing at jokes, reading inspiring quotes, or simply writing down 10 things you are thankful for. It can make a huge difference!
- **Reflection:** Everyone makes mistakes, and if you are lucky enough to be a nurse educator your mistakes will likely be pointed out to you in a large classroom full of people who expect perfection. Embarrassing, yes, but it happens to everyone. The key is to learn from it. And why stop there? Learn from everything that you do. Think critically about your actions, not just at New Years' resolution time or in the therapist's office, but everyday. Your job as a nurse educator is to be constantly learning. When you are looking in the mirror, you are looking at the problem. But, remember, you are also looking at the solution.
- **Confidence:** Teaching is a tough job, especially when your students are adults. After all, they have grown minds, so why should they listen to you? Your sense of confidence is what gives your students confidence in you. If you are constantly second-guessing yourself, you will be a mess in the classroom even if you have got 25 years of nursing experience under your belt. As they say, sometimes even the best nurses cannot be nurse educators—it takes a special level of confidence in your own talent and ability in order to teach others how it is done. If that sounds scary, well,

that is because teaching can be scary. The good news? The more you start to teach others, the more you realize how much you still have to learn yourself. In turn, the more you desire further learning, the better teacher you become. The ability to recognize one's own opportunities for growth is of paramount importance. And when you finally realize that you are always a student (and like it!) that is when you are a real nurse educator.

- **Humor:** You cannot even think about functioning as a nursing teacher when you do not have a sense of humor. With all the disgusting body functions, bad tempers, big egos and whirlwind pace of the nursing world, there is not a lot of tolerance for someone who cannot handle it all in stride with a quick joke and a smile. Your students will appreciate it, and your stress levels (and the people you take your stress out on) will thank you.
- **Passion:** Passion, of course, tops the list. Simply put, if you do not want to be a nurse educator, then you will not make a good nurse educator. It is a difficult and challenging job that is not for everyone, but those who really love nursing and teaching will thrive. Passion shows through in all aspects of teaching: in the lesson plan, attention to detail, and especially in the attention paid to students. It is passion that really makes a great teacher.

Teaching Principles

Teaching is a complex entity. Teaching requires teachers to be multitasking personalities with high level brilliance and critical thinking and analytical abilities. To get the name of 'Efficient teacher' teachers must adopt and practice certain principles:

Acquiring relevant knowledge about students

Knowing the clients is very important for any profession. Nursing faculty knows how to learn their students. Here, the teacher puts more efforts to learn students that would help her to become an efficient teacher. Knowing the students start from the first contact or meeting. For example, students' cultural and generational backgrounds influence how they see the world; disciplinary backgrounds lead students to approach problems in different ways; and students' prior knowledge shapes new learning.

(a) Learning objectives (i.e. the knowledge and skills that we expect students to demonstrate by the end of a course); (b) the instructional activities (e.g. case studies, labs, discussions, readings) support these learning objectives by providing goal-oriented practice; and (c) the assessments (e.g. tests, papers, problem sets, performances) provide opportunities for students to demonstrate and practice the knowledge and skills articulated in the objectives, and for instructors to offer targeted feedback that can guide further learning.

Efficiency in Aligning the three Major Concepts of Instruction

Articulating explicit expectations regarding learning objectives and policies: Being clear about our expectations and communicating them explicitly helps students learn more and perform better. Articulating our learning objectives (i.e. the knowledge and skills that we expect students to demonstrate by the end of a course) gives students a clear target to aim for and enables them to monitor their progress along the way. Orienting the students to the policies of the college is added responsibility of the teacher.

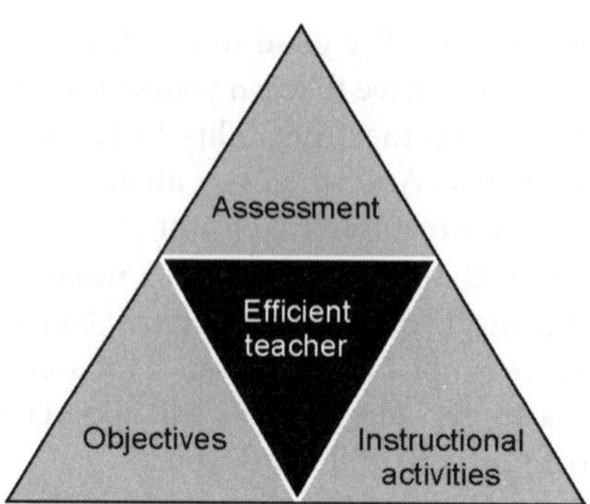

Prioritizing the knowledge and skills we choose to focus on: This involves (a) recognizing the parameters of the course (e.g., class size, students' backgrounds and experiences, course position in the curriculum sequence, number of course units), (b) setting our priorities for student learning, and (c) determining a set of objectives that can be reasonably accomplished.

Recognizing and overcoming our expert blind spots: We often skip or combine critical steps when we teach. Students do not yet have sufficient background and experience to make these leaps and can become confused. We need to identify and explicitly communicate to students the knowledge and skills we take for granted.

- Adopting appropriate teaching roles to support our learning goals.
- We can take on a variety of roles in our teaching (e.g., synthesizer, moderator, challenger, commentator). This would help the students to a great extent.
- Progressively refining our courses based on reflection and feedback.
- Teaching requires adapting. We need to continually reflect on our teaching and be ready to make changes when appropriate.

Characteristics of Teaching Models

Teaching models are specific approaches to instruction that have three characteristics:

- Goals: They are designed to help students develop critical-thinking abilities and acquire deep understanding of specific forms of content.
- Phases: They include a series of steps—often referred to as 'phases'—that are intended to help students reach specific learning goals.
- Foundations: They are supported by theory and research on learning and motivation.

> A holistic orientation uses social constructivist approaches of learning that focus on the development of the individual while fostering awareness and understanding of education in the broader context–community and world. Teacher education pedagogy builds on this broader perspective of the 'whole teacher' and emphasizes reflective practice, critical inquiry and the engagement of candidates in learning communities. (Sleeter, 2004; Taylor & Sobel, 2001).

Preparation of professional teacher

Several different approaches and models of teacher education and development are found in peer reviewed research literature.

The Applied Science Model: Put forward by Michael J. Wallace in 1991. The model derives its authority from the achievements of empirical science. The Applied Science Model is based on the following assumptions: Teaching is a science and as such can be examined rationally and objectively. Teachers learn to be teachers by being taught research-based theories. These theories are being conveyed to the students only by those who are considered to be the experts in the particular field. Teachers are said to be educated when they become proficient enough to apply these theories in practice.

The Craft Model: It is the oldest form of professional education and is still used today in teacher education, albeit rather limitedly. Its conceptual basis, however, is widely utilized in practicum courses in which students work with classroom teachers, often called cooperating teachers. The basic assumptions underlying this model are as follows. In its most basic form, Craft Model consists of the trainee or beginner working closely with the expert teacher. The practitioner is supposed to learn by imitating all the teaching techniques used by the experienced teacher. Knowledge is acquired as a result of observation, instruction, and practice.

> **Total of 103 teaching** skills have been identified necessary for an effective teacher.
> Out of these 103 skills, 20 skills have been tested by Stanford University which can be easily mastered through microteaching.

The Reflective Model: It is not an innovation in teaching. It has its roots in the work of a number of educational theorists and practitioners. The reflective model is based on the assumption that teachers develop professional competence through reflecting on their own practice. In other words, a teaching experience is recalled and considered to reach an evaluation and to provide input into future planning and action.

Twelve Qualities of a Teacher as a Mentor

Committed to the work

- Focuses on educational needs of the students
- Works with passion
- Keen to uphold the university's values
- Enthusiastic about work and about teaching

Encourages and appreciates diversity

- Does not stereotype or speak negatively of others
- Nurtures and encourages diversity
- Seeks and encourages understanding of, and respect for, people of diverse backgrounds

Interacts and communicates respect

- Communicates effectively with others
- Encourages input from others, listening deeply and giving credit for their contributions
- Acts with integrity
- Provides a model of high ethical standards
- Shows a caring attitude

Motivates students and co-workers

- Encourages students to achieve their goals
- Provides constructive feedback
- Monitors progress of students and fosters their success

Brings a wide range of skills and talents to teaching

- Teaching is clearly presented and stimulates high-order thinking skills
- Presents difficult concepts comprehensibly
- Brings appropriate evidence to the critique
- Teaches memorably

Demonstrates leadership in teaching

- Contributes to course design and structure
- Contributes to publications on education
- Evidence of self-development in an educational context
- Demonstrates creativity in teaching strategies
- Committed to professional development in education

Important 10 skills for teacher

- Planning
- Set induction
- Presentation
- Questioning
- Encouraging the students to question
- Exemplification
- Communication
- Methodology
- Judging the students problems
- Summing up

Encourages an open and trusting learning environment

- Creates a climate of trust
- Encourages students to learn from mistakes
- Helps students redefine failure as a learning experience
- Encourages student questions and engagement in the learning process
- Encourages student growth with appropriate behavior-based feedback

Fosters critical thinking

- Teaches students how to think, not what to think
- Encourages students to organize, analyze and evaluate
- Explores with probing questions
- Discusses ideas in an organized way
- Helps students to focus on key issues
- Trains students in strategic thinking

Encourages creative work

- Motivates students to create new ideas
- Fosters innovation and new approaches

Emphasizes teamwork

- Builds links at national and international levels in education
- Encourages students to work in teams
- Encourages collaborative learning

Seeks continually to improve teaching skills

- Seeks to learn and incorporate new skills, and information teaching
- Seeks feedback and criticism
- Keeps up to date in specialty

Provides positive feedback

- Listens to students and discovers their educational needs
- Values students, never belittles
- Provides constructive feedback
- Helps and supports people to grow
- Teaches the students how to monitor their own progress.

TEACHER DEVELOPMENT

Nurses are expected to incorporate teaching in all aspects of their practice. Teaching is one activity that reportedly gives nurses a great deal of professional satisfaction.

- Program or curriculum-based models that are designed to implement a specific instructional program or a new curriculum that includes new learning objectives, suggested or required learning activities and/or student assessment techniques. This is sometimes referred to as a 'cascade' model where knowledge is passed down from experts, usually through workshops and training sessions.
- Skills-based models that focus on general or specific teaching skills such as interactive teaching, classroom management, student questioning, lesson planning and many more. These models often use a scaffolding approach, where the skills are developed over time in a planned sequence, going from dependence on experts to independence.
- Concerns-based Adoption Models
- Mentoring or Coaching Models
- Thoughtful or reflective teaching models
- Social-professional networking models
- Site/organization-based models where teachers work in teams on individually on long-term plans
- Self-directed models where the teacher determines the goals, plans and activities
- Action-research models where teachers use data and student/parent feedback to improve their practice
- Multi-level or comprehensive models where teacher development is part of a system-wide approach that develops the skills of school principals, support staff, such as guidance counselors and school psychologists
- Comprehensive, inter-sectorial models that develop teacher competencies in partnership programs with other sectors that employ professionals, such as public health nurses, social workers, addictions workers, etc.

Standards for Effective Teacher Educators

Numerous distinguished teacher education organizations with decision-making power (i.e. accreditation or certification) have set standards applicable to teacher educators throughout the world. The National Professional Standards outline seven key elements for effective teacher educators (identified as 'lead teachers'), which are summarized below (AITSL).

Standard 1. Know the students and how they learn. Lead teachers are expected to select, develop, evaluate and revise teaching strategies 'to improve student learning using knowledge of the physical, social and intellectual development and characteristics of students' in order to meet the needs of students from diverse cultural and economic backgrounds.

Standard 2. Know the content and how to teach it. Lead teachers must be able to 'lead initiatives [...] to evaluate and improve knowledge of content and teaching strategies,' as well as to 'monitor and evaluate the implementation of teaching strategies to expand learning opportunities and content knowledge for all students'.

Standard 3. Plan for and implement effective teaching and learning. Qualified lead teachers should 'demonstrate exemplary practice and high expectations [...] and lead colleagues to plan, implement and review the effectiveness of their learning and teaching programs'.

Standard 4. Create and maintain supportive and safe learning environments. Lead teachers are expected to be active in 'the development of productive and inclusive learning environments,' as well as to 'lead and implement behavior management initiatives' in order to ensure students' well-being.

Standard 5. Assess, provide feedback and report on student learning. Lead teachers are required to 'evaluate school assessment policies and strategies' to diagnose learning needs and to coordinate student performance and program evaluation using internal and external student assessment data to improve teaching practice.

Standard 6. Engage in professional learning. Lead teachers should 'initiate collaborative relationships to expand professional learning opportunities, engage in research, and provide quality opportunities and placements for pre-service teachers'.

Standard 7. Engage professionally with colleagues, parents/careers and the community. Lead teachers are expected to 'model exemplary ethical behavior and exercise informed judgments in all professional dealings with students, colleagues and the community,' as well as taking a 'leadership role in professional and community networks and supporting the involvement of colleagues in external learning opportunities'.

Functions of teacher educators: Standards within a profession are often associated with the necessary functions of individuals within that profession. Koster, Korthagen, Wubbels & Hoornweg (1996) discusses several general functions that teacher educators fulfill.

- **Facilitators of the learning process for student teachers:** Effective teacher educators play a major role in facilitating and supporting the reflective learning process student teachers develop (see, Richards and Lockhart, 1994). This, however, needs be accomplished by sharing not only their theoretical knowledge, but also by putting this knowledge into their own practice, in other words, by 'making tacit knowledge explicit' (Korthagen and Kessels, 1999, p. 31).
- **Developers of new knowledge and curricula:** Teacher educators are expected to create new knowledge, consisting of practical knowledge in the form of new curricula and learning programs for teacher education and schools, as well as theoretical knowledge generated from research.
- **Assessors and Gatekeepers:** Another key function of teacher educators is assessment; both formative assessment enhancing learning, as well as summative assessment that requires teacher educators to act as gate-keepers and decide who has the necessary training and skills to become a teacher. In this sense, teacher educators not only provide support to candidates seeking enter the profession, but also act as their judges before they can do so, a dual role some have found to be problematic (e.g. Wilson, Darling-Hammond, & Berry, 2001).
- **Collaborators and team members:** Efficient teacher educators are collaborators with members of the university and other higher educational institutions and decision makers (Koster, Korthagen, and Wubbels, 1998), as well as with teachers and school administrators where teacher candidates' student-teaching takes place. Thus, it is essential that teacher educators help student teachers to develop the skill of being good team members through involvement with the respective contexts they serve (university and school); by promoting partnership in

their relationships with others (i.e. with student teachers, or other faculty); and by encouraging student teachers to take part in joint efforts, such as group-work and research projects.

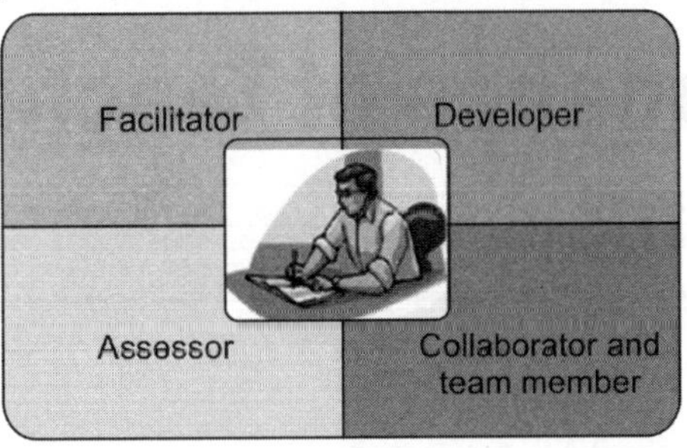

14

Interdependence of Teaching and Learning

Chapter Highlights

- Elements in a Students' Relationship to a Teacher
- Teachers' Responsibility to Students
- Definitions-Education Process, Teaching, Instruction and Learning
- Teachers' Beliefs about Learners, Learning and Themselves
- Six Major Categories of Effective Teaching
- Key Elements of Learning and Their Relationship with the Curriculum
- Different Phases of Teaching
- Different Teaching Models

Learning Objectives

Upon completion of this chapter, the students will be able to:

- Describe the elements in a students' relationship to a teacher
- Describe teachers' responsibility to students
- Define the terms education process, teaching, instruction and learning
- Describe teachers' beliefs about learners, learning and themselves
- Identify six major categories of effective teaching
- Describe the key elements of learning and their relationship with the curriculum
- Describe different phases of teaching
- Apply different teaching models

Teaching learning system is a purposeful complex system composed of interdependent interacting parts:

- The parts are on continuous interaction with each other.
- The parts are dependent on each other.
- The parts put together form a whole. Each component or part complements the other parts. Teacher and learner relationship is mutual relationship. The relationship between student and teacher, if it is to be maximally productive, must reflect certain attitudes and commitments of each to the other.

ELEMENTS IN A STUDENT'S RELATIONSHIP TO A TEACHER

Respect to Teacher

The student must respect his or her teacher and hold him in the highest esteem, for this is a necessary prerequisite to accepting his advice. Regarding someone who is only giving factual information, and not assuming the role of mentor, this condition becomes less critical.

Trust Your Teacher

The student must trust the teacher's concern. The student must believe that the teacher always has his or her best interests in mind. If the student would sense some ulterior motive, some self-interest, or even carelessness in the teacher's instruction, he or she would not be able to surrender wholeheartedly to the teacher's advice, and this would make the entire exchange meaningless.

Commitment: The student must commit himself or herself to following the instruction with utmost discipline, for only then can the intended effect be realized. Just as a doctor's orders must be followed precisely, since failure to do so could cause more harm than good, so a teacher's 'prescription' must be obeyed with equal conscientiousness and deference to his superior knowledge and authority.

TEACHER'S RESPONSIBILITY TO STUDENTS

Know Your Student

The first is fulfillment of the prerequisite of getting to know his students individually, to probe the innermost depths of their hearts as well as examining the outer details of their lives. As the teacher's familiarity grows, so the potency of his advice deepens proportionately.

Affection

The teacher must express love and affection toward his or her students. It is this affection that dissolves the students' natural tendency to resist being told what to do. Thus, the advice can penetrate more deeply and effectively.

Give Time

The teacher must take time to reflect upon his her students' progress, refining and adjusting his vision of how best to influence them toward positive change. This is an ongoing requirement because students quickly 'outgrow' old advice, and the categories of what is beautiful and what is ugly change with each new stage of growth.

TEACHING AND LEARNING

The **education process** is a systematic, sequential, planned course of action consisting of two major interdependent operations, teaching and learning. This process forms a continuous cycle that also involves two interdependent players, the teacher and the learner.

Teaching is a specialized communication process in which desired behavior changes are achieved. The goal of all teaching is learning. Learning is thought to mean gaining knowledge, comprehension, or mastery.

Teaching is a deliberate intervention that involves the planning and implementation of instructional activities and experiences to meet intended learner outcomes according to a teaching plan. The actual act of teaching is merely one component of the education process. Education process includes the acts of teaching and instruction.

> My experience on education indicates that the concept of effective learning is derived from the understanding of many elements that influence learning. Studies on philosophy of education, curriculum, instruction and evaluation support the idea that these factors have their individual strengths to affect how a person learns (Wong and Watkins, 1998)

Instruction, a term often used interchangeably with teaching, is one aspect of teaching.

Learning is defined as a change in behavior (knowledge, skills, and attitudes) that can occur at anytime or in any place as a result of exposure to environmental stimuli. Learning is a process of assimilating new information that promotes a permanent change in behavior.

Teaching learning process is not a linear sequence of events but a dynamic phenomenon, whereby the teacher, who is more knowledgeable, is called upon to act, among other things, as a mediator, influencing and being influenced by the students, who happen to lack this knowledge. Teachers in the real world come in all shapes and sizes, exhibiting a wide range of different personalities, beliefs and ways of thinking and working.

Teachers' Beliefs

Beliefs cannot be defined or evaluated, but there are a number of things that we should know about them. Beliefs are culturally bound and, since they are formed early in life, they tend to be resistant to change. By virtue of the fact that they are difficult to measure, we almost always have to infer people's beliefs from the ways in which they act rather than from what they say they believe.

BELIEFS ABOUT LEARNERS

Teachers hold any or a combination of beliefs about their students. Roland Meighan (1990) suggests that there are at least seven different ways in which teachers construe learners and that such evaluative constructions have a profound influence on their classroom practice. So, according to him, learners may be construed as:

- Resisters
- Receptacles
- Raw material
- Clients
- Partners
- Individual explorers
- Democratic explorers

These constructs are seen in terms of a continuum which mirrors the nature of the teacher-learner power relationship. Thus, the first three constructs are teacher dominated, whereas the latter involve learner participation.

BELIEFS ABOUT LEARNING

Teaching is not indivisible from learning. We can be good teachers only if we know what we mean by learning because only then can we know what we expect our learners to achieve. If our goal is to prepare our students to pass an exam, then this will affect the way in which we teach.

Gow and Kember (1993) suggest that most approaches to learning can be subsumed under any of the following points:

- A quantitative increase in knowledge
- Memorization
- The acquisition of facts and procedures which can be retained and/or used in practice
- The abstraction of meaning
- An interpretative process aimed at the understanding of reality
- Some form of personal change.

TEACHERS' BELIEFS ABOUT THEMSELVES

For humanistic teachers, teaching is essentially a personal expression of the self, which has particular implications with regard to teachers' views of themselves, since a teacher who lacks self-esteem will not be able to build the self-esteem of others. The teacher who does not accept his learners for who they are makes it difficult for them to accept themselves.

Teaching is not merely information or knowledge, but mainly an expression of values and attitudes. What teachers usually get back from their students is what they themselves have brought to the teaching-learning process. The nurse as a teacher seeks to transmit information in such a way that the student demonstrates a relatively permanent change in behavior. After learning, students are capable of doing something that they could not do before learning took place. Effective teaching is a cause; learning becomes the effect. To teach effectively, in various educational settings nursing faculty need to understand the various domains of learning and related learning theories. This would be helpful for gaining confidence in teaching as well to function as an effective teacher using excellent measurement and evaluation strategies.

EFFECTIVE TEACHING IN NURSING

Jacobson (1966) identified six major categories of effective teaching in nursing.

- **Professional competence:** Professional competence means maintenance of thorough knowledge and skills throughout the career. Research reports that the teacher who enjoys nursing would show genuine interest in patients and displays confidence in professional abilities. Such teachers will be creative and stimulating the students can excite student interest in learning.
- **Interpersonal relationships with students**: This include personal interest in learners, sensitive to their feelings and problems, conveying respect, alleviating anxieties, accessible for conferences, being fair, permitting learners to express different points of view, Creating good atmosphere with sense of warmth. Nursing students and patients often lack self-confidence and fear of making mistakes while learning, leads to stress. Teachers can help learners maintain self-esteem and minimize anxieties by using three basic therapeutic approaches of 1. Empathic listening, 2. Acceptance and 3. Honest communication.

  Therapeutic approaches: Empathic listening-listen and try to see the world through the learners' eyes.

  Acceptance: Whether or not you like them-accept them as they are; Learners are different from each other.

  Honest communication: Openness between teacher and learners
- **Personal characteristics:** Qualities such as:
  - Authenticity
  - Enthusiasm
  - Cheerfulness
  - Self-control
  - Patience
  - Flexibility
  - Sense of humor
  - Good speaking voice
  - Caring attitude are desirable personal characteristics of teacher.

- **Teaching practices:** Teaching practices is defined as the mechanics, methods and skills in class room and clinical teaching. Students and colleagues value a teacher who has thorough knowledge of the subject and can present material in an interesting, clear and organized manner.
- **Evaluation practices:** Communicate the expectations, alert them then and there when expectation are not met and use fairness in evaluation.

KEY ELEMENTS OF LEARNING AND RELATIONSHIPS WITH CURRICULUM

Key elements within the curriculum and the relationships between them are shown in diagram below. Staff and students are at the heart of curriculum. The relationships between them are shaped by the answers to key questions about:

- Assessment
- Content
- Learning interactions
- The connections between those elements.

In the diagram the top question in each pair is a design question for staff. The lower set of questions is commonly asked by students to shape their approach to learning. Curriculum design should help ensure alignment between the answers staff build into their design and those that students find through their experience of the curriculum.

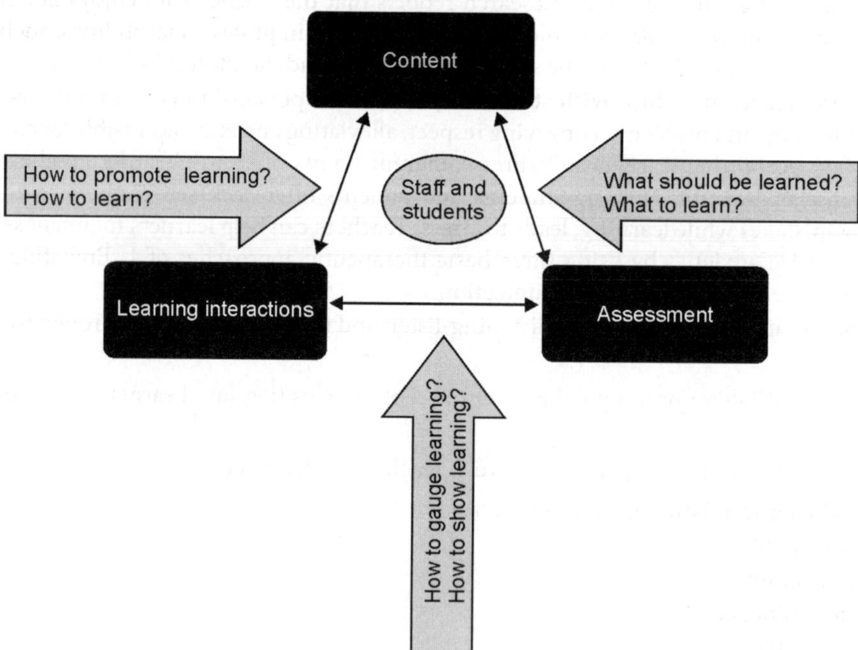

These elements and relationships of course are all context bound. In current systemic approaches to curriculum design, a major element of the educational context is the intended learning outcomes for students of a topic or course.

Intended learning outcomes frame and influence the detail and alignment of assessment, learning interactions and content (Biggs, 1999). Intended learning outcomes describe the characteristics that a student should be able show on successful completion of a course or topic. Assessment gauges the extent of students' achievement of the intended outcomes, learning interactions and content should help to build towards students' achievement of those outcomes.

ADDITIONAL IMPORTANT ELEMENTS IN CONTEMPORARY TEACHING

Significance of Reflection in Teaching

You are not a brilliant teacher if you feel proud for simply walking through the three phases of teaching. The most important aspect of teaching and learning process is 'reflection'. After you have taught a lesson, you will want to reconsider your planning and the decisions you have made. Reflection, whether written or mental, is an effective tool for refining professional thoughts, ideas, and beliefs. Reflection enables us to evaluate our experiences, learn from mistakes, repeat successes, and revise and plan for the future Specifically, reflection tries to answer questions such as the following:

- How appropriate were the topics—that is, should they be taught again?
- Was the sequence of topics appropriate? If not, how should they be re-sequenced?
- Was my goal(s) appropriate for my students?
- Was my instruction aligned? Did my lesson plans facilitate my unit plan? Were the procedures and assessments I specified consistent with my goals?
- Were the procedures I used as effective as they might have been? If not, what procedures might have been better?
- Did the materials I used adequately represent the topic?
- What representations or resources would have made the topic more understandable?
- Is there a way I could have made the overall environment more conducive to learning?

Technology in the Classroom

Our modern world is often characterized as having been profoundly shaped by a technological revolution, a change that has, among other things, drastically altered the way in which we both live and teach. With specific regard to education, today's teachers need to be knowledgeable about the hardware, primarily computers; the software, disks, programs, and other resources available and the appropriate applications of technology to classroom instruction. From a constructivist perspective, the implementation of technology in the classroom enhances the facilitating role of the teacher, who becomes the 'guide on the side' rather than the 'sage on the stage'. Technology can support many classroom strategies, including the following (Armstrong, Henson, and Savage, 2005):

- Presenting content effectively
- Re teaching and reinforcing content
- Providing enrichment experiences for talented learners
- Individualizing assignments
- Promoting global perspectives by using Websites and encouraging.

PHASES OF INSTRUCTION

The conceptual frame for teaching flows in three phases. A teacher, in developing any learning activity, first plans, then implements those plans, and finally assesses the activity's success. In addition to its role as an organizational framework for classroom instruction, this approach provides a focus for connecting learning experiences with the standards set in the country or region. These three phases are sequential and interrelated. The basic steps in the three-phase approach to instruction are:

- Planning
- Implementing
- Assessing

Planning

Teaching begins with planning, in which a teacher finds himself as the initiator of the teaching process. Teacher always starts with the questions like: What exactly I want my students to learn, understand, appreciate and perform in an appropriate manner? What should be my role in it and to do that what do I need to have in my brain and hands. The answer to this question is the teacher's goal, and the first step in the planning phase is the establishment of some kind of goal. Whatever the intent, the establishment of some type of goal or purpose is a first priority in teaching. What determines a teacher's goals? The answer to this question can be philosophical or practical. Subsequent steps in the planning phase are selecting an instructional strategy, organizing learning activities, and gathering supporting materials. Effective instructional planning extends well beyond establishing learning goals, Constructivist classrooms emphasize creating classroom rules collaboratively with students as a meaningful learning experience, leading to the following (Castle, 1993):

- Active involvement
- Reflection
- Meaningful connections
- Respect for rules
- Sense of community
- Problem-solving through negotiation
- Cooperation
- Higher-order thinking skills
- Ownership.

Implementing

Having determined a goal and selected an appropriate means to reach that goal, a teacher then implements that strategy. Selecting the most appropriate method depends on the goal, students' backgrounds and needs, available materials, and the teacher's personality, strengths, and style.

In addition to teaching strategies classroom management is an another essential component of the implementing phase. Management ranges from something as simple as a verbal reminder to a student to pay attention to the creation of a complex set of rules and procedures to create productive learning environments. Conducive environment enhances smooth learning. Without attending to the learning task, students cannot learn, and organizing a learning activity invariably requires the teacher to consider management issues.

Assessing

This phase or component beautifies and gives meaning to the entire process of teaching and learning. This gives lays the base for our future planning phase. This can be done in many ways, including administering tests or quizzes, grading individual project/group project, written or spoken seminars, conference or simply noting students' reactions to questions or comments. The teacher can use each of these methods to make decisions concerning whether the goal established in the planning stage was reached.

Teaching Models

There are literally hundreds of models of teaching and learning. **Models deal with the ways in which learning environments and instructional experiences can be constructed, sequenced, or delivered**. They may provide theoretical or instructional frameworks, patterns, or examples for any number of educational components — curricula, teaching techniques, instructional groupings, classroom management plans, content development, sequencing, delivery, the development of support materials, presentation methods, etc. **Models of teaching and learning are critical pieces to instructional planning and delivery.**

Uses of Teaching Models

- Develop highly tuned and more varied professional repertoires
- To reach larger numbers for students more effectively
- To create either more uniform, or varied, or effective instructional events, guided by targeted subjects, content, or processes
- To understand curricular foci better, especially as different models can be matched specifically to both learning outcomes and/or targeted learning populations
- Gain insights into why some methods work with some learners. while others do not
- Radically modify or redesign existing methods of teaching and instructional delivery so that emerging or modified instructional techniques may better meet the needs of tomorrow's students.

Types of Teaching Models

Traditionally, models of teaching are represented by a broad array of teaching systems, each system containing a distinctive philosophical foundation, or theory of learning basis, with related pedagogical methodologies. Most models can be loosely fitted into one of four or five distinct families of educational psychology—*social; information-processing; personal; behavioral* systems are the traditional ones, with *constructivist* added lately.

Basically there are two types of models of teaching—ones that can be cleanly categorized and placed into one of the classic philosophical orientation groupings—*social; information-processing; personal; or behavioral* systems; or ones that are hybrid/mixed models that have combined elements from different families of learning like those that can be labeled as *constructivist.*

Traditional Teaching Models

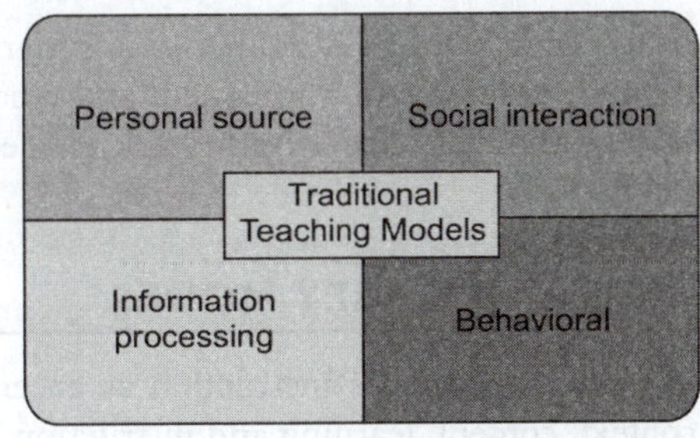

Personal source: This group of approaches acknowledges the uniqueness of each learner. Methods in this category foster the importance of individuals in creating, directing, and structuring personal meaning. Also models in this area are often targeted to foster things like self-esteem, self-efficacy, emotional and personal understanding and acceptance. Carl Roger's *Nondirective Teaching Model* would be a good example for this group.

Social interaction: This group of methods aims at building learning communities and purports to develop productive ways of interacting in a democratic setting. These models also emphasize that human learning occurs in social settings and through modeled behaviors and social exchanges. The Schaftel's *Role Playing Model* is one of the more popular models in this group. Donald Oliver's The *Jurisprudence Model* also exemplifies a form of social learning.

Information processing: This is the largest grouping of approaches aimed at emphasizing ways of learning specific information and of acquiring and organizing data, solving problems, and developing concepts and language. Models confined to this category deal with intellectual development, powers of reasoning and logic, aiding students in organizing and retaining information, and in enhancing their meta- cognitive functions. Primary examples designate in this area might be David Ausubel's *Advanced Organizers*, or Jerome Bruner's *Concept Attainment* models.

Behavioral: Behavioral techniques are amenable to highly structured outcomes that concentrate on observable objectives such as learning to read, physical skills, behavioral and emotional adaptations and restructuring. These models are highly structured with finite goals toward specific predetermined ends. B. F. Skinner is one of the more well know developers of behavioral techniques like his *Operant Conditioning*.

EXAMPLES OF INSTRUCTIONAL DESIGNS BY DIFFERENT SCHOLARS

There are many researchers contributed various teaching models to teaching. The selection of teaching model is totally based on the institutional policy on curriculum and teaching style of individual teacher.

Backward Design

The idea of Backward Design comes from Wiggins and McTighe and suggests that learning experiences should be planned with the final assessment in mind. One starts with the end—the desired results (goals or standards)—and then derives the curriculum from the evidence of learning (performances) called for by the standard and the teaching needed to equip students to perform' (Wiggins and McTighe, 2000, page 8) By beginning with the end in mind, teachers are able to avoid the common problem of planning forward from unit to another, only to find that in the end some students are prepared for the final assessment and others are not.

Three Stages of Backward Design

Stage 1: Identify Desired Results

Stage 2: Determine Acceptable Evidence of Learning Stage

Stage 3: Design Learning Experiences and Instruction

Instructional Design is defined as 'a systematic process that is employed to develop education and training programs in a consistent and reliable fashion' (Reiser and Dempsey, 2007). In addition, it may be thought of as a framework for developing modules or lessons that (Merrill, Drake, Lacy, Pratt, 1996).

DICK AND CAREY MODEL

The model addresses instruction as an entire system, focusing on the interrelationship between context, content, learning and instruction. According to Dick and Carey, 'Components such as the instructor, learners, materials, instructional activities, delivery system, and learning and performance environments interact with each other and work together to bring about the desired student learning outcomes'. The components of the Systems Approach Model, also known as the Dick and Carey Model.

The Dick and Carey Model includes the 9 step process:
Stage 1: Identify Instructional Goals
Stage 2. Conduct Instructional Analysis
Stage 3. Identify Entry Behaviors and Learner Characteristics
Stage 4: Write Performance Objectives
Stage 5. Develop Criterion-Referenced Test Items
Stage 6. Develop Instructional Strategy
Stage 7: Develop and Select Instructional Materials
Stage 8: Develop and Conduct Formative Evaluation
Stage 9: Develop and Conduct Summative Evaluation.

The Kemp Design Model

- Identify instructional problems, and specify goals for designing an instructional program
- Examine learner characteristics that should receive attention during planning
- Identify subject content, and analyze task components related to stated goals and purposes
- State instructional objectives for the learner
- Sequence content within each instructional unit for logical learning
- Design instructional strategies so that each learner can master the objectives
- Plan the instructional message and delivery
- Develop evaluation instruments to assess objectives
- Select resources to support instruction and learning activities.

ASSURE Model

The ASSURE model is an ISD (Instructional Systems Design) process that was modified to be used by teachers in the regular classroom. The ISD process is one in which teachers and trainers can use to design and develop the most appropriate learning environment for their students. You can use this process in writing your lesson plans and in improving teaching and learning. The ASSURE model incorporates Robert Gagne's events of instruction to assure effective use of media in instruction.

A —Analyze learners
S — State standards and objectives
S — Select strategies, technology, media and materials
U —Utilize technology, media and materials
R — Require learner participation
E — Evaluate and revise.

15

Learning Theories

Chapter Highlights

- Classification of Major Learning Theories
- Behavioral Learning Theory
- Contiguity Theory
- Classical or Respondent Conditioning Theory
- Basic Principles of the Process of Classical Conditioning
- Operant or Instrumental Conditioning Theory
- Cognitive Theory
- Main Issues Studied and Discussed by Cognitive Psychologists
- Gestalt Psychology
- Constructivism Principles of Constructivist Theory
- General Educational Applications of Constructive Theory
- Thorndike's Laws of Learning
- Social Learning Theory
- Principles of Social Learning Theory
- Perspectives Upon Learning Theories
- Deep and Surface Learning
- Characteristics and Factors that Encourage Deep and Surface Approaches to Learning

Learning Objectives

Upon completion of this chapter, the students will be able to:

- List major learning theories
- Explain behavioral learning theories and cognitive learning theories
- List down the principles of constructivist's theory
- State the meaning of deep and surface learning
- List down the factors encouraging deep and surface approaches to learning
- List the educational applications of constructivist's theory for designing instruction

There are many learning theories given by many scholars to perpetuate the teaching learning practices. Each theory has its own contribution for the reshaped system of education today. Nursing profession always tried pulling out the best concepts from behavioral and social sciences to make a platform for teaching and learning. Though there are many criticisms about learning theories but no teacher denies specific contribution to teaching and learning. Theories of learning, whether explicit or tacit, informed by study or intuition, well-considered or not, play a role in the choices instructors make concerning their teaching.

Learning theories take concepts and prepositions (statements of relationship between concepts) and fit them together to explain why people learn and predict under what circumstances they will learn.

CLASSIFICATION OF MAJOR LEARNING THEORIES

A. Behaviorist theories

B. Cognitive theories

Behavioral Learning Theory

According to the behaviorists, learning can be defined as 'the relatively permanent change in behavior brought about as a result of experience or practice' Behaviorists recognize that learning is an internal event. However, it is not recognized as learning until it is displayed by overt behavior. The behavioral learning theory is represented as an S-R paradigm. The organism is treated as a 'black box.' We only know what is going on inside the box by the organism's overt behavior.

Behavioral learning theories:

1. Contiguity theory
2. Classical or respondent conditioning theory
3. Operant or instrumental conditioning theory

Stimulus (S) → Organism (O) → Response (R)

There are three types of behavioral learning theories:

- **Contiguity theory:** Contiguity theory is based on the work of E R Guthrie. It proposes that any stimulus and response connected in time and/or space will tend to be associated.
- **Classical or respondent conditioning theory:** Classical conditioning was the first type of learning to be discovered and studied within the behaviorist tradition (hence the name 'classical'). Classical conditioning is a type of learning that had a major influence on the school of thought in psychology known as behaviorism. Discovered by Russian physiologist Ivan Pavlo, classical conditioning is a learning process that occurs through associations between an environmental stimulus and a naturally occurring stimulus.

Assumptions

- Behaviorism is based on the assumption that learning occurs through interactions with the environment.
- The environment shapes behavior.
- Consideration to internal mental states, such as thoughts, feelings, and emotions are useless in explaining behavior.

It is important to note that classical conditioning involves placing a neutral signal before a naturally occurring reflex. In Pavlov's classic experiment with dogs, the neutral signal was the sound of a tone and the naturally occurring reflex was salivating in response to food. By associating the neutral stimulus with the environmental stimulus (the presentation of food), the sound of the tone alone could produce the salivation response.

Basic principles of the process of classical conditioning

Unconditioned Stimulus

The unconditioned stimulus is one that unconditionally, naturally, and automatically triggers a response. For example, when you smell one of your favorite foods, you may immediately feel very hungry. In this example, the smell of the food is the unconditioned stimulus.

Unconditioned Response

The unconditioned response is the unlearned response that occurs naturally in response to the unconditioned stimulus. In our example, the feeling of hunger in response to the smell of food is the unconditioned response.

Conditioned Stimulus

The conditioned stimulus is previously neutral stimulus that, after becoming associated with the unconditioned stimulus, eventually comes to trigger a conditioned response. In our earlier example, suppose that when you smelled your favorite food, you also heard the sound of a whistle. While the whistle is unrelated to the smell of the food, if the sound of the whistle was paired multiple times with the smell, the sound would eventually trigger the conditioned response. In this case, the sound of the whistle is the conditioned stimulus.

Conditioned Response

The conditioned response is the learned response to the previously neutral stimulus. In our example, the conditioned response would be feeling hungry when you heard the sound of the whistle.

It can be helpful to look at a few examples of how the classical conditioning process operates both in experimental and real-world settings:

A stimulus will naturally (without learning) elicit or bring about a reflexive response. Unconditioned Stimulus (US) elicits > Unconditioned Response (UR).

Neutral Stimulus (NS) does not elicit the response of interest. For example, if air is blown into your eye, you blink. You have no voluntary or conscious control over whether the blink occurs or not.

Important elements in understanding the classical conditioning process

Acquisition: Acquisition is the initial stage of learning when a response is first established and gradually strengthened. For example, imagine that you are conditioning a dog to salivate in response to the sound of a bell. You repeatedly pair the presentation of food with the sound of the bell. You can say the response has been acquired as soon as the dog begins to salivate in response to the bell tone. Once the response has been acquired, you can gradually reinforce the salivation response to make sure the behavior is well learned.

Extinction: Extinction is when the occurrences of a conditioned response decrease or disappear. In classical conditioning, this happens when a conditioned stimulus is no longer paired with an unconditioned stimulus. For example, if the smell of food (the unconditioned stimulus) had been paired with the sound of a whistle (the conditioned stimulus), it would eventually come to evoke the conditioned response of hunger. However, if the unconditioned stimulus (the smell of food) were no longer paired with the conditioned stimulus (the whistle), eventually the conditioned response (hunger) would disappear.

Spontaneous recovery: Spontaneous recovery is the reappearance of the conditioned response after a rest period or period of lessened response. If the conditioned stimulus and unconditioned stimulus are no longer associated, extinction will occur very rapidly after a spontaneous recovery.

Stimulus generalization: Stimulus generalization is the tendency for the conditioned stimulus to evoke similar responses after the response has been conditioned. For example, if a child has been conditioned to fear a stuffed black monkey, the child will exhibit fear of objects similar to the conditioned stimulus.

Discrimination: Discrimination is the ability to differentiate between a conditioned stimulus and other stimuli that have not been paired with an unconditioned stimulus. For example, if a bell tone were the conditioned stimulus, discrimination would involve being able to tell the difference between the bell tone and other similar sounds.

Operant or instrumental conditioning theory

Operant conditioning was devised by behaviorist BF Skinner and referred to as Skinnerian conditioning. Changes in behavior are the result of an individual's response to events (stimuli) that occur in the environment. A response produces a consequence, such as defining a word, hitting a ball, or solving a math problem. When a particular Stimulus-Response (S-R) pattern is reinforced (rewarded), the individual is conditioned to respond. Operant conditioning (sometimes referred to as instrumental conditioning) is a method of learning that occurs through rewards and punishments for behavior. Through operant conditioning, an association is made between a behavior and a consequence for that behavior.

When a particular Stimulus-Response (S-R) pattern is reinforced (rewarded), the individual is conditioned to respond. The distinctive characteristic of operant conditioning relative to previous forms of behaviorism is that the organism can emit responses instead of only eliciting response due to an external stimulus.

- ***Reinforcement*** is the key element in Skinner's S-R theory. A reinforcer is anything that strengthens the desired response. There are two kinds of reinforcers:
  - ***Positive reinforcers*** are favorable events or outcomes that are presented after the behavior, such as praise or a direct reward. It could be verbal praise, a good grade or a feeling of increased accomplishment or satisfaction.

    Negative reinforcers are any stimulus that results in the increased frequency of a response when it is withdrawn (different from aversive stimuli—punishment—which result in reduced responses). Negative reinforcers involve the removal of an unfavorable event or outcome after the display of a behavior. In these situations, a response is strengthened by the removal of something considered unpleasant. In both of these cases of reinforcement, the behavior increases.

Cognitive Theory

This school was heavily influenced by Ivan Pavlov and BF Skinner. They proposed that psychology could only become an objective science if it is based on observable behavior in test subjects. Since mental events are not publicly observable, behaviorist psychologists avoided description of mental processes or the mind in their literature.

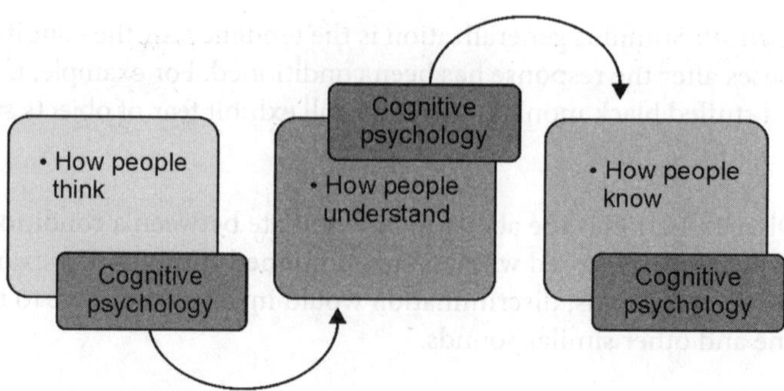

Cognitive psychology focuses on the study of how people think, understand, and know. They emphasize on learning and how people comprehend and represent the outside world within themselves and how our ways of thinking about the world influence our behavior. Cognitive theory attempts to explain human behavior by understanding the thought processes. 'Information processing' is a commonly used description of the mental process, comparing the human mind to a computer. Information process explains the way that information is handled once it enters the senses and how it is organized and stored. From a cognitive learning perspective, learning involves the transformation of information in the environment into knowledge that is stored in the mind. Cognitive learning theory includes several well-known perspectives, such as gestalt, information processing, human development, social constructivism, and social cognition theory.

Main issues studied and discussed by cognitive psychologists

The cognitive theories present a positive view of development, emphasizing conscious thinking.

The cognitive theories (especially Piaget's and Vygotsky's) emphasize on the individual's active construction of understanding.

Piaget's and Vygotsky's theories underscore the importance of examining developmental changes in children's thinking.

The information processing theory offers detailed descriptions of cognitive processes.

Gagne and his colleagues outlined nine events and their corresponding cognitive processes that activate effective learning (Gagne, Briggs, and Wagner, 1992):

- Gain the learner's attention (reception)
- Inform the learner of the objectives and expectations (expectancy)
- Stimulate the learner's recall of prior learning (retrieval)
- Present information (selective perception)
- Provide guidance to facilitate the learner's understanding (semantic encoding)
- Have the learner demonstrate the information or skill (responding)
- Give feedback to the learner (reinforcement)
- Assess the learner's performance (retrieval)
- Work to enhance retention and transfer through application and varied practice (generalization)

GESTALT PSYCHOLOGY

Gestalt psychologhy is a perspective focusing on the belief that human consciousness cannot be broken down into its elements. This approach to psychology was founded on the concept of the gestalt, or whole. Gestalt psychologists led by Max Wertheimer (1880–1943), Wolfgang Kohler (1887–1967) and Kurt Koffka (1886–1941) have made substantial contributions to our understanding of perception. Gestaltists pointed out that perception has meaning only when it is seen as a whole.

The word Gestalt in German literally means 'shape' or 'figure'. Gestaltists performed many researches on perception and human learning. They believed learning is the result from good perception, which enables an individual to form correct concept in their mind. Later on, they proposed the principles or law for perceptual organization. Gestalt psychology (also Gestalt of the Berlin School) is a theory of mind and brain that proposes that the operational principle of the brain is holistic, parallel, and analog, with self-organizing tendencies, or that the whole is different from the sum of its parts.

Gestalt's principles:

- Good form
- Figure or ground
- Similarity
- Proximity
- Closure
- Continuity

Law of Good Form or Pragnanz

The word 'Gestalt' means 'form' or 'shape'. Gestalt psychologists were of the view that psychological organization will always be as 'good' as prevailing conditions allow. For Gestalt psychologists, form is the primitive unit of perception. When we perceive, we will always pick out form. Our perceptions are influenced by our past experiences. This principle is also called Pragnanz Law. (Tan Oon Seng et al., 2003).What did you see in this picture? A saxophone player or a lady?

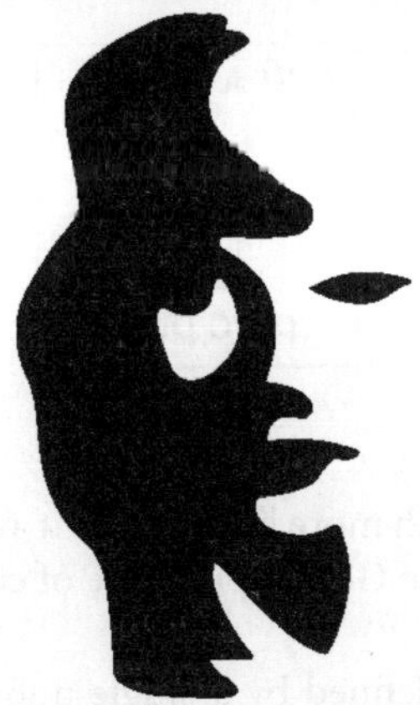

Law of Figure (Ground Discrimination)

The Rubin Vase shown is an example of this tendency to pick out form. We do not simply see black and white shapes, we also see two faces and a vase.

The problem here is that we see the two forms of equal importance. If the source of this message wants us to perceive a vase, then the vase is the intended figure and the black background is the ground. The problem here is a confusion of figure and ground.

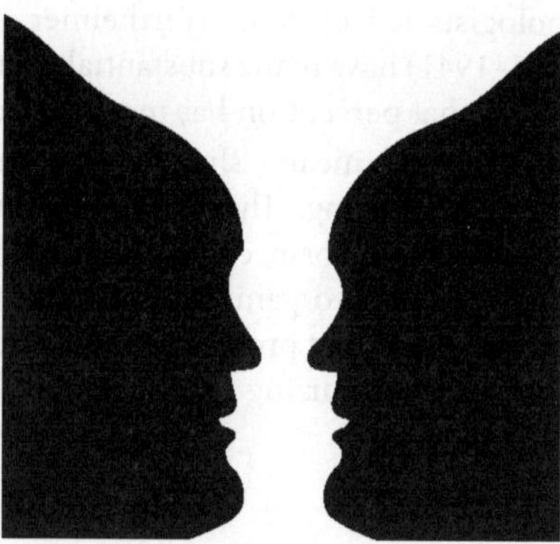

Law of Proximity

Things, which are close together in space or time, tend to be perceived as grouped together. Thus, if you want your audience to associate the product with the presenter, put them close together; if you want them to perceive two ideas as associated, present them in close proximity.

Law of Similarity

Things that are similar are likely to form 'Gestalten' as groups.

Law of Closure

Perceptually, we have the tendency to fill in the gaps. In other words, we can still read WASHO, see the square and read 'perception' despite the missing information.

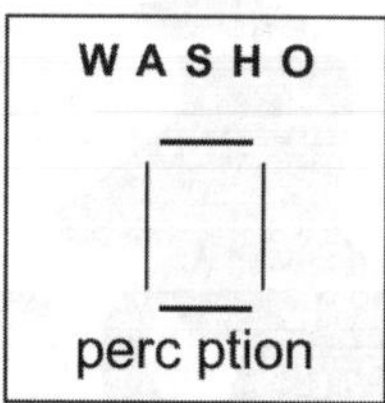

Law of Continuity

When you see this figure, you are much more likely to see it as consisting of two lines like (1a), rather than of the two shapes (1b).This is the Gestalt principle of continuity which saw a single unbroken line is likely to be seen as an entity.

Perceptually, where figures are defined by a single unbroken line, they tend to be seen as an entity. This principle is, of course, of particular importance in teaching. Even something, as simple as drawing a squiggle to link up apparently disparate elements on a page, can be helpful in suggesting to the reader that they are parts of a whole.

Constructivism

A cognitive learning theory proposes that individual learners actively construct their own learning on the basis of their prior knowledge and experiences and interactions with their environment. In the view of constructivist, learning is a constructive process in which the learner is building an internal illustration of knowledge, a personal interpretation of experience.

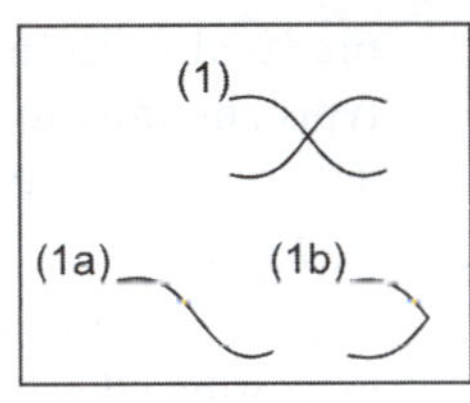

Learning is an active process in which meaning is accomplished on the basis of experience. This view of knowledge does not necessarily reject the existence of the real world, and agrees that reality places constrains on the concepts that are, but contends that all we know of the world are human interpretations of our experience of the world.

They have claimed that objectives should be negotiated with students based on their own felt needs, that programmed activities should emerge from within the contexts of their lived worlds, that students should work together with peers in the social construction of personally significant meaning and that evaluation should be a personalized ongoing, shared analysis of progress (Hanckbarth S, 1996, p.11). Learning through cognitive apprenticeship, mirroring the collaboration of real world problem-solving, and using the tools available in problem-solving situations are keys.

Principles of Constructivist Theory

- Instruction must be concerned with the experiences and contexts that make the student willing and able to learn (readiness).
- Instruction must be structured so that it can be easily grasped by the student (spiral organization).
- Instruction should be designed to facilitate extrapolation and/or fill in the gaps (going beyond the information given).

Educational applications of constructive theory for designing instruction

If learning depends on how information is mentally processed, then students' cognitive processes should be a major concern to educators. For example, while learning, disabled children process information less effectively than nondisabled children (Swanson, 1987).

- Teachers must become aware not only of what students learn, but also of how they attempt to learn it.
- Educators must consider students' levels of cognitive development when planning topics and methods of instruction.
- Students organize the information they learn. Teachers can help students learn by presenting organized information and by helping students see how one thing relates to another.
- New information is most likely acquired when people can associate it with things they have already learned. Therefore, teachers should help students learn by showing them how new ideas relate to old ones. When students are unable to relate new information to anything with which they are familiar, learning is likely to be slow and ineffective.
- Students must actively respond if they are to learn. If students control their own cognitive process, it is ultimately the students themselves who decide what information will be learned, and how.

THORNDIKE'S LAWS OF LEARNING

Law of Readiness

First primary law of learning, according to him, is the 'Law of Readiness' or the 'Law of Action Tendency', which means that learning takes place when an action tendency is aroused through preparatory adjustment, set or attitude. Readiness means a preparation of action. If one is not prepared to learn, learning cannot be automatically instilled in him. For example, unless the typist, in order to learn typing, prepares himself to start, he would not make much progress in a lethargic and unprepared manner.

Law of Exercise

The second law of learning is the 'Law of Exercise', which means that drill or practice helps in increasing efficiency and durability of learning and, according to Thorndike's S-R Bond Theory, the connections are strengthened with trail or practice and the connections are weakened when trial or practice is discontinued. The 'Law of Exercise', therefore, is also understood as the 'Law of Use and Disuse' in which case connections or bonds made in the brain cortex are weakened or loosened. Many examples of this case are found in case of human learning. Learning to drive a motor-car, typewriting, singing or memorizing a poem or a mathematical table, and music, etc. need exercise and repetition of various movements and actions many times.

Law of Effect

The third law is the 'Law of Effect', according to which the trial or steps leading to satisfaction stamp in the bond or connection. Satisfying states lead to consolidation and strengthening of the connection, whereas dis-satisfaction, annoyance or pain lead to the weakening or stamping out of the connection. In fact, the 'Law of Effect' signifies that if the responses satisfy the subject, they are learnt and selected, while those which are not satisfying are eliminated. Teaching, therefore, must be pleasing. The educator must obey the tastes and interests of his pupils. In other words, the greater the satisfaction, the stronger will be the motive to learn. Thus, intensity is an important condition of 'Law of Effect'.

Besides these three basic laws, Throndike also referred to five subordinate laws, which further help to explain the learning process:

Law of Multiple—Response

According to it, the organism varies or changes its response till an appropriate behavior is hit upon. Without varying the responses, the correspondence for the solution might never be elicited. If the individual wants to solve a puzzle, he is to try in different ways rather than mechanically persisting in the same way. Throndike's cat in the puzzle box moved about and tried many ways to come out till finally it hit the latch with her paw, which opened the door and it jumped out.

Law of Set or Attitude

Learning is guided by a total set or attitude of the organism, which determines not only what the person will do but what will satisfy or annoy him. For instance, unless the cricketer sets himself to make a century, he will not be able to score more runs. A student, similarly, unless he sets to get first position and has the attitude of being at the top, would while away the time and would not learn much. Hence, learning is affected more in the individual if he is set to learn more or to excel.

Prepotency of Elements

According to this law, the learner reacts selectively to the important or essential in the situation and neglects the other features or elements which may be irrelevant or nonessential. The ability to deal with the essential or the relevant part of the situation makes analytical and insightful learning possible. In this law of prepotency of elements, Thorndike is really anticipating insight in learning, which was more emphasized by the Gestatians.

Law of Response by Analogy

According to this law, the individual makes use of old experiences or acquisitions while learning a new situation. There is a tendency to utilize common elements in the new situation as existed in a similar past situation. The learning of driving a car, for instance, is facilitated by the earlier acquired skill of driving a motor cycle or even riding a bicycle because the perspective or maintaining a balance and controlling the handle helps in stearing the car.

Law of Associative Shifting

According to this law, we may get a response, of which a learner is capable, associated with any other situation to which he is sensitive. Thorndike illustrated this by the act of teaching a cat to stand up at a command. A fish was dangled before the cat while he said ' stand up'. After a number of trials by presenting the fish after uttering the command 'stand up', he later ousted the fish and the overall command of 'stand up' was found sufficient to evoke the response in the cat by standing up on her hind legs.

Principles of Thorndike's Laws of Learning

- According to this theory, the task can be started from the easier aspect towards its difficult side. This approach will benefit the weaker and backward students.
- A small child learns some skills through trial and error method only, such as sitting, standing, walking, running, etc. In teaching also, the child rectifies the writing after committing mistakes.
- In this theory, more emphasis has been laid on motivation. Thus, before starting teaching in the classroom, the students should be properly motivated.
- Practice leads a man towards maturity. Practice is the main feature of trial and error method. Practice helps in reducing the errors committed by the child in learning any concept.
- Habits are formed as a result of repetition. With the help of this theory, the wrong habits of the children can be modified and the good habits strengthened.
- The effects of rewards and punishment also affect the learning of the child. Thus, the theory lays emphasis on the use of reward and punishment in the class by the teacher.
- The theory may be found quite helpful in changing the behavior of the delinquent children. The teacher should cure such children making use of this theory.
- With the help of this theory, the teacher can control the negative emotions of the children, such as anger, jealousy, etc.
- The teacher can improve his teaching methods making use of this theory. He must observe the effects of his teaching methods on the students and should not hesitate to make necessary changes in them, if required.
- The theory pays more emphasis on oral drill work. Thus, a teacher should conduct oral drill of the taught contents. This helps in strengthening the learning more.

Social Learning Theory

The social learning theory of Bandura emphasizes the importance of observing and modeling the behaviors, attitudes, and emotional reactions of others. Bandura (1977) states that learning would be exceedingly laborious, not to mention hazardous, if people had to rely solely on the effects of their own actions to inform them what to do. Fortunately, most human behavior is learned observationally through modeling—from observing others one forms an idea of how new behaviors are performed, and, on later occasions, this coded information serves as a guide for action.

Social learning theory explains human behavior in terms of continuous reciprocal interaction between cognitive, behavioral, and environmental influences. The component processes underlying observational learning are: Attention, Retention, Motor Reproduction and Motivation.

Because it encompasses attention, memory and motivation, social learning theory spans both cognitive and behavioral frameworks. Social learning theory has been applied extensively to the understanding of aggression (Bandura, 1973) and psychological disorders, particularly in the context of behavior modification (Bandura, 1969). It is also the theoretical foundation for the technique of behavior modeling which is widely used in training programs. In recent years, Bandura has focused his work on the concept of self-efficacy in a variety of contexts.

Principles of Social Learning Theory

- The observer will imitate the model's behavior if the model possesses characteristics (such as talent, intelligence, power, good looks, or popularity) that the observer finds desirable.
- Individuals are more likely to adopt a modeled behavior if the model is similar to the observer, has admired status, and the behavior has functional value.
- The observer will react to the way the model is treated and then imitate the model's behavior. If the model is rewarded then the observer is more likely to perform the behavior. If the model is punished, then the observer is less likely to repeat the behavior.
- There is a difference between an observer's 'acquiring' a behavior and 'performing' a behavior. By observing, the observer can acquire the behavior and not perform the behavior. The observer may then choose to perform the behavior later on if the situation seems right.
- Coding modeled behavior into labels, words or images results in better retention than just observing.
- Learning by observation involves four different processes—attention, retention, motor production, and motivation/reinforcement.
- Attention and retention account for learning a model's behavior. Whereas, motor production and motivation control the performance of the behavior.
- Human development reflects the complex interaction of the person, the person's behavior, and the environment. A lot of what a person knows comes from the environmental resources, such as television, parents, and books. The environment also affects behavior: what a person observes can powerfully influence what he or she does. But a person's behavior can also contribute to his or her environment.

PERSPECTIVES UPON LEARNING THEORIES

Deep and Surface Learning

One perspective upon learning theory identifies two types of learning, deep and surface learning. Deep learning involves the critical analysis of new ideas, linking them to already known concepts and principles, and leads to understanding and long-term retention of concepts so that they can be used for problem-solving in unfamiliar contexts. Deep learning promotes understanding and application for life.

In contrast, surface learning is the tacit acceptance of information and memorization as isolated and unlinked facts. It leads to superficial retention of material for examinations and does not promote understanding or long-term retention of knowledge and information. Following table compiled by Warren Houghton (Higher Education Academy—Engineering Subject Centre 2004) from the work of Entwistle (1988), Ramsden (1992) and Biggs (1999) provides some very valuable characteristics of the two approaches and illustrates the importance of how teaching impacts on the learning process.

Characteristics and factors that encourage deep and surface approaches to learning:

	Deep learning	Surface learning
Definition	Examining new facts and ideas critically, and tying them into existing cognitive structures and making numerous links between ideas.	Accepting new facts and ideas uncritically and attempting to store them as isolated, unconnected, items.
Characteristics	Looking for meaning. Focusing on the central argument or concepts needed to solve a problem. Interacting actively. Distinguishing between argument and evidence. Making connections between different modules. Relating new and previous knowledge. Linking course content to real life.	Relying on rote learning. Focusing on outward signs and the formulae needed to solve a problem. Receiving information passively. Failing to distinguish principles from examples. Treating parts of modules and programs as separate. Not recognizing new material as building on previous work. Seeing course content simply as material to be learnt for the exam.
Encouraged by students	Having an intrinsic curiosity in the subject. Being determined to do well and mentally engaging when doing academic work. Having the appropriate background knowledge for a sound foundation. Having time to pursue interests through good time management. Positive experience of education leading to confidence in the ability to understand and succeed.	Studying a degree for the qualification and not being interested in the subject. Not focusing on academic areas, but emphasizing others (e.g. social, sport). Lacking background knowledge and understanding necessary to understand material. Not enough time/too high a workload. Cynical view of education, believing that factual recall is what is required. High anxiety.
Encouraged by teachers	Showing personal interest in the subject. Bringing out the structure of the subject. Concentrating on and ensuring plenty of time for key concepts. Confronting students' misconceptions. Engaging students in active learning. Using assessments that require thought, and require ideas to be used together.	Conveying disinterest or even a negative attitude to the material. Presenting material so that it can be perceived as a series of unrelated facts and ideas. Allowing students to be passive. Assessing for independent facts (short-answer questions). Rushing to cover too much material.

Contd...

Contd...

	Deep learning	Surface learning
	Relating new material to what students already know and understand. Allowing students to make mistakes without penalty and rewarding effort. Being consistent and fair in assessing declared intended learning outcomes, and, hence, establishing trust.	Emphasizing coverage at the expense of depth. Creating undue anxiety or low expectations of success by discouraging statements or excessive workload. Having a short assessment cycle.

16

Adult as a Learner

Chapter Highlights

- Knowles' 5 Assumptions of Adult Learners
- Adult Learning Principles
- Principles of Knowles in Application to Nursing Education
- Knowles' Adult Learning Principles
- Adults Bring Life Experiences and Knowledge to Learning Experiences
- Barriers to Learning
- Learning Style
- Visual Learners
- Characteristics of Visual Learners
- Tips for Visual Learners
- Auditory Learners
- Characteristics of Auditory Learners
- Study Hints for Auditory Learners
- Kinesthetic Learners
- Strategies for Kinesthetic Learners
- Strengths of Kinesthetic Learners

Learning Objectives

Upon completion of this chapter, the students will be able to:

- Explain the process of Kolb's learning theory
- Describe the adult learning principles of Knowles and its application to nursing education
- Demonstrate skills in categorizing the learners based on VAK learning style of Fleming
- State Knowles' 5 assumptions about adult learners
- List down the barriers to learning
- Describe various used to teach visual, auditory and kinesthetic learners

Adult learners, as they climb in educational process and progress through their education, often question and reevaluate their original assumptions and motivation as they use education to re-create their lives. As such, learning will be more successful if the learner 1. Take an active role in planning, monitoring, and evaluating his/her education, 2. Discard preconceived notions about what college-what it is and what it is not. 3. Choose subjects and courses that are most relevant to each ones job/profession or personal life.

Kolb (1984), an adult learning specialist provided a descriptive model on adult learning process. David Kolb has described the learning process as a four-phase cycle.

Kolb's Learning Process as a Four-Phase Cycle

1. Does something concrete or has a specific experience that provides a basis for, 2. The learner's observation and reflection on the experience and his or her own response to it. These observations are then 3. Assimilated into a conceptual framework or related to other concepts in the learner's past experience and knowledge from which implications for action can be derived; and 4. Tested and applied in different situations.

Stage I: Concrete Experience

Learning initially occurs when a person encounters a new concrete experience and deals with it in terms of observations, feelings, and reactions. Accordingly, the most profound way to promote Stage I learning is by providing the student with exploratory tools e.g. concrete experiences and materials. Learners should become actively involved in the exploration of the learning experience if they are to get the most out of it. This can involve drawing up a checklist of things the learner should try to do: actively observing what is going on, producing a log or record of some sort, and formulating appropriate questions.

Stage II: Observation and Reflection

As the student observes the new situation in Stage I, the student adds to or adjusts his or her perceptions based on previous learning. This process compels the student to reflect on past experiences and to think about the current experience as either fitting into previous patterns or not. This is generally acknowledged as the most difficult stage of the Kolb cycle, but is probably the most crucial of all. Students and practitioners should reflect on what they learned, how they learned it, why they learned it, whether the learning experience could have been more effective, and so on. Discussion of these reflections with an instructor can prove extremely helpful, as can peer-to-peer discussions, either informally or at a formal debriefing session of some sort.

Stage III: Concept Formation

If the experience fits a pattern, then the student can form a generalization and a set of concepts to define the situation. As the student develops these concepts and generalizations, his or her thinking includes imagining other discrete concrete experiences that invariably raise new questions. The answers to these questions require further learning experimentation and the accompanying development of new concepts. Accordingly, the most profound way to promote

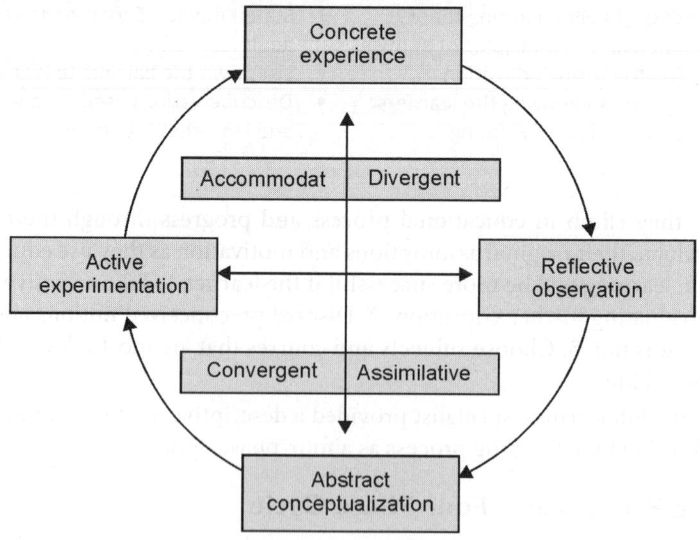

Kolb's Learning Cycle

Stage III learning is by introducing the student to key concepts, e.g. subject vocabulary and relationship diagrams. This stage is very often left out of experiential learning programs, but is extremely important if learners are to gain the maximum possible benefit from such programs. The main object of this stage is to link the actual learning experience with the theories that describe it, and/or with a greater understanding of the theories that the learning experience was designed to illustrate. Again, discussion with an instructor or advisor can prove extremely helpful during this stage of the Kolb cycle, as can discussion with peers.

Stage IV: Testing Implications in New Situations

When the student realizes that the answers constructed in Stage III are not necessarily complete, further testing is required. The student proposes new concrete experiments and restarts the learning cycle. Accordingly, the most profound way to promote Phase IV learning is by helping the student formulate new situations to be tested. Kolb believes that the learner must be involved in the planning of the learning experience if experiential learning is to be fully effective. This can be done in a variety of ways—through action planning or preparing a learning contract. The former may involve nothing more than jotting down a set of things to do, or discussing the proposed procedure with the instructor. In either case, it is useful for individual learners to set their own objectives for the action plan. If a formal learning contract is used, this should be drawn up using a standard checklist.

The four elements are drawn from two dimensions, each of which forms a dialectic and represents the two things that can be done with information. The first is to grasp the information, i.e., to become aware of it. The dialectic lies between grasping information by first-hand experience (concrete experience), which Kolb refers to as apprehension, and grasping by calling up a memory (abstract conceptualization), which Kolb refers to as comprehension. Apprehension is external; the information is only available in the 'here and now.' For example, only when you are touching a piece of ice does it feel cold. Comprehension is an internal process and is not bound by the instant of time. The second is to transform the information. Similarly, there is dialectic between the external process of active experimentation and the internalized reflective.

Important facts learned through the learning theories

- What is the role of the environment?
- How do the internal dynamics of a person respond to the external environment?
- What is the influence of educator on learner and learning process?
- What motivates the learner to learn?
- What encourages a learner to transfer and apply the learning in new situations?

Knowles adult learning

Malcolm Shepherd Knowles (1913–1997) was an American educator well-known for the use of the term andragogy as synonymous to the adult education. According to Malcolm Knowles, andragogy is the art and science of adult learning, thus andragogy refers to any form of adult learning. (Kearsley, 2010). Six characteristics of adult learners were identified by Knowles (1970) He advocated creating a climate of mutual trust and clarification of mutual expectations with the learner. In other words, a cooperative learning climate is fostered.

Knowles' 5 assumptions of adult learners

In 1980, Knowles made 4 assumptions about the characteristics of adult learners (andragogy) that are different from the assumptions about child learners (pedagogy). In 1984, Knowles added the 5th assumption.

Self-concept

As a person matures his/her self concept moves from one of being a dependent personality toward one of being a self-directed human being.

Adult learner experience

As a person matures he/she accumulates a growing reservoir of experience that becomes an increasing resource for learning.

Readiness to learn

As a person matures his/her readiness to learn becomes oriented increasingly to the developmental tasks of his/her social roles.

Orientation to learning

As a person matures his/her time perspective changes from one of postponed application of knowledge to immediacy of application, and accordingly his/her orientation toward learning shifts from one of subject-centeredness to one of problem centeredness.

Motivation to Learn

As a person matures the motivation to learn is internal (Knowles 1984:12).

Characteristics of adult learners (Knowles 1970)

- Autonomous and self-directed
- Accumulated a foundation of experiences and knowledge
- Goal oriented
- Relevancy oriented
- Practical
- Need to be shown respect

Adult learning principles

Knowles identified the six principles of adult learning outlined below.

- Adults are internally motivated and self-directed
- Adults bring life experiences and knowledge to learning experiences
- Adults are goal oriented
- Adults are relevancy oriented
- Adults are practical
- Adult learners like to be respected

Principles of Knowles (1984) in application to nursing education

- Adults must take part in the planning and assessment of their own education. Each lesson must be explained. Students must be aware and understand the rationale behind certain procedures or information.
- Experience (both right and wrong) offers the foundation for learning activities. Instead of memorization, instruction must be task-oriented (learning activities must be in line with the usual tasks done). *'Experience is the best teacher'*. Nursing education is not only a matter of memorization but also of understanding, internalization and application.

- Adults give more attention in learning instruction that have immediate importance to their personal life or career. Lessons must consider the learners' big array of diverse backgrounds. Learning activities and materials must enable for varied types/stages of previous experiences.
- Instead of focusing on content, adult learning is problem-oriented. Being self-directed, adults must be allowed to learn things on their own, giving assistance in times of mistakes so as to prevent similar occurrences to happen. In nursing, committing mistakes is a very good way to learn. However, this is not so in life-and-death situations.

Knowles' Adult Learning Principles

- **Adults are internally motivated and self-directed:** Adult learners resist learning when they feel others are imposing information, ideas or actions on them (Fidishun, 2000). Teachers' role is to facilitate a students' movement toward more self-directed and responsible learning as well as to foster the student's internal motivation to learn.
  - Set up a graded learning program that moves from more to less structure, from less to more responsibility and from more to less direct supervision, at an appropriate pace that is challenging yet not overloading for the student.
  - Develop rapport with the student to optimize your approachability and encourage asking of questions and exploration of concepts.
  - Show interest in the student's thoughts and opinions. Actively and carefully listen to any questions asked.
  - Lead the student toward inquiry before supplying them with too many facts.
  - Provide regular constructive and specific feedback (both positive and negative)
  - Review goals and acknowledge goal completion
  - Encourage use of resources such as library, journals, internet and other department resources.
  - Set projects or tasks for the student that reflect their interests and which they must complete and 'tick off' over the course of the placement. For example, to provide an in-service on topic of choice; to present a case study based on one of their clients; to design a client educational handout; or to lead a client group activity session.
  - Acknowledge the preferred learning style of the student.
- **Adults bring life experiences and knowledge to learning experiences**
  - Adults like to be given opportunity to use their existing foundation of knowledge and experience gained from life experience, and apply it to their new learning experiences. As a nursing faculty you can:
  - Find out about your student—their interests and past experiences (personal, work and study related)
  - Assist them to draw on those experiences when problem-solving, reflecting and applying clinical reasoning processes.
  - Facilitate reflective learning opportunities which Fidishun (2000) suggests can also assist the student to examine existing biases or habits based on life experiences and 'move them toward a new understanding of information presented' (p4).
- **Adults are goal oriented:** Adult students become ready to learn when 'they experience a need to learn it in order to cope more satisfyingly with real-life tasks or problems' (Knowles, 1980

p 44, as cited in Fidishun, 2000). Facilitate a student's readiness for problem-based learning and increase the student's awareness of the need for the knowledge or skill presented:

- Provide meaningful learning experiences that are clearly linked to personal, client and fieldwork goals as well as assessment and future life goals.
- Provide real case-studies (through client contact and reporting) as a basis from which to learn about the theory, functional issues implications of relevance.
- Ask questions that motivate reflection, inquiry and further research.

- **Adults are relevancy oriented:** Adult learners want to know the relevance of what they are learning to what they want to achieve. One way to help students to see the value of their observations and practical experiences throughout their placement, is to:
  - Ask the student to do some reflection on for example, what they expect to learn prior to the experience, on what they learnt after the experience, and how they might apply what they learnt in the future, or how it will help them to meet their learning goals.
  - Provide some choice of fieldwork project by providing two or more options, so that learning is more likely to reflect the student's interests.
- **Adults are practical:** Through practical fieldwork experiences, interacting with real clients and their real life situations, students move from classroom and textbook mode to hands-on problem solving where they can recognize firsthand how what they are learning applies to life and the work context. As a clinical educator you can:
  - Clearly, explain your clinical reasoning when making choices about assessments, interventions and when prioritising client's clinical needs.
  - Be explicit about how what the student is learning is useful and applicable to the job and client group you are working with.
  - Promote active participation by allowing students to try things rather than observe. Provide plenty of practice opportunity in assessment, interviewing, and intervention processes with ample repetition in order to promote development of skill, confidence and competence.
- **Adult learners like to be respected**

  Respect can be demonstrated to your student by:
  - Taking interest
  - Acknowledging the wealth of experiences that the student brings to the placement;
  - Regarding them as a colleague who is equal in life experience
  - Encouraging expression of ideas, reasoning and feedback at every opportunity.

Barriers to learning: Some of these barriers include (a) lack of time, (b) lack of confidence, (c) lack of information about opportunities to learn, (d) scheduling problems, (e) lack of motivation, and (f) 'red tape' (Lieb, 1991). If the learner does not see the need for the change in behavior or knowledge, a barrier exits.

Learning style: Most adult learners develop a preference for learning that is based on childhood learning patterns (Edmunds, Lowe, Murray, and Seymour, 1999). Several approaches to learning styles have been proposed, one being based on the senses that are involved in processing information. Three different learning styles are popularized by Neil D. Fleming in his VAK model of learning. According to this model, most people possess a dominant or preferred learning style; however some people have a mixed and evenly balanced blend of the three styles:

Visual learners

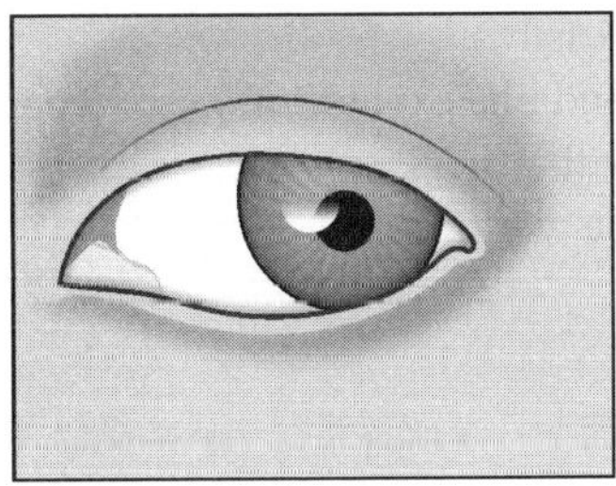

Visual learners prefer seeing what they are learning. Pictures and images help them understand ideas and information better than explanations (Jezierski, 2003). Phrase you may hear these learners use is 'The way I see it is.' The teacher needs to create a mental image for the visual learner as this will assist in the ease of holding on to the information. If a visual learner is to master a skill, written instructions must be provided.

Behaviors/Characteristics of Visual Learners

- Remember what they see rather than what they hear
- Remember diagrams and pictures
- Prefer to read and write rather than listen
- Have trouble remembering verbal instructions
- Need an overall view and purpose before beginning a project
- Like art more than music
- Sometimes tune out when trying to pay attention

Tips for Visual Learners

- Create graphic organizers such, as diagrams and concept maps that use visual symbols to represent ideas and information.
- When trying to remember information, close your eyes and visualize the information.
- Include illustrations as you take notes in class.
- Use highlighter pens of contrasting colors to color code different aspects of the information in your textbooks.
- Sit in the front of the class so that you can clearly see the teacher. This will allow you to pick up facial expressions and body language that provide cues that what your teacher is saying is important to write in your notes.

To address this type of learner in a classroom, use a lot of visual stimuli. Most teachers like to write on the board; this will help the visual learner a lot. Note taking, illustrations, and handouts are also some things that can help the visual learner succeed in classroom.

Auditory learners

Auditory learners prefer to hear the message or instruction being given. These adults prefer to have someone talk them through a process, rather than reading about it first. A phrase they may use is 'I hear what you are saying.' Some of these learners.

May even talk themselves through a task, and should be given the freedom to do so when possible. Adults with this learning style remember verbal instructions well and prefer someone else read the directions to them while they do the physical work or task.

Characteristics of auditory learners:

- Can follow verbal instructions easily
- Like to hear someone explain and like explaining to someone else
- Like debating and discussing with others
- Tend to talk to themselves while working
- Enjoy reading aloud
- Like music more than art.

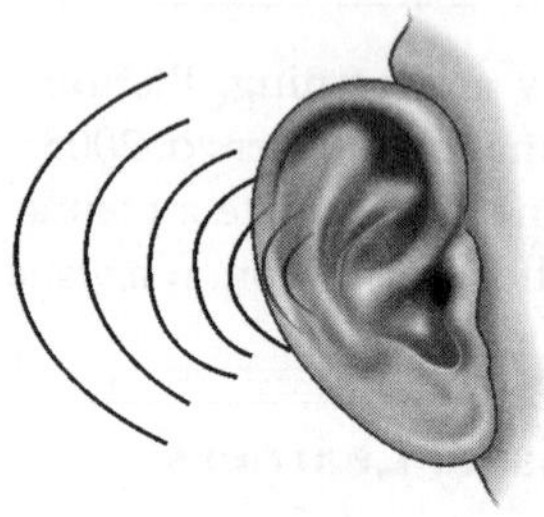

Study hints for auditory learners:

- Start or join a study group
- Say things aloud to remember information
- Use a tape recorder. Record yourself reading texts and/or discussing issues with others
- Read notes aloud when studying and after you have read something summarize it out loud.
- Explain or 'retell' something you have learnt to someone else
- If possible listen to pod casts of lectures.

Kinesthetic learners

Kinesthetic learners want to sense the position and movement of the skill or task. These learners generally do not like lecture or discussion classes, but prefer those that allow them to 'do something.' Basically, it means that the learner needs to be actively doing something while learning. Often, those with a kinesthetic learning style are going to have a hard time learning during sedentary things like lectures because the body does not make the connection that they are doing something when they are listening. Much of the time, they need to get up and move to put something into memory.

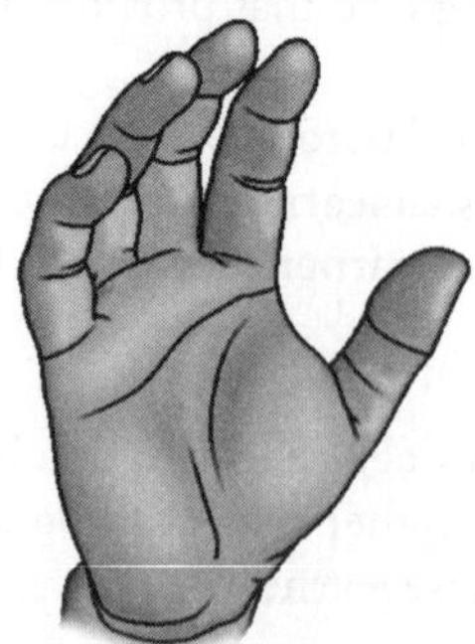

Strengths of kinesthetic learners

- Great hand-eye coordination
- Quick reactions
- Excellent motor memory (can duplicate something after doing it once)
- Excellent experimenters
- Good at sports
- Performs well in art and drama
- High levels of energy

Students with this learning style are often called fidgety, problematic, antsy or hyper, merely because their bodies need to be in action in order to learn.

Strategies to deal kinesthetic learners in classroom

- During a lecture, allow the kinesthetic learners to stand, bounce their legs or doodle.
- Offer various methods of instruction—lectures, paired readings, group work, experiments, projects, plays, etc.
- Involve them perform tasks during the lecture like filling out a worksheet on the material or taking notes.
- Allow those students to perform movement tasks before and after lectures like passing back assignments, handing out quizzes, writing on the chalkboard, or even rearranging desks.
- If you feel the kinesthetic learners slipping away from you in class, stop everyone and have the whole class do something energetic like marching, stretching, switching desks just the act of moving can flip a switch in a learner's brain and help them regain focus.
- Keep your lectures short and sweet. Be mindful of all your different learners when planning.

17

Learning Domains and Taxonomy of Education

Chapter Highlights

- Learning Domains
- Taxonomy of Education
- Bloom's Taxonomy of Education—Old Version (1956)
- Revised Taxonomy
- Uses of Taxonomy of Education
- Writing Learning Objectives
- The Affective Domain of Learning
- Krathwohl's Taxonomy of Affective Domain
- The Psychomotor Domain of Learning
- Other Popular Psychomotor Domain Version by Dave (1975) and Harrow (1972)
- Integrated Framework by Miller et al
- Competence-Based Education (CBE)
- Outcome-Based Education (OBE)
- Microteaching
- Syllabus
- Lesson Planning
- Assessment of Teaching

Learning Objectives

Upon completion of this chapter, the students will be able to:

- State the meaning of learning domains and taxonomy of education
- Recognize and interpret the changes made in new version of Bloom's taxonomy of education
- List down principles of writing clear behavioral learning objectives
- Describe competency-based and outcome-based education
- Demonstrate skills writing lesson plan
- List the six major categories of Bloom's old version of taxonomy of education
- Identify the uses of taxonomy of education
- Develop skills in writing learning objectives
- Describe the components of affective and psychomotor domain
- Describe the principles of microteaching
- Three major purposes of a syllabus
- Assess teaching

LEARNING DOMAINS

There are significant differences in the way learning occurs in the different domains. For example, students memorize information in a different way from the way their attitudes are formed, and they learn to apply cognitive skills in problem solving in a different way again. This means that if learning outcomes are to be achieved in the different domains of learning, different teaching strategies that are appropriate for those types of learning must be used. The domains of learning can be categorized as cognitive domain (knowledge), psychomotor domain (skills) and affective domain (attitudes).

TAXONOMY OF EDUCATION

This categorization is best explained by the Taxonomy of Learning Domains formulated by a group of researchers led by Benjamin Bloom in 1956. The original Taxonomy provided the six major categories in the cognitive domain. The categories were *Knowledge, Comprehension, Application, Analysis, Synthesis,* and *Evaluation.* With the exception of *Application,* each of these was broken into subcategories. The categories were ordered from simple to complex and from concrete to abstract. Further, it was assumed that the original Taxonomy represented a cumulative hierarchy; that is, mastery of each simpler category was prerequisite to mastery of the next more complex one. One of the most frequent uses of the original Taxonomy has been to classify curricular objectives and test items.

Cognitive (Knowledge, 'Head')

The cognitive domain involves knowledge and the development of intellectual skills. This includes the recall or recognition of specific facts, procedural patterns, and concepts that serve in the development of intellectual abilities and skills.

Affective (Attitudes, 'Heart')

This domain includes the manner in which we deal with things emotionally, such as feelings, values, appreciation, enthusiasms, motivations, and attitudes.

Psychomotor (Skills, 'Hands')

The psychomotor domain includes physical movement, coordination, and use of the motor-skill areas. Development of these skills requires practice and is measured in terms of speed, precision, distance, procedures, or techniques in execution.

Six major categories of blooms taxonomy of education—old version (1956)			
1.0	**Knowledge**	2.2	Interpretation
1.10	Knowledge of specifics	2.3	Extrapolation
1.11	Knowledge of terminology	**3.0**	**Application**
1.12	Knowledge of specific facts	**4.0**	**Analysis**
1.20	Knowledge of ways and means of dealing with specifics	4.1	Analysis of elements
		4.2	Analysis of relationships
1.21	Knowledge of conventions	4.3	Analysis of organizational principles
1.22	Knowledge of trends and sequences	**5.0**	**Synthesis**
1.23	Knowledge of classifications and categories	5.1	Production of a unique communication
1.24	Knowledge of criteria	5.2	Production of a plan, or proposed set of operations
1.25	Knowledge of methodology		
1.30	Knowledge of universals and abstractions in a field	5.3	Derivation of a set of abstract relations
		6.0	**Evaluation**
1.31	Knowledge of principles and generalizations	6.1	Evaluation in terms of internal evidence
1.32	Knowledge of theories and structures	6.2	Judgments in terms of external criteria
2.0	**Comprehension**		
2.1	Translation		

Three categories based on hierarchy:

Level 1. Recall—Knowledge and comprehension
Level 2. Interpretation—Application and analysis
Level 3. Problem-solving—Synthesis and evaluation

The categories were ordered from simple to complex and from concrete to abstract. This also means the cumulative hierarchy. Objectives requiring only recognition or recall of information fall in the *Knowledge* category. This is basic or lower level of cognition.

Objectives that involve the understanding and use of knowledge would be classified in the categories from *Comprehension* to *Synthesis;* considered the most important goals of education provide a basis for moving curricula and tests toward objectives that would be classified in the more complex categories.

REVISED TAXONOMY

In the original Taxonomy, the *Knowledge* category embodied both noun and verb aspects. This anomaly was eliminated in the revised Taxonomy by allowing these two aspects, the noun and verb, to form separate dimensions, the noun providing the basis for the Knowledge dimension and the verb forming the basis for the Cognitive Process dimension. Revised Bloom's taxonomy of education concentrates on 1. Knowledge dimension and 2. Cognitive process dimension.

Knowledge Dimension

The revised Bloom's Taxonomy cut across subject matter lines. Just like the original one. The new Knowledge dimension contains four instead of three main categories. Three of them include the substance of the subcategories of Knowledge in the original framework. But they were reorganized to use the terminology, and to recognize the distinctions of cognitive psychology that developed since the original framework was devised. A fourth and new category, ***Metacognitive Knowledge,*** provides a distinction that was not widely recognized at the time the original scheme was developed.

Cognitive Process Dimension

The original number of categories, six, was retained, but with important changes. Three categories were renamed, the order of two was interchanged, and those category names retained were changed to verb form to fit the way they are used in objectives. The verb aspect of the original *Knowledge* category was kept as the first of the six major categories, but was renamed ***Remember.*** *Comprehension* was renamed because one criterion for selecting category labels was the use of terms that teachers use in talking about their work.

Because *understand* is a commonly used term in objectives, its lack of inclusion was a frequent criticism of the original Taxonomy. So, *Comprehension,* the second of the original categories, was renamed ***Understand.*** *Application, Analysis,* and *Evaluation* were retained, but in their verb forms as *Apply, Analyze, and Evaluate. Synthesis* changed places with Evaluation and was renamed *Create*

Structure of the cognitive process dimension of the revised—Bloom's taxonomy

1.0	**Remember:** Retrieving relevant knowledge from long-term memory.
1.1	Recognizing
1.2	Recalling
2.0	**Understand:** Determining the meaning of instructional messages, including oral, written, and graphic communication.
2.1	Interpreting
2.2	Exemplifying
2.3	Classifying
2.4	Summarizing
2.5	Inferring
2.6	Comparing
2.7	Explaining
3.0	**Apply:** Carrying out or using a procedure in a given situation.
3.1	Executing
3.2	Implementing
4.0	**Analyze:** Breaking material into its constituent parts and detecting how the parts relate to one another and to an overall structure or purpose.

Contd...

Contd...

Structure of the cognitive process dimension of the revised—Bloom's taxonomy	
4.1 Differentiating 4.2 Organizing 4.3 Attributing **5.0 Evaluate:** Making judgments based on criteria and standards. 5.1 Checking	5.2 Critiquing **6.0 Create:** Putting elements together to form a novel, coherent whole or make an original product. 6.1 Generating 6.2 Planning 6.3 Producing

Knowledge Dimension of the Revised Bloom's Taxonomy of Education

A. Factual knowledge: The basic elements that students must know to be acquainted with a discipline or solve problems in it.
- Aa. Knowledge of terminology
- Ab. Knowledge of specific details and elements

B. Conceptual knowledge: The interrelationships among the basic elements within a larger structure that enable them to function together.
- Ba. Knowledge of classifications and categories
- Bb. Knowledge of principles and generalizations
- Bc. Knowledge of theories, models, and structures

C. Procedural Knowledge: How to do something; methods of inquiry, and criteria for using skills, algorithms, techniques, and methods.
- Ca. Knowledge of subject-specific skills and algorithms
- Cb. Knowledge of subject-specific techniques and methods
- Cc. Knowledge of criteria for determining when to use appropriate procedures

D. Metacognitive Knowledge: Knowledge of cognition in general as well as awareness and knowledge of one's own cognition
- Da. Strategic knowledge
- Db. Knowledge about cognitive tasks, including appropriate contextual and conditional Knowledge
- Dc. Self-knowledge

USES OF TAXONOMY OF EDUCATION

The taxonomies provide a framework for the teacher to plan instruction and design assessment strategies at different levels of learning:
- From simple to complex in the cognitive domain
- From awareness of a value to developing a philosophy of practice based on a value system in the affective domain
- Increasing psychomotor competency, from imitation of the skill to performance as a natural part of care.

WRITING LEARNING OBJECTIVES

Taxonomy of education provides the base for writing outcome oriented objectives that are beneficial to learners as well for the instructors. It is important to be able to differentiate the course description from the course objectives. A course description simply tells what the course is about. You might consider the GOALS of the course to be linked to the course description; they are broad educational statements fitting the mission and description of the course. Specific measurable objectives, however, tell what the learner will be able to do upon successful completion of the course. Goals are appropriate for an entire course or a curriculum of study, while objectives are written for individual units of study. Always begin with the end in mind.

Importance of well Written Objectives

- Provide some basis and guidance for the selection of instructional content and procedures.
- Help in evaluating the success of the instruction.
- Help the student organize his/her efforts to accomplish the intent of the instruction.

Principles of Writing Clear Behavioral Learning Objectives

- When writing behavioral objectives, stick to the words that leave less room for interpretation.

There are words that we often use that are open to many interpretations, and there are words that we can use that leave less to the imagination.

Words open to many interpretations: *To understand, to really understand, to appreciate, to fully appreciate, to grasp the significance of, to enjoy, to believe, to have faith in.*

Words open to fewer interpretations: *To write, to recite, to identify, to sort, to solve, to construct, to build, to compare, to contrast.*

- There are three characteristics that help communicate intent when writing an objective: Performance, Conditions, and Criterion.

  Performance: An objective always states what a learner is expected to be able to *DO*.

  Conditions: An objective often describes the conditions under which a student is able to *DO* or perform the task.

  Criterion: If possible, an objective clarifies how well the student must perform the task, in order for the performance to be acceptable.

Other ways to of writing instructional objectives:

1. Who? 2. Will do? 3. How much (how well) ? 4. of what? 5. by when?

ABCDs of Writing Objectives

The ABCD method of writing objectives is similar to the theory explained here; the terminology is just slightly different. *A* is the audience, always the student. *B* is the behavior or the action verb. *C* is the condition for the objective and *D* is the degree of achievement or acceptable criteria.

Conditions describe the relevant factors associated with the desired performance. For example:

- After attending a lecture session on
- Following a demonstration
- Given a specific instrument.

Criteria

The criteria are specified as the acceptable level of achievement desired. They tell how well the learner must perform. For example:

- Percent of correct responses

- Within a given time period
- In compliance with criteria presented by the faculty.

Preferred order and tense when writing objectives

The condition is usually placed first, followed by the behavior or verb, and then the criteria. Objectives are written in the future tense.

For example:

Recall: After attending lecture and reading the assigned materials, the student will state the function of a thermometer.

AFFECTIVE DOMAIN OF LEARNING

The affective domain describes learning objectives that emphasize a feeling tone, an emotion, or a degree of acceptance or rejection. Affective objectives vary from simple attention to selected phenomena to complex but internally consistent qualities of character and conscience. We found a large number of such objectives in the literature expressed as interests, attitudes, appreciations, values, and emotional sets or biases (Krathwohl et al, 1964).

We want our students respond to what they learn, to value it, to organize it and maybe even to characterize themselves as nurses, nurse educators and academicians and whatever they are aiming to achieve. There are some basic skills which we stress in apart from core curriculum: good attitudes, motivation, effective verbal and non-communication, patience, respect for self and others, adjustment, teamwork, leadership-managerial abilities, Empathy, self and cultural awareness, pleasing manners, interpersonal relationships, emotional stability, etc. All these are belonging to affective domain.

Student is not just a machine who will memorize and recite what a teacher teaches. Rather he is a social animal who is built with elements of feeling or affect. As teachers we must show great concern to affective domain. Affective domain must be given equal importance that would enhance students learning.

KRATHWOHL'S TAXONOMY OF AFFECTIVE DOMAIN

Receiving refers to the student's willingness to attend to particular phenomena of stimuli (classroom activities, textbook, music, etc.). Learning outcomes in this area range from the simple awareness that a thing exists to selective attention on the part of the learner. Receiving represents the lowest level of learning outcomes in the affective domain.

Verbs to use-asks, chooses, describes, follows, gives, holds, identifies, locates, names, points to, selects, sits erect, replies, uses.

For example, listening to discussions of controversial issues with an open mind. Respecting the rights of others.

Listen for and remember the name of newly introduced people.

Responding refers to active participation on the part of the student. At this level he or she not only attends to a particular phenomenon but also reacts to it in some way. Learning outcomes in this area may emphasize acquiescence in responding (reads assigned material), willingness to respond (voluntarily reads beyond assignment), or satisfaction in responding (reads for pleasure or enjoyment). The higher levels of this category include those instructional objectives that are commonly classified under "interest"; that is, those that stress the seeking out and enjoyment of particular activities.

Valuing is concerned with the worth or value a student attaches to a particular object, phenomenon, or behavior. This ranges in degree from the simpler acceptance of a value (desires to improve group skills) to the more complex level of commitment (assumes responsibility for the effective functioning of the group). Valuing is based on the internalization of a set of specified values, but clues to these values are expressed in the student's overt behavior. Learning outcomes in this area are concerned with behavior that is consistent and stable enough to make the value clearly identifiable. Instructional objectives that are commonly classified under "attitudes" and "appreciation" would fall into this category.

Affective learning is demonstrated by behaviors indicating attitudes of awareness, interest, attention, concern, and responsibility, ability to listen and respond in interactions with others, and ability to demonstrate those attitudinal characteristics or values which are appropriate to the test situation and the field of study.

***Organization i**s* concerned with bringing together different values, resolving conflicts between them, and beginning the building of an internally consistent value system. Thus, the emphasis is on comparing, relating, and synthesizing values. Learning outcomes may be concerned with the conceptualization of a value (recognizes the responsibility of each individual for improving human relations) or with the organization of a value system (develops a vocational plan that satisfies his or her need for both economic security and social service). Instructional objectives relating to the development of a philosophy of life would fall into this category.

Characterization by a value or value set. The individual has a value system that has controlled his or her behavior for a sufficiently long time for him or her to develop a characteristic "lifestyle." Thus, the behavior is pervasive, consistent, and predictable. Learning outcomes at this level cover a broad range of activities, but the major emphasis is on the fact that the behavior is typical or characteristic of the student. Instructional objectives that are concerned with the student's general patterns of adjustment (personal, social, emotional) would be appropriate here.

The affective domain can significantly enhance, inhibit or even prevent student learning. The affective domain includes factors such as student motivation, attitudes, perceptions and values. Teachers can increase their effectiveness by considering the affective domain in planning courses, delivering lectures and activities, and assessing student learning.

PSYCHOMOTOR DOMAIN OF LEARNING

The psychomotor domain (Simpson, 1972) includes physical movement, coordination, and use of the motor-skill areas. Development of these skills requires practice and is measured in terms of speed, precision, distance, procedures, or techniques in execution. The seven major categories are listed from the simplest behavior to the most complex:

Perception (awareness): The ability to use sensory cues to guide motor activity. This ranges from sensory stimulation, through cue selection, to translation.

Set: Readiness to act. It includes mental, physical, and emotional sets. These three sets are dispositions that predetermine a person's response to different situations (sometimes called mindsets)

Guided Response: The early stages in learning a complex skill that includes imitation and trial and error. Adequacy of performance is achieved by practicing.

Mechanism (basic proficiency): This is the intermediate stage in learning a complex skill. Learned responses have become habitual and the movements can be performed with some confidence and proficiency.

Complex Overt Response (Expert): The skillful performance of motor acts that involve complex movement patterns. Proficiency is indicated by a quick, accurate, and highly coordinated performance, requiring a minimum of energy. This category includes performing without hesitation, and automatic performance. For example, players are often utter sounds of satisfaction or expletives as soon as they hit a tennis ball or throw a football, because they can tell by the feel of the act what the result will produce.

Adaptation: Skills are well developed and the individual can modify movement patterns to fit special requirements.

Origination: Creating new movement patterns to fit a particular situation or specific problem. Learning outcomes emphasize creativity based upon highly developed skills.

OTHER POPULAR PSYCHOMOTOR DOMAIN VERSION BY DAVE (1975) AND HARROW (1972)

Imitation: Observing and patterning behavior after someone else. Performance may be of low quality.

Manipulation: Being able to perform certain actions by memory or following instructions.

Precision: Refining, becoming more exact. Performing a skill within a high degree of precision

Articulation: Coordinating and adapting a series of actions to achieve harmony and internal consistency.

Naturalization: Mastering a high level performance until it becomes second-nature or natural, without needing to think much about it.

INTEGRATED FRAMEWORK BY MILLER ET AL

One other framework that could be used to classify objectives was developed by Miller et al. (2009, pp. 54–55). This framework integrates the cognitive, affective, and psychomotor domains into one list and can be easily adapted for nursing education:

- **Knowledge** (knowledge of terms, facts, concepts, and methods)
- **Understanding** (understanding concepts, methods, written materials, and problem situations)
- **Application** (of factual information, concepts, methods, and problem-solving skills)
- **Thinking skills** (critical and scientific thinking)
- **General skills** (laboratory, performance, communication, and other skills)
- **Attitudes** (and values, for example, reflecting standards of nursing practice)
- **Interests** (personal, educational, and occupational)
- **Appreciations** (literature, art, and music; scientific and social achievements)
- **Adjustments** (social and emotional).

COMPETENCE-BASED EDUCATION (CBE)

Competency-based education turns the traditional model on its head. Instead of awarding credits based on how much time students spend learning, this model awards credits based on whether students can prove they have mastered *competencies*—the skills, abilities, and knowledge required in an area of study. Competency-based education is about what the students know and are able to do than simply finishing the fixed credit hours or required hours spent in theory and practice.

Nature and Scope of CBE

Although competency-based education offers returning adult learners a real opportunity to earn a college degree while balancing commitments to work and family, this innovative model is not for everyone. In competency-based education, students work at their own pace to acquire competencies that are assessed for mastery. This is known as direct assessment. The scope of the curriculum reaches beyond core competencies and focuses on knowledge, attitudes and skills that encompass professional nursing practice. The curriculum is not standardized, but the model aims to reach standardized outcomes. Students use a variety of Open Education Resources (textbooks, videos, simulations) to acquire knowledge and complete assignments that are reviewed by faculty members. With their time freed-up from teaching and grading mass assignments, faculty are able to provide in-depth, quality feedback to the students.

Competency-based education is very desirable for working adult students. It is self-paced and not tied to the traditional credit hour. This means the student can work as quickly as they want and achieve competencies—and their degree—in a short time period. In addition, if a student already has knowledge or work experience in the competency, they can just choose to take the assessment to show their mastery. There are no set classes, and the pace of your learning is entirely up to you. But if you are the right kind of student—experienced, self-directed, and motivated to succeed—then competency-based programs such as the Flexible Option may be just what you've been waiting for.

Competency-based education is based on six critical components (Van der Horst & McDonald 1997):

1. Explicit learning outcomes with respect to the required skills and concomitant proficiency (standards for assessment).
2. A flexible time frame to master these skills.
3. A variety of instructional activities to facilitate learning.
4. Criterion-referenced testing of the required outcomes.
5. Certification based on demonstrated learning outcomes.
6. Adaptable programs to ensure optimum learner guidance.

Features of Competency-based Education

- **Flexible:** The Flexible Option lets you start when you want, the first of any month, and work toward your degree online, on your own time, when and where your schedule allows.
- **Personalized**: The flexible option recognizes and rewards prior learning by giving you the opportunity to pass assessments using knowledge you already have. You study only the material you need to master and never spend time or money revisiting things you already know. In addition, an Academic Success Coach will work with you to customize your learning plan based on your knowledge and goals.
- **Self-paced**: Take assessments whenever you are ready. Practice first to make sure. As soon as you prove mastery, you receive credit and move on, without having to wait for the next lesson or semester. Move quickly through material you know or take more time if you need it.
- **Supportive**: Receive personalized mentoring and advising from an Academic Success Coach who will help you prepare for assessments and point you to learning resources you need to succeed, such as textbooks, web pages, and even free online resources offered by other universities.
- **Skills-based**: You make progress by passing assessments that show you have mastered the skills essential to your degree—not by accumulating credit hours, either in the classroom or online.

- **Respected**: By measuring and assessing your mastery of competencies, the flexible option provides proof to employers that you have the skills and knowledge your field requires.
- **Affordable**: Instead of paying by course or by credit, the Flexible Option lets you pay a flat rate for a subscription period of your choice. If you are rightly motivated you may be able to accelerate your progress and shorten your time to graduation, saving time and money.

Advantages of Competency-based Education

- Individualized path to learning and completing a degree
- Based on mastery not credit hour
- Affordable and flexible for working adult students
- Use of multiple instructional materials/methods to match different learning styles and preferences
- Allows one to skip a course and just take assessment if they have knowledge/work experience on the subject (so prior learning assessment is built in)
- Students can move through quickly if they prefer and shorten graduation time
- Faculty can provide timely and higher quality feedback as they have more without teaching or everyone submitting assignments at same time.

Disadvantages of Competency-based Education

- Finding a way to standardize the definitions of competencies and develop reliable assessments.
- Uncertainty about scaling to large universities especially due to the fact that this type of education challenges the traditional credit hour (and the revenue associated with it).
- Traditional students and unmotivated students may not benefit as much as adult students.

Outcome-based Education (OBE)

Education is aimed at creating teaching and learning environments that would bring about desired changes in learners, whether to be more knowledgeable, better skilled or to influence their attitudes and values positively. An outcome is a culminating demonstration of learning. It is what the student should be able to do at the end of a course. It is an approach to education in which decisions about the curriculum are driven by the exit learning outcomes that the student should display at the end of the course. Here the product defines the process (Harden et al). It is the transformational way of doing business in education.

OBE Definition

Spady (1994) defines OBE as a ... *comprehensive approach to organizing and operating an education system that is focused on and defined by the successful demonstrations of learning sought from each student.*

Outcomes are ... *clear learning results that we want students to demonstrate at the end of significant learning experiences* ... and ... *are actions and performances that embody and reflect learner competence in using content, information, ideas, and tools successfully* (Spady, 1994).

Regarding the OBE paradigm, Spady (1994) states: ... *WHAT and WHETHER students learn successfully is more important than WHEN and HOW they learn something.*

At best OBE may be described as an eclectic philosophy which takes the best from several past educational approaches and incorporating them in a new system that is appropriate to the needs and demands of a country.

Claassen (1998) states that *OBE is a transformational perspective on the curriculum.*

It offers a dialogue between learner and the curriculum where the learner interacts with sources of knowledge, reconstructs knowledge, and takes responsibility for his or her own learning outcomes. In the same way the teacher becomes a facilitator in the teaching and learning situation instead of acting as a source of information transferring content to learners. From this viewpoint the transformational character of OBE is influenced by the mastery learning and competency-based education movements.

Ten key components that underlie OBE as a transformation approach (Spady 1994):

1. Outcomes-defined,
2. Expanded opportunities for learners,
3. Performance 'credentialing',
4. Concept integration,
5. Instructional coaching,
6. Culminating achievement,
7. 'Inclusionary' success,
8. Cooperative learning,
9. Criterion
10. Validation and collaborative structures.

MICROTEACHING

Microteaching is a technique that is used in teacher education where a teacher candidate teaches a small portion of a lesson to a small group of his classmates and teaching competencies are carried out under strict supervision. After teaching a small group, to begin to teach a whole class is one of the techniques that improves teacher education. Also, teaching a whole lesson can be a useful option in teacher education.

History

The history of microteaching goes back to the early and mid 1960s, when Dwight Allen and his colleagues from the Stanford University developed a training program aimed to improve verbal and nonverbal aspects of teacher's speech and general performance. The Stanford model consisted a three-step (teach, review and reflect, re-teach) approach using actual students as an authentic audience. The model was first applied to teaching science, but later it was introduced to language teaching. A very similar model called Instructional Skills Workshop (ISW) was developed in Canada during the early 1970s as a training support program for college and institute faculty. Both models were designed to enhance teaching and promote open collegial discussion about teaching performance.

Nature and Scope of Microteaching

The teacher education involves training for a practice that should be planned around designing a total teaching practice. This total teaching practice requires, e.g. the mastery of a number of teaching skills. The ideal way to really master a teaching skill is to execute it in practice under controlled circumstances. (Louw, 1981) Microteaching provides an opportunity to develop instructional skills in a positive, learner-centered environment.

In a microteaching session, each participant gives a five-minute mock teaching lesson on a chosen subject with explicit pedagogical goals and then receives feedback on his/her teaching style in general and his/her effectiveness in achieving the stated goals. These sessions are usually conducted in a small group (four presenters) within a department. Each participant has an opportunity to see how others perceive his/her teaching style, to observe and evaluate a variety of teaching approaches, and to learn how to share observations constructively with others.

Purposes of Microteaching Sessions

- To strengthen our approach to teaching;
- To identify our personal strengths and areas for improvement;
- To encourage an empathic understanding of students as learners;
- To enhance our understanding for a variety of effective teaching styles
- To improve your ability to provide and receive effective feedback.

Definitions

Olivero (1971:1), one of the original co-workers at Stanford, defines it as follows: "Microteaching is a scaled-down sample of actual teaching which generally lasts ten to thirty minutes and involves four to ten students. A microteaching session simulates a regular classroom instructional period in every way except that both time and number of students are reduced".

"Microteaching is a teaching situation which is scaled down in terms of time and number of students. The lesson is scaled down to reduce some of the complexities of the teaching act, thus allowing the teacher to focus on selected aspects of teaching" (Cooper and Allen 1970).

In Kieviet's (1972:61) "Microteaching is a method for training teachers where explicit use is made of the principle of feedback and where the teacher-learning situation remains limited with respect to:

- The number of students to whom the lesson is given;
- The duration of the lesson;
- The extent of the lesson in terms of contents and didactic presentation".

Principles of Conducting Microteaching

- *Less number of students:* Five is accepted as the most appropriate number of persons for group work of any nature whatever. This makes the situation less threatening, easy to manage and disciplined; gain self-confidence in using the particular teaching skill before he is confronted with the management of a large number of pupils.
- *Amount of teaching time:* The teaching time in a micro-lesson is limited to between five and ten minutes. It elevates the learning effect for the students because the short period of time limits the possibility of getting entangled in the management of more than one teaching skill.
- *One teaching skill:* The number of teaching skills practiced during a microteaching situation is limited to only one. The student is evaluated only on this skill
- *Amount of learning content:* The limitation of the amount of learning content that is unlocked during the microteaching situation ultimately is a logical consequence especially of the limitation of teaching time. So content is considerably reduced to match the time.

Uses

- Microteaching helps develop skills to prepare lesson plans, choose teaching goals, speak in front of a group, and to ask questions and use evaluation techniques.
- Teachers' self-confidence grows in a comfortable environment.

- It provides an opportunity to learn multiple skills that are important for teaching in a short time. It is a useful experience to learn how to realize teaching goals through planning a model lesson. It shows how preparation, organization, and presentation are important in learners' learning. Choosing activities, putting them in a logical order, maintaining improvement make it possible to become a whole with the content.
- Receiving immediate feedback is a means to determine productivity and using teaching strategies.
- By asking appropriate questions a strong learning environment can be established.
- Allows for asking questions at various difficulty levels. Also, it makes it possible to create an environment that involves thinking differently and interaction.

Stages of Microteaching

This comprises of five stages which are decision making, planning, application, evaluation and reflection. Every stage involves reflection.

- *Decision-making:* At this stage the teacher candidate decides on what kind of a prior preparation and what content will be presented by using thinking processes, different method and techniques.
- *Planning:* By considering the content and the teaching behaviors together teaching plans and teaching materials are prepared. The lesson plan is devised by taking the advise of other teacher
- *Application:* Presentation is done according to the plan devised. This stage involves a presenter and a teacher candidate observer. Both candidates participate in the learning process actively. The teacher candidate observers take notes by observing the presentation while the presenter is giving the presentation. In classroom teaching, learner-centered active question and answer, observation, problem solving, role-playing, and discussion can be done (Baytekin, 2004).
- *Evaluation:* Evaluation involves two assessments: one after each presentation and one at the end of all presentations. After each presentation both the presenter and the observer is asked to evaluate themselves. After all the presentations are made everybody evaluates themselves and the lesson in general and determines the progress made.
- *Reflection:* Reflection involves for the presenters the decisions made based on the feedback received from the peers and the teacher at every stage of the activities. For the observer candidates the presentation is part of the reflection stage. Viewing the tapes and the peers' observations and notes are the components of reflection.

SYLLABUS

A course syllabus is essentially a *contract* between the instructor and the student and is a vital tool for communicating expectations between students and faculty. A well-constructed syllabus provides a road map for the course, answers frequently asked questions, can help to lessen student anxiety, and allows the faculty member to concentrate on instruction. Syllabus is the embodiment of your philosophy of teaching and learning. Implicit in every assignment, every choice of textbook, every discussion topic should be an indication of what you want your students to learn from your course and why you want them to learn it. Syllabi in any form (hard copy or syllabi digitally uploaded in blackboard system of learning) should be available on or before the first day of class to all students.

Purposes

Syllabi seem to vary in two fundamental areas—the apparent reason for writing the syllabus and the material that it contains. The purpose of the syllabus should drive the decision as to what content to include (Parkes & Harris, 2002).

Three Major Purposes of a Syllabus

Three major purposes that a syllabus should serve as described by Parkes and Harris (2002):

1. Syllabus as a contract
2. Syllabus as a permanent record
3. Syllabus as a learning tool

1. Syllabus as a contract—Makes clear what the rules are:

- Sets forth what is expected to happen during the semester
- Delineates the responsibilities of students and of the instructor
- Describes appropriate procedures and course policies
- Content required for a syllabus to serve as a contract:
  - Clear and accurate course calendar
  - Grading policies: components and weights
  - Attendance policy
  - Late assignment policy, policies on incompletes and revisions
  - Academic dishonesty and academic freedom policies
  - Accommodation of disabilities policy.

2. Syllabus as a permanent record—Serves accountability and documentation functions

- Contains information useful for evaluation of instructors, courses, and programs
- Documents what was covered in a course, at what level, and for what kind of credit-hours (useful in course equivalency transfer situations, accreditation procedures, and articulation)
- Content required for a syllabus to be useful as a permanent record:
  - Title and semester of course (program), department offering the course, credit hours earned, (hours of teaching theory and practice) meeting time and place
  - Name, title, qualification and designation/rank of instructor(s)
  - Pre- or co-requisites (means the vertical and horizontal alignment of the curriculum)
  - Required texts and other materials
  - Course objectives (linked to professional standards if appropriate)
  - Description of course content
  - Description of assessment procedures (Allocation of marks for internal and external examinations).

3. Syllabus as a learning tool

- Helps students become more effective learners in the course
- Inform students of the instructor's beliefs about teaching, learning, and the content area
- Focuses on students and what they need to be effective learners
- Places the course in context (how it fits in the curriculum, how it relates to students' lives)
- Content required for a syllabus that serves as a learning tool for students:
  - Instructor's philosophy about the course content, teaching and learning
  - Relevance and importance of the course to students
  - Information on how to plan for the semester including self-management skills, guidance on time to spend outside of class, tips on how to do well on assessments, common misconceptions or mistakes, and specific study strategies

- Prerequisite courses or skills
- Availability of instructor (s) and teaching assistants
- Campus resources for assistance and offices that aid students with disabilities.

How Important the Syllabus is? Syllabus is the Backbone

A syllabus is often thought of as "that apparently benign document instructors assemble and distribute to students at the start of the semester." Whether it is intended or not, the quality of the syllabus is a fairly reliable indicator of the quality of teaching and learning that will take place in a course (Woolcock, 2003). Therefore, it behooves instructors to make the effort to construct a high-quality syllabus.

The process of developing a syllabus can be a reflective exercise, leading the instructor to carefully consider his or her philosophy of teaching, why the course is important, how the course fits in the discipline, as well as what topics will be covered, when assignments will be due, and so on (Eberly, Newton, & Wiggins, 2001; Grunert, 1997). This can be an enlightening experience that results in an improved course. In addition, by making sure expectations are clearly communicated, instructors can circumvent a whole host of student grievances and misunderstandings during the semester.

The syllabus is, thus, both a professional document and a personal document, one that reflects the instructor's feelings, attitudes, and beliefs about the subject matter, teaching, learning, and students, as well as setting out the "nuts and bolts" of the course. When so constructed, the syllabus can serve as a guide to the instructor as much as a guide to the class (Parkes & Harris, 2002).

A syllabus lets students know what the course is about, why the course is taught, where it is going, and what will be required for them to be successful in the course (Altman & Cashin, 2003). The well-designed syllabus provides a solid beginning to the semester, sets the tone for the course, provides a conceptual framework for the course, serves as a "virtual handshake" between the instructor and students, and becomes a resource that is referred to over the course of the semester. It also shows students that you take teaching seriously (Davis, 1993).

Components of a Syllabus

Owner Credentials of the Intellectual Property: Name of the council/university or institution who formulated and published the syllabus.

Title That Specifies the Discipline: There may be so many programs run by the university from various disciplines. For example, Baccalaureate program in nursing, Baccalaureate program in medical laboratory sciences, Baccalaureate program in occupational therapy, etc.

Course/Program Code: Assigned numbers for a particular program/discipline/course.

Course Description: A brief introduction to the course: scope, purpose and relevance of the material.

Course Objectives: Skills and knowledge you want students to gain.

Course Organization: Explanation of the topical organization of the course

Materials: Required (and/or optional) books (with authors and editions), reserve readings, course readers, software, and supplies with information about where they can be obtained.

Prerequisites and co-requisites—Before joining the course/program what credentials you should have in your hand. How does the course run by organizing certain subjects/courses prior or simultaneously with the other courses? This is mainly to follow the educational principles of vertical and horizontal relationships in organizing.

Course Requirements: What students will have to do in the course: assignments, exams, projects, performances, attendance, participation, etc.? Describe the nature and format of assignments and the expected length of written work. Provide due dates for assignments and dates for exams.

Evaluation and Grading Policy: What will the final grade be based on? Provide a breakdown of components and an explanation of your grading policies (e.g. weighting of grades, curves, extra-credit options, the possibility of dropping the lowest grade).

Course Policies and Expectations: Policies concerning attendance, participation, tardiness, academic integrity, missing homework, missed exams, recording classroom activities, food in class, laptop use, etc. Describe your expectations for student behavior (e.g. respectful consideration of one another's perspectives, open-mindedness, creative risk-taking). Let students know what they can expect from you (e.g. your availability for meetings or e-mail communication).

Course Calendar: A day-to-day breakdown of topics and assignments (readings, homework, project due-dates)

LESSON PLANNING

A lesson plan is the road map or framework used to plan and conduct every class from first meeting to final exam. In addition, lesson plans ensure you have created a logical, systematic learning process essential to making sure your students achieve the most learning in the least time. Lesson planning is a professional activity, either formal or informal, which is beneficial to our teaching practice (Harmer 1998).

A lesson is a single activity or a series of activities designed by the instructor so as to achieve one or more instructional objectives determined, or desired in promoting positive change in the learner. Richard Pregent (1994) observes that "professors who have carefully prepared lesson plans save an enormous amount of time when you teach a course again; you have a written record of everything you have done."

A lesson plan is designed for a specific set of learners during a single class period. The class period may vary in length from one to four hours and provides learners with instruction on skills needed to accomplish an objective from the unit plan. It may be a theoretical a practical one.

The lesson plan breaks the unit plan down into detail and is the direction for the class period. Adult learners appreciate instruction that is well planned and want to know the objective for the class period. Writing a lesson plan requires thinking about the skills to be taught, the objectives, timing, and procedures for the class.

Preparation to Write a Lesson Plan

Contact the appropriate administrative office at your college or university and ask for a course outline, syllabus, and course catalog description for the course(s) you will teach. It is a must for the new teachers to orient themselves to teaching. Some institutions also can provide you with a faculty or instructor handbook. In addition, ask if a course specification sheet is available that includes information on course objectives and expected student performance outcomes and/or competencies. In addition, ask if a course specification sheet is available that includes information on course objectives and expected student performance outcomes and/or competencies. Countries where the centrally administered syllabus in practice would advise the faculty buy a syllabus book from the university or from the nursing council. Rest of the items like mission, vision, philosophy, teaching and learning strategies, Duration of course delivery would be guided by the institution.

Importance of Lesson Planning

- Provides a framework or an overall shape.
- Teachers feel certain, confident and purposeful about the whole class from the beginning, throughout the middle stages and to the ending.

- Planning allows teachers to think about the lesson, which helps to create ideas for dynamic and meaningful classroom teaching.
- Plan helps to remind the teacher of what to do next in class. Glancing at their plan will solve this problem.
- Formal plan helps teachers to become professional.
- Well prepared plan can promote teachers' image in students' eyes. Students can feel their teachers' commitment and responsibility, which can build up students' trust in and cooperation with teachers.

Types of Lesson Plan

There are different types of lesson planning according to its nature and styles:

1. Mental and written 2. Formal and informal, 3. Personal and professional, 4. Short-term and long-term lesson plans.

Mental lesson plan	Written lesson plan
A lesson plan can be mental, i.e. the teacher thinks about how to teach the lesson without writing his/her ideas down.	A written lesson plan is the one that the teacher writes down what he/she is going to do for the lesson.
A mental plan can be hard work or a little work, which is unseen but revealed in the teacher's material selection, activities design and effective instruction.	A written plan cannot record the teacher's entire mental work.
We cannot say that the mental planners are not committed	A written plan, in some degree, reveals clearly whether the teacher devotes his/her time to plan writing.
Formal lesson plan	**Informal lesson plan**
A formal plan is of high professionalism, including required components of a plan and with professional language expressions	An informal lesson plan is of casual nature. Focuses on content of classroom teaching: language or tasks, but it lacks professionalism
Time consuming; the teacher may pay more attention to how to write a plan than how to teach a lesson	Time saving
The teacher might be restricted by his/her teaching plan in teaching.	Teacher can be flexible in teaching
Personal lesson plan	**Professional lesson plan**
For personal use with no intention of being seen or read by others.	A formal one
For self	For administrative and managerial inspections
Short-term lesson plans	**Long-term lesson plans**
Immediate lesson for tomorrow or the day after tomorrow.	A long-term plan is one to be made by the teacher over time.
There is a clear picture of what to teach, what material to use and what activities to design	The teacher is thinking about his/her teaching almost all the time. Over time planning greatly helps teachers to do successful teaching.

General Principles for Writing a Lesson Plan

Knowledge: In order to make a good lesson plan, teachers should have a clear picture of the students, the syllabus, activities, language skills, language types, subject and content, and institution and its restrictions (Harmer1993:265).

Variety: Classroom variety refers to different activities ranging from listening, speaking, reading, and writing, each of which has further varieties

Coherence and Cohesiveness: All activities serve common objectives and each activity should be connected by teachers using connective devices to make the lesson a wholeness of harmoniousness. Good lesson plan is the art of mixing techniques, activities and materials in such a way that an ideal balance is created for the class" (Harmer 1993:259).

Flexibility: Many experienced teachers comment that they do not look at the lesson plan while teaching and that they often make impromptu changes in actual teaching

Essential Components of a Lesson Plan

Each specific lesson plan forms a comprehensive course lesson plan a specific lesson plan consisting of goals, objectives, materials and equipment, procedures, follow-up notes or evaluation (Brown 2003).

- **Goal(s):** This part is general aims, which means overall purposes that the teacher attempts to accomplish by the end of the class. Usually the aims are the same for several lessons.
- **Objectives:** This part is to concretize goals to specific aims that teachers have for the students and are written in terms of what the students will do and achieve specifically. They can refer to activities, skills, vocabulary, functions, etc.
- **Materials and Equipment:** Materials refer to the textbook and other materials for students to study in the class. Equipment can be a tape recorder, a poster or other items of regalia. Writing down what materials and equipment to use can make the plan appear professional and also function as a reminder for the teacher before the class.
- **Procedures:** This part is the main contents of a plan, which have tremendous variations for different teachers.

  Usually this part includes sequential steps:

  - Opening step or warming-up part;
  - Middle steps: a set of activities and techniques to be used in the class with time allocation;
  - Closure, which is usually about assignments.
- **Evaluation:** This part is of reflective nature. Teachers look back at the lesson and assess its efficiency, points out problems and work out in order to make adjustments for the next class or classes. Evaluation helps teachers to theorize their experience through which teachers develop their analytical, critical and conceptual power.
- **Assignments:** Teacher assigns some work to the learners to get the feedback by announcing the timelines for the learners.
- **References:** These are resources from which the teachers as well as the learners obtain or extract the content to be taught or learnt. They include all audiovisual materials (textbooks, library books, dictionaries, newspapers, periodicals, internet and online sources etc.) And online sources.

GUIDELINES TO TEACH THE PLANNED LESSON

Introduction

Any lesson hour starts with a good introduction. Introduction gives life to the lesson session. Grabbing the attention of the students lie on how the lesson begins. Introduction is assures the students that they have a good teacher with them to deliver the session. Opening the topic by starting with the principle of "Known to unknown". Life related example at start holds the attention of the students. Registering in mind that the students too know something would take you to heights. An introduction of 3 to 5 minutes would do better.

Body: The session takes into full swing. The teacher maintains the interest of the students using various strategies. The teacher delivers the content based on the specific objectives formulated from the central objective.

Summary/Conclusion

The teacher summarizes the content in a systematic way to make the students remember and recollect.

Points to Remember for the Teacher

- Read through the previous lesson to review a bit before you could start. Be thorough about the lesson what you are planning to teach
- Give importance to extra reading
- Do not restrict yourself only with the prescribed textbook
- Remember your objectives for each of the element you are planning to teach because at the end of the session you need to look whether the learner objectives are attained
- Be sure about the specific strategies you are going to adopt for each part of your content
- Please remember that you use various strategies of teaching to keep up the interest of your students.
- Get ready with your baseline questions to alert the students and hold them with you through the session. Your extra reading will help you tackle the students. At same time be conscious about your time.
- Ensure that you have suitable instructional materials to deliver the components. Better use visual as well electronic media for your teaching
- Some teachers prefer to give handouts; Many prefer to give outline, essential references and suggested references.
- If you are a novice teacher need to read and learn so much about communication, professional relationship etc.
- Do not look at your lesson plan. You do not have to follow your lesson plan. Make any on-the-spot adjustments based on the classroom situation.

ASSESSMENT OF TEACHING

It is a common practice in the nursing colleges to wait until the end of the term to get the course evaluation done by the stakeholders. An alternative approach is to request informal constructive criticism throughout the term. Instructors can gather information about the effectiveness of their teaching strategies, the usefulness of instructional materials, and other features of the course that can be changed during the semester.

Typically, when teachers want to assess students' learning, they tend first to think of giving tests or quizzes; however, there are alternatives to the standard test or quiz. Informal ways can be used to determine whether students are learning the material throughout the term. Some suggestions (see, for example, Davis 1993; Silberman, 1996) to try are to:

- Ask questions during class. Give the students time to respond. Try to get a sense of whether students are keeping up by asking questions for which answers require students to apply a given concept or skill to a new context.
- Ask students for their questions. Rather than ask, "Do you have any questions?," ask instead "What questions do you have?" This implies that you expect questions and are encouraging students to ask them.
- Give frequent, short, in-class assignments or quizzes. Pose a question or problem on an overhead or the board, give students time to respond, perhaps in writing and have students compare answers with their neighbors.
- Ask students to write a "minute paper." Just before the end of a class session, ask: "What is the most significant thing you learned today?" and, perhaps in addition, "What question is uppermost in your mind at the end of today's class?" These "minute papers" should be collected as students leave class. Reading these will help you to evaluate how well your students are grasping the material, and you can respond, if needed, during the next class period.
- Ask students to jot down three or four key concepts or real-world connections about a recent topic, then start a class discussion by having students compare their lists.
- Ask students to keep a learning journal in which they write, once or twice a week, about things they disagree with or how what they are learning is reflected in other things they read, see, or do. Collect and comment on the learning journals periodically.

Portfolio to Assess the Teacher and Course

Teaching portfolios composed of work samples and self-evaluative commentary. A portfolio might include copies of syllabi, assignments, handouts, and teaching notes; copies of students' lab notebooks or assignments; descriptions of steps taken to evaluate and improve one's teaching (such as exchanging course materials with colleagues or using fast-feedback techniques); and information from students (such as student rating forms).

Portfolios can also include a statement of teaching philosophy. Less comprehensive than portfolios are self-evaluations that ask faculty to comment on their courses: How satisfied were you with this course? What do you think were the strong points of the course and your teaching? The weak points? What did you find most interesting about this course? Most frustrating? What would you do differently if you taught this course again?

Evaluating your own teaching: Videotaping is one way to view and listen to the class as your students do; you can also observe your students' reactions and responses to your teaching. You can also check the accuracy of your perceptions of how well you teach and identify those techniques that work and those that need improvement. You may want someone from the professional development office/expert to view the tape with you to avoid focusing on your appearance or mannerisms.

Watching yourself (teacher) on Videotape

- What are the specific things I did well?
- What are the specific things I could have done better?
- What kept the students engaged?
- When did students get lost or lose interest?
- If I could do this session over again, what three things would I change?
- How would I go about making those changes?

As you watch the tape, try the technique of stopping every five seconds and putting a check in the following columns: teacher talk, student talk, silence. Or look at your lecture in terms of organization and preparation: Did I give the purpose of the session? Emphasize or restate the most important ideas? Make smooth transitions from one topic to another? Summarize the main points? Include neither too much nor too little material in a class period? Seem at ease with the material? Begin and end class promptly?

Peer Evaluation

Most universities use this method to give feedback about teaching The peer teaching evaluation is intended to be not just an evaluative process but also an opportunity to receive constructive feedback to improve teaching effectiveness. Peer review of teaching is a form of evaluation designed to provide feedback to instructors about teaching and learning. Peer review may be used either as a way to help instructors improve teaching and learning in their courses, known as a formative review; or it may be part of a formal reward system used in tenure and pay decisions, known as a summative review.

In general, peer review is a collaborative process in which the instructor under review works closely with a colleague or group of colleagues to discuss his or her teaching. Formative peer observation assists in the improvement of teaching. Summative peer observation involves the evaluation of teaching effectiveness used for merit, promotion, and/or tenure decisions. Both formative and summative observations can be based on the same observation instruments.

Peer Observation Guidelines

- The observer should arrive at least 10 minutes before class. "Walking into class late is poor practice and inconsiderate" (Seldin, 1999, p. 81).
- The observer can be briefly introduced to the students, with an equally brief explanation of why the observer is present. Then move on!
- Observers are not to ask questions or participate in activities during class; such behavior can detract from and invalidate the observations.
- An effective observation requires an observation instrument designed to accurately and reliably portray the teacher's behavior.

Observation Instruments

The three most common instruments are checklists, rating scales, and open-ended narratives (written analysis). Seldin recommends a combination of two instruments. When choosing observation instruments, keep in mind that

- Forms and checklists help standardize observations, making the observation more reliable;
- Viewing a videotape of one's teaching and then completing an observation instrument is a feasible option;
- The blank sheet observation is not reliable and therefore is not recommended for summative purposes. However, for formative purposes, copious notes about what is taking place during the class can be the most useful prompt for discussion.

Postobservation Conference Guidelines

- Schedule this conference within a week of the observation.
- Review results from the completed classroom observation instrument(s).
- Begin the conference with a positive comment (i.e. "I really enjoyed your class...").

Provide Honest, Constructive Feedback. Observable Characteristics of Effective Teachers

- Begins class promptly and in a well-organized way
- Treats students with respect and caring
- Provides the significance/importance of information to be learned
- Provides clear explanations
- Holds attention and respect of students, practices effective classroom management
- Uses active, hands-on student learning
- Varies his/her instructional techniques
- Provides clear, specific expectations for assignments
- Provides frequent and immediate feedback to students on their performance. Praises student answers and uses probing questions to clarify/elaborate answers
- Provides much concrete, real life, practical examples
- Draws inferences from examples/models and uses analogies
- Creates a class environment which is comfortable for student... allows students to speak freely
- Teaches at an appropriately fast pace, stopping to check student understanding and engagement
- Communicates at the level of all students in class
- Has a sense of humor!
- Uses nonverbal behavior, such as gestures, walking around, and eye contact to reinforce his/her comments
- Presents him/herself in class as 'real people.'
- Focuses on the class objective and does not let class get sidetracked
- Uses feedback from students (and others) to assess and improve teaching
- Reflects on own teaching to improve it.

Process

I. Pre visit preparatory meeting

The Peer evaluator and faculty member meet prior to the scheduled peer evaluation in order to:

- Review course syllabus for course objectives, teaching, and assessment methods
- Discuss the types of learners in class
- Discuss methods of instruction selected for class, and class format
- Discuss how feedback is provided to students
- Discuss areas of focus for the evaluation
- Go over peer evaluation forms to be used during class observation
- Other areas, as requested by the faculty member being evaluated.

II. Peer evaluation visit

A peer evaluation form should be completed as part of the class observation (a sample one can be found at the end of this document). Upon completion of the visit, the faculty member being evaluated should do a self-appraisal that can be used as part of a post-evaluation meeting.

III. Post-evaluation meeting

The Peer evaluator and faculty member should meet following the class visit to go over the peer evaluation and the self-appraisal. Following the review and discussion, a summary should be jointly developed by the peer evaluator and the faculty member. This summary may include strategies for improvement as appropriate.

1. Course content

- Does the instructor demonstrate command of subject matter?
- Does content reflect current research/knowledge of discipline?
- Is the purpose of the session evident?
- Is the content consistent with the course syllabus?
  - Successful elements
  - Elements to refine

2. Teaching methods

- Are transitions between ideas smooth?
- Are relevant examples given and used to clarify concepts?
- Is the presentation organized?
- Is the instructor enthusiastic about the subject?
- Is material adapted to student needs?
- Are supplemental materials/visual aids/technology used effectively?
- Does the instructor notice and adapt to student feedback accordingly?
- Given the type and size of class, are the methods selected appropriate?
- Is there an assessment tool/strategy integrated into the lesson?

3. Learning environment

- Is the classroom atmosphere participatory?
- Do students seem engaged with the topic?
- Does the instructor encourage questions and check-in with students?
- Is the instructor attentive to cues of boredom or confusion?
- Was the session thought provoking and stimulating?
- Was the environment conducive to critical thinking and student-centered learning?
- Is the instructor sensitive to issues of diversity and inclusiveness in order to promote a safe learning environment for students?
  - Successful elements
  - Elements to refine
  - General comments
  - Recommendations for improvement.

18

Learning to Care: Nursing and Clinical Teaching

Chapter Highlights

- Clinical Teaching
- Significance of the Word 'Clinical'
- Principles of Clinical Teaching
- What is Clinical Teaching?
- The Process of Clinical Teaching
- Guidelines for Observing Students in Clinical Practice
- Qualities of Effective Clinical Teacher
- Pressure on Clinical Educators
- Clinical Teaching Models
- How should a Clinical Instructor Herself Conduct in the Clinical Area?
- Types of Students' Assignments
- Guidelines for Using Rating Scales for Clinical Evaluation

Learning Objectives

Upon completion of this chapter, the students will be able to:

- State what is 'clinical teaching'
- Identify the significance of the word 'clinical'
- List the principles of clinical teaching
- Identify the steps in the process of clinical teaching
- Identify the guidelines for observing students in the clinical practice
- List the qualities of an effective clinical instructor
- Enumerate the criteria to be followed to conduct self in the clinical area
- State the types of students' assignments
- List the guidelines for clinical evaluation

Infante (1985) took the position that nursing students are *learning to care* for patients; they are not nurses with *responsibility for patient care.*

CLINICAL TEACHING

Every man lives with a philosophical principle developed within him. Nurses are no exceptions. Philosophy determines that the teacher understands his or her role, approaches to clinical teaching, selection of teaching and learning activities, use of evaluation processes, and relationships with learners and others in the clinical environment. Philosophical statements serve as a guide for examining issues and determining the priorities of a discipline (Haynes, Boese, and Butcher, 2004, p. 77; Iwasiw et al., 2009, p. 172). Although a philosophy does not prescribe specific actions, it gives meaning and direction to practice, and it provides a basis for decision making and for determining whether one's behavior is consistent with one's beliefs. Without a philosophy to guide choices, a person is overly vulnerable to tradition, custom, and fad (Fitzpatrick, 2005; Tanner and Tanner,

2006). Because the context is different for each nursing education program, each curriculum is somewhat unique (Iwasiw, Goldenberg, and Andrusyszyn, 2009, p. xi).

SIGNIFICANCE OF THE WORD 'CLINICAL'

Therefore, the practice of clinical teaching differs somewhat from program to program clinical evaluation. The word 'clinical' is an adjective, derived from the noun clinic. Clinical means involving direct observation of the patient. We routinely hear nursing faculty members say, 'The students are in clinical today' or 'They will be in clinical tomorrow.' Examples of correct use include 'clinical practice,' 'clinical instruction,' and 'clinical evaluation.' Though we say 'we provide' clinical experience to the students, actually it is not so. Literature states that our faculty can provide only opportunity for learning and gaining experience. We provide plan for entire activities within the curriculum and we function as facilitators for learning to take place; rest lies with the student nurse. Her learning principles, philosophy, goal, interest, self motivation, competitive spirit, hard work, adjustment and adaptability and intellectual ability and whom she perceived as her role models, etc. The teacher's role is to plan and provide appropriate activities that will facilitate learning. However, each student will experience an activity in a different way.

Clinical practice requires critical thinking and problem-solving abilities, specialized psychomotor and technological skills, and a professional value system. Practice in clinical settings exposes students to realities of professional practice that cannot be conveyed by a textbook or a simulation (Oermann and Gaberson, 2009). Clinical setting is the place where the rubber meets the road. Means the students are exposed to actual place of their practice where they get hands on experience.

Because professional practice occurs within the context of society, it must respond to social and scientific demands and expectations. Therefore, the knowledge base and skill repertoire of a professional nurse cannot be static. What nurses and nursing students do in clinical practice is more important than what they can demonstrate in a classroom. Nursing profession solely lies on the hands on experience to take care of ill and debilitated people no matter in hospital, community or home.

Principles of Clinical Teaching

- Clinical education should reflect the nature of professional practice
- Clinical teaching is more important than classroom teaching the nursing student in the clinical setting is a learner, not a nurse
- Quality is more important than quantity
- Sufficient learning time should be provided before performance is evaluated
- Clinical teaching is supported by a climate of mutual trust and respect
- Clinical teaching and learning should focus on essential knowledge, skills, and attitudes.

What is Clinical Teaching?

Clinical teaching is a series of deliberate actions on the part of the teacher to guide students in their learning. It involves a sharing and mutual experience on the part of both teacher and student and is carried out in an environment of support and trust. Here the teacher is not a lecturer who simply lectures and at the same time the students are not simply passive listeners but they do be considered as doers or performers who would satisfy the needs of people who are in agony physically and mentally. Your magical words (effective communication) and empathy matters to gain confidence from patients.

The Process of Clinical Teaching Includes Five Steps

- Identifying the outcomes for learning
- Assessing learning needs
- Planning clinical learning activities
- Guiding students
- Evaluating clinical learning and performance

Guidelines for Observing Students in Clinical Practice

- Examine own values and biases that may influence observations of students in clinical practice and judgments about clinical performance.
- Do not rely on first impressions for these might change significantly with further observations of the student (Nitko and Brookhart, 2007).
- Make a series of observations before drawing conclusions about clinical performance.
- Share with students on a continual basis observations made of clinical performance and judgments about whether students are meeting the clinical competencies.
- Focus observations on the outcomes of the clinical course or competencies to be achieved.
- When the observations reveal other aspects of performance that need further development, share these with students and use the information as a way of providing feedback on performance.
- Discuss observations with students, obtain their perceptions of performance, and be willing to modify judgments when a different perspective is offered (Oermann and Gaberson, 2009).

Qualities of Effective Clinical Teacher

Knowledge

Teachers must update their clinical knowledge. Practices are not static. Everyday we happen to meet new challenges in the field of healthcare. Accordingly clinical nursing instructors must be current in their knowledge and practice. In clinical teaching, this means that educators are knowledgeable about the types of patient problems in the clinical setting, how to manage them, new technologies in patient care, and related research (Beitz & Wieland, 2005; Gignac-Caille & Oermann, 2001; Tang, Chou, & Chiang, 2005).

Clinical Competence

An instructor cannot teach her students if she is not competent enough. Clinical competence is an important characteristic of effective clinical teaching in nursing (Gignac-Caille & Oermann, 2001; Tang et al., 2005). A competent instructor doesn't feel low and does not get angry on students for her mistakes. Competent persons walk with eyes and ears open and always looking for opportunity to learn. Lifelong learner only can be current in clinical field.

Skill in Clinical Teaching

In a study by Berg and Lindseth (2004), the instructional skills of the teacher were ranked second highest when students (n = 171) were asked to describe characteristics of an effective teacher in nursing.

- Be specific about the learning objectives
- No bias
- Note the individual difference

- Ensure that all the students get the chance to practice under guidance and observation
- Maintain good interpersonal and professional relationship with all the departments in the clinical area.
- Develop a good rapport
- Assesses learning needs of students, recognizing and accepting individual differences
- Plans assignments that help in transfer of learning to clinical practice, meet learning needs, and promote acquisition of knowledge and development of competencies
- Honest communication to students on learning and expectations and evaluation of students in clinical practice
- Explain clearly concepts and theories applicable to patient care
- Demonstrate effectively clinical skills, procedures, and use of technology
- Provides opportunities for practice of clinical skills, procedures, and technology and recognize differences among students in the amount of practice needed.

Pressure on Clinical Educators

- Coping with the many expectations associated with clinical teaching
- Feeling exhausted at the end of a clinical teaching experience with students
- Job demands that interfere with activities of personal importance
- Too heavy a workload
- Pressure to maintain clinical competence or a clinical practice without time to do so
- Feeling unable to satisfy the demands of students, clinical agency personnel, patients, and others
- Teaching inadequately prepared students (Oermann, 1998).

Clinical Teaching Models

Traditional Model

In this model the instructor or educator provides clinical instruction and training for the students who are assigned under her in an appropriate clinical setting. (Hospital, community, etc.)

Advantages

- Assists students in using the concepts and theories learned in class,
- The teacher can select clinical activities that best meet the students' needs and are consistent with course goals and objectives faculty member may be more
- Teacher implements the philosophy of the nursing program than preceptors or clinicians hired only for clinical teaching, often on a short-term basis.

Disadvantages

- The large number of students for whom faculty members may be responsible; not being accessible to students when needed because of demands of other students in the group;
- Teaching procedures, clinical skills, and use of technologies for which the faculty member may lack expertise; the time commitment of providing on-site clinical instruction for faculty members with multiple other roles
- High costs for the nursing program
- The educator and students may not be part of the health care system in which students have clinical practice.

Preceptor Model

In the preceptor model of clinical instruction, the faculty member from the nursing program serves as the course coordinator, liaison between the nursing education program and clinical setting, and resource person for the preceptor. The faculty member, however, is typically not on site during the clinical practicum. In a preceptor-based nursing course, students can transition into independent practice, become socialized into their professional role, and develop their clinical competencies (Blum, 2009; Kim, 2007).

Strengths

Consistent one-to-one relationship of the student and preceptor, providing an opportunity for the student to work closely with a role students are able to work closely with a clinical expert in the field, develop self-confidence.

Weaknesses

- Lack of integration of theory, research, and practice
- Lack of flexibility in reassigning students to other preceptors if needed
- Time and other demands made on the preceptors.
- Although preceptors should be prepared educationally for this role, some preceptors may lack clinical teaching skills.

Partnership Model

In some programs, the partnership model is a collaborative relationship between a clinical agency and nursing program that involves sharing an Advanced Practice Nurse (APN) and academic faculty member. The APN teaches students in the clinical setting, with the faculty member serving as course coordinator, and the faculty member in turn contributes to the clinical agency. Through partnerships patients may get care they otherwise would not receive, students gain learning experience, and nursing faculty members also get practical experience (Yeh, Rong, Chen, Chang, and Chung, 2009).

The teacher should select a model considering these factors:

- Educational philosophy of the nursing program
- Philosophy of the faculty about clinical teaching
- Goals and intended outcomes of the clinical course and activities
- Level of nursing student
- Type of clinical setting
- Availability of preceptors, expert nurses, and other people in the practice setting to provide clinical instruction
- Willingness of clinical agency personnel and partners to participate in teaching students and other educational activities.

Clinical area: Where the rubber meets the road

Though the nursing students learn the theory in the classrooms, the actual nursing profession starts when a nurse starts to care her patients. To provide such hands on experience to nursing students the clinical instructors must have thorough knowledge and skills in clinical area. Otherwise the instructor may not be able to provide quality clinical education to her nursing students.

How Should a Clinical Instructor Herself Conduct in the Clinical Area?

Eden Zabat Kan and Susan Stabler-Haas (2009) have stated the following advises for the nursing clinical instructors on how should they conduct them in the clinical area:

- Think more like a teacher and less like a nurse
- Maintain the boundary of teacher and student.
- Keep personal information out of the clinical setting
- Focus instead on the 'aha' moments of your students—moments when your clinical thinking questions led to further student inquiry and successful application of concepts! Once you experience this moment, you will be hooked on teaching. You will realize that friendships and being 'liked' cannot replace this feeling of accomplishment
- You are not there to teach the nurses or other ancillary staff
- Become familiar with the unit and the staff before the arrival of your students
- Encourage students to be responsible by thoroughly reading each patient's chart, medication list, and care plan
- You cannot be everywhere all of the time
- Financial gain should not motivate you to become a clinical instructor. Rather, your motive should be to skillfully and effectively teach students to be successful nurses
- You are helping to educate nurses whom you would want to care for you and your family.

Clinical Learning

In some nursing education programs, one set of course objectives applies to both the classroom and clinical learning outcomes; in others, separate but related sets of objectives are created to reflect the different emphasis of 'knowing that' (classroom learning outcome) and 'knowing how' (clinical learning outcome) (O'Connor, 2006, p. 114). Depending on the level of the learner, students may have difficulty envisioning how broad program or course outcomes can be achieved in the context of a specific clinical environment. It is the instructor's role to translate these outcomes into specific clinical objectives and to select and structure learning activities so that they relate logically and sequentially to the goals (Case and Oermann, 2004).

The teacher must consider these individual differences; all learners do not have the same needs, so it is unreasonable to expect them to have the same learning assignments on any given day.

Clinical instructor must consider patients' need as well students' needs; she must be careful in assigning the patients to the students with the learning objectives in the mind.

Traditional clinical assignment for nursing students is to give total care to one or more patients. However, not all learning objectives require students to practice total patient care. Depending on their individual learning needs, some students might be engaged in activities that focus on developing a particular skill, while others could be practicing more integrative activities such as providing total patient care. For example, if students are learning physical assessment skills, some students could be assigned to practice auscultation by listening to breath, heart, and abdominal sounds of a variety of patients without having the responsibility of performing other patient care activities (O'Connor, 2006, p. 120).

Types of Students' Assignments

One student/one patient. One student is responsible for certain aspects of care or for comprehensive care for one or more patients. The student works alone to plan, implement, and evaluate nursing care.

This type of assignment is advantageous when the objective is to integrate many aspects of care after the student has learned the individual activities.

Multiple students/one patient. Two or more students are assigned to plan, implement, and evaluate care for one patient. Each learner has a defined role, and all collaborate to meet the learning objective.

Multiple student/patient aggregate. A group of students is assigned to complete activities related to a community or population subgroup at risk for certain health problems.

Administrative assignments

Master's and doctoral students may be preparing for management and administrative roles in health care organizations; their clinical activities might focus on enacting the roles of first-level or middle manager, patient care services administrator, or case manager.

Research Link: Needs of the clinical instructor

Kathleen M. Davidson & Liam Rourke (2012). Surveying the Orientation Learning Needs of Clinical Nursing Instructors. International Journal of Nursing Education Scholarship, Vol. 9, Iss. 1, Art. 3

The purpose of this study was to describe the knowledge and skills nurses need to be successful clinical instructors. A formal learning needs assessment was conducted to measure the orientation learning needs of new part-time clinical nursing faculty at one university. The respondents (n = 44; 16.6%) unanimously identified five essential learning needs for nursing clinical instructors, thus providing sound justification upon which to base an instructor orientation program. This literature search revealed only one validated learning needs assessment tool for the orientation of clinical nursing instructors (Seal-Whitlock, 2000). Other learning needs assessments have been conducted and published; however, these tools were not directly applicable to the learning needs of part time clinical nursing instructors. The CNI respondents unanimously identified five areas: 1) accessing and using the program website and intranet, university email accounts and instructional software; 2) key clinical policies and procedures; 3) information about the correlation of clinical experience with the theory component of concurrent courses; 4) all aspects of student evaluation; 5) the role of the CNI in clinical simulation experiences.

Guidelines for Using Rating Scales for Clinical Evaluation (Oermann, MH, and Gaberson, K 2006)

- Be alert to the possible influence of your own values, attitudes, beliefs, and biases in observing performance and drawing conclusions about it.
- Use the clinical outcomes, competencies, or behaviors to focus your observations. Give students feedback on other observations made about their performance.
- Collect sufficient data on students' performance before drawing conclusions about it.
- Observe the student more than once before rating performance. Rating scales when used for clinical evaluation should represent a pattern of the students' performance over time.
- If possible, observe students' performance in different clinical situations, either in the patient care or simulated setting. If that is not possible, develop other strategies for evaluation so performance is evaluated with different methods and at different times.
- Do not rely on first impressions; they may not be accurate.
- Always discuss observations with students; obtain their perceptions of performance; and be willing to modify your own judgments and ratings when new data are presented.

- Review the available clinical learning activities and opportunities in the simulation and learning laboratories. Do they provide sufficient data for completing the rating scale? If not, new learning activities may need to be developed or behaviors may need to be modified to be more realistic considering the clinical teaching circumstances.
- Avoid using rating scales as the only source of data about a student's performance use multiple evaluation methods for clinical practice.
- Rate each outcome, competency, or behavior individually, based on your observations of performance and conclusions drawn. If you have insufficient information about achievement of a particular competency, do not rate it—leave it blank.
- Do not rate all students high, low, or in the middle; similarly, do not let your general impression of the student or personal biases influence the ratings.
- If the rating form is ineffective for judging student performance, then revise it. Consider these questions: Does the form yield data that can be used to make valid decisions about students' competence? Does it yield reliable, stable data? Is it easy to use? Is it realistic for the types of learning activities students complete and available in clinical settings?

19

Teaching Methods

Chapter Highlights

- Grouping Various Instructional Methods
- Teaching Methods Under Different Family Names
- Distinct Phases of Learning
- Five First Principles Stated in the Most Instructional Models
- Approaches to Select Teaching and Learning Methods and Strategies
- Selecting Teaching and Learning Methods
- Lecture Method
- Discussion
- Demonstration
- Clinical Laboratory
- Project Method
- Workshop
- Role-play
- Panel Discussion
- Conference
- Symposium
- Seminar
- Programmed Instruction
  - Linear Programming
  - Branching Programming
  - Mathetics Programming
- Questioning

Learning Objectives

Upon completion of this chapter, the students will be able to:

- Classify various ways of grouping the instructional methods
- Describe distinct phases of learning
- List first five principles stated in the most instructional models
- State different approaches to select teaching and learning methods and strategies
- Describe various teaching methods and their advantages and disadvantages

A well-rounded class should be exposed to multiple teaching methods, not just one. Different students learn better in different ways – there are visual learners, tactile learners, and auditory learners. Also, different subjects and topics are often more understandable when taught in different ways. Teaching methods are the complement of content, just as the instructions that complement the curriculum. All students are not the same, yet they have some commonalities. We have learned quite a bit about accommodating the variability of students through research into instructional methods and learning styles. If we vary our methods, we have learned, we accommodate a wider range of learning styles than if we used one method consistently.

GROUPING VARIOUS INSTRUCTIONAL METHODS

Instructional strategy is the overall plan for a learning experience. It involves the use of one or several methods of teaching, and it encompasses both the content and the process that will be used to achieve the desired outcomes of instruction (Rothwell and Kazanas, 1992).

Instructional methods are the techniques or approaches the teacher uses to bring the learner into contact with the content to be learned. Methods are a way, an approach, or a process to communicate information, whereas instructional materials or tools are the actual vehicles by which information is shared with the learner.

Literature evidence shows that there are many ways of classifying the teaching or instruction:

Didactic: Direct teaching; verbal and typically in the form of a lecture or presentation.

Modeling: Direct teaching; visual and typically in the form of demonstration and practice.

Managerial: Indirect or interactive teaching; facilitation, individualization and group management.

Dialogic: Indirect interactive teaching; Socratic technique of dialogue, questions and thought provocations.

In the ***Direct instruction models***, the teacher imparts knowledge or demonstrates a skill. In the ***Indirect instruction models***, the teacher sets up strategies, but does not teach directly; the students make meaning for themselves. In the ***Interactive instruction models***, the students interact with each other and with the information and materials; the teacher is the organizer and facilitator. ***Experiential learning models*** mean that the students experience and feel; they are actively involved. In ***Independent study models***, the students interact with the content more or less exclusive of external control of the teacher.

Some of the other theorists classify it into three categories as follows:

1. ***Transmissive teaching***, or direct instruction, means that the teacher delivers *status quo* content *via* some method, such as lecturing or demonstrating.
2. ***Transactive teaching***, or indirect instruction, means that the teacher and students arrive at *status quo* content to be learned though transactions and dialogue.
3. ***Transformative teaching***, or a combination of direct and indirect instructions, means that the teacher and students reject *status quo content* and focus on a transformation of themselves or their world.

TEACHING METHODS UNDER DIFFERENT FAMILY NAMES

Joyce and Well group the teaching methods under different family names by considering the characteristics of the teaching methods:

- **Social Interaction Family**

  It emphasizes the relationship of the individual to society or to other persons. It gives priority to the individual's ability to relate to others. Examples for this family:
  - Partner and Group Collaboration
  - Role Playing
  - Jurisprudential Inquiry
- **Information Processing Family**

  It emphasizes the information processing capability of students. It gives priority to the ways students handle stimuli from their environment, organize data, generate concepts and solve problems. Examples related to this family:

- Inductive investigation and inquiry
- Deductive investigation and inquiry
- Memorization
- Synectics (Techniques for creativity)
- Design and problem-solving
- Projects and Reports

- **Personal Family**

It emphasizes the development of individuals, their emotional life and self-hood. It gives priority to self-awareness. Examples:

- Indirect Teaching
- Awareness training and values clarification
- Role modeling
- Self-reflection

- **Behavioral Modification Family**

It emphasizes the development of efficient systems for sequencing learning tasks and shaping behavior. It gives priority to the observable behavior of students. Examples:

- Direct instruction (Demonstrations and presentations)
- Anxiety reduction
- Programmed instruction
- Simulations.

DISTINCT PHASES OF LEARNING

Many current instructional models suggest that the most effective learning products or environments are those that are problem-centered and involve the student in four distinct phases of learning: (a) activation of prior experience, (b) demonstration of skills, (c) application of skills, and (d) integration of these skills into real-world activities.

FIVE FIRST PRINCIPLES STATED IN THE MOST INSTRUCTIONAL MODELS

1. Learning is promoted when learners are engaged in solving real-world problems
2. Learning is promoted when existing knowledge is activated as a foundation for new knowledge
3. Learning is promoted when new knowledge is demonstrated to the learner
4. Learning is promoted when new knowledge is applied by the learner
5. Learning is promoted when new knowledge is integrated into the learner's world.

APPROACHES TO SELECT TEACHING AND LEARNING METHODS AND STRATEGIES

Cranton (2000) recommends the following steps while selecting the teaching and learning methods:

1. *Determine learning outcomes* : Outcomes are statements of what the student is expected to learn and be able to do after the instruction.
2. *Methods should be congruent with the learning outcome first and foremost*: Methods must 'match' the learning objectives or outcomes.

3. *Determine sequence*: Sequencing is the process of organizing content in the order that is most conducive to learning. Sequencing instructions/objectives helps ensure that learners are introduced systematically to what they must know and do to perform competently. The approach used depends on the learning objectives and the instructional environment and, at times, the learners themselves. There are many different sequencing strategies. Sequencing can vary among units of instruction considering the topic, the learners' and instructors' experience regarding the sequencing strategy selected.

Examples of sequencing strategies:

- ***Chronological sequencing:*** In order of occurrence, like history.
- ***Topical:*** Start with a topic for discussion, or a problem, then look at how it originated.
- ***Whole to part:*** Start with the big picture, the whole and then break down into parts.
- ***Part to whole:*** Like whole to part but starting with the components and moving to the bigger picture, i.e. pulling apart the components in a lesson plan template, then moving to the design process itself.
- ***Known to unknown:*** Start there and then move on to what is not known.
- ***Unknown to known:*** Disoriented at the beginning with what is not known. Motivates learners to see how much they do not know.
- ***Step-by-step:*** Learners are introduced to a task by either the steps in the task itself or the knowledge they must possess to perform competently. For example, superficial to superficial, then back to original for more in-depth look.
- ***General to specific:*** Business where first year is base topics, and second year specializes in marketing, sales, etc.

Determine the method:

- Instructor-centered or student-centered
- Interactive
- Individualized
- Experiential.

SELECTING TEACHING AND LEARNING METHODS

- Selecting methods based upon student characteristics
- Keep general characteristics of a learner in mind
- Clarify goals of the program and course
- Incorporate learner experiences into the learning
- Consider the diverse needs of the learner group and ensure that selection of methods is suitable to all learners
- Set a positive climate to encourage tolerance and acceptance of all
- Those with practical knowledge learn best with interaction and experiential methods, and individual projects for those with specific learning in mind
- Be aware that everyone learns differently and we should build variety into our teaching to challenge students and ourselves
- Consider developmental stages of learners and make sure they have the preknowledge, skills and attitudes that are required to learn a new skill
- Selecting methods based upon teacher styles

- All teachers have preferences just as learners have learning style preferences
- Teacher-centered strategies imply that the focus is on the teacher rather than the student. An example of a teaching-centered strategy is Lecture method. Though the inclination is to do what works best for you as a teacher, research suggests that students learn best when the focus is on learning rather than teaching!
- Selecting methods based upon context
- May be limited by facility, size of group, time of day, resources
- Be aware of the effects they may have and try to be creative to work around limitations.

Teaching methods might be classified into the following three categories:

1. *Controlled*: Teacher dominates the teaching learning process.
2. *Semi-controlled*: It is joint teacher-student participation.
3. *Uncontrolled*: The students are the main participants in the classroom activities.

LECTURE METHOD

The lecture can be an immensely effective tool in the classroom, allowing an instructor to provide an overarching theme that organizes material in an illuminating and interesting way. The instructor must take care, however, to shape the lecture for the specific audience of students who will hear it and to encourage those students to take an active and immediate part in learning the material. It is essential to see lectures as a means of helping students learn to think about the key concepts of a particular subject, rather than primarily as a means of transferring knowledge from instructor to student.

What is the Lecture Method?

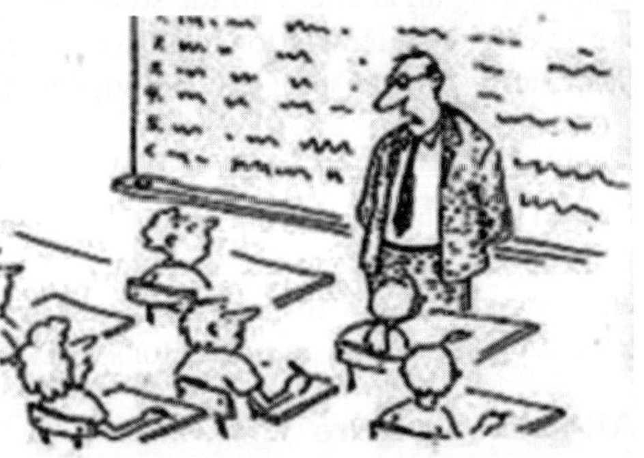

The word 'lecture' comes from the Latin word 'lectus', from the 14th century, which translates roughly into 'to read.' It was not until the 16th century that the word was used to describe oral instruction given by a teacher in front of an audience of learners. Today, lecturing is a teaching method that involves, primarily, an oral presentation given by an instructor to a body of students.

Many lectures are accompanied by some sort of visual aid, such as a slideshow, a word document, an image, or a film. Some teachers may even use a

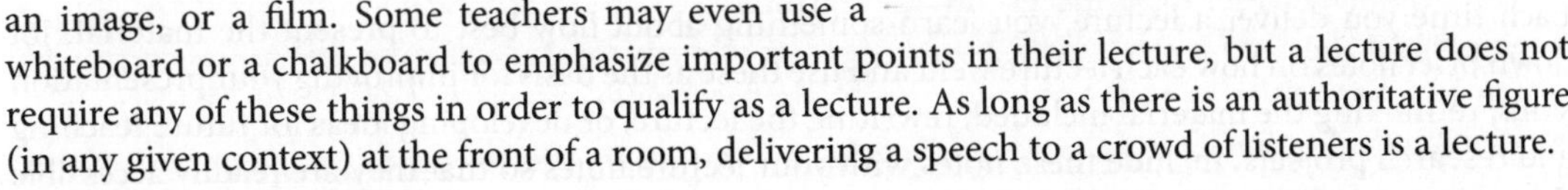

whiteboard or a chalkboard to emphasize important points in their lecture, but a lecture does not require any of these things in order to qualify as a lecture. As long as there is an authoritative figure (in any given context) at the front of a room, delivering a speech to a crowd of listeners is a lecture.

During the Lecture

Interact with your students

The more an instructor interacts with the students during a lecture, the more active the learning will be. The judicious use of questions throughout a class session can move the lecture forward, engage the students, increase the use of higher-order thinking processes, and make the lecture more interesting.

Provide students a clear sense of the day's topics and their relation to the course as a whole.

Write an outline on the board before the class begins. This strategy will help students organize the material you are presenting. An outline can also help students when they are studying to identify ideas and connections that they did not grasp during the lecture itself. Take time at the beginning of the class to connect the day's ideas, concepts, or problems to the material that you presented in the previous class and to the overarching themes of the course.

Show Passion for the Subject

Tell students what you find fascinating about what you are teaching. If you are teaching a course that you have taught many times, recall what is interesting about the subject to someone learning about it for the first time. Find new applications and examples that will enable you to communicate why the topic should be studied and understood. Speak clearly so that all the students can hear you.

Project Your Voice

When lecturing in a large room, use a microphone. Ask students to tell you if they cannot hear you; some may feel too intimidated to speak up unless you ask. Speak with an animated tone, but more slowly than you would in an informal conversation.

Use gestures, eye contact and movement around the room to engage student attention.

Make eye contact with students in all areas of the room, not just with those students who routinely answer your questions or otherwise appear engaged.

When Asking Questions, Do not be Afraid of Silence

Give students 5–10 seconds to think and formulate a response. If 10–15 seconds pass without anyone volunteering an answer and the students are giving you puzzled looks, rephrase your question. Do not give in to the temptation to answer your own questions, which will condition students to hesitate before answering to see if you will supply 'the answer'. Patience is key; do not be afraid of silence.

Demonstrate Respect for, and Interest in, Student Ideas and Questions

Make it clear that you are interested in what and how students are thinking about the material. Show that you value their questions and insights by referring back to these responses later in the lecture or on a subsequent day. This strategy is especially important in a large group. It is common for students to be very sensitive to an instructor's reaction.

After the Lecture

Rethink, Retool, Revise

Each time you deliver a lecture, you learn something about how best to present the material. Jot down brief notes on how each lecture went and use these as the basis for improving your presentation skills, rethinking the material included, rewriting the lecture, or developing ideas for future teaching and research projects. Include these notes with your lecture notes so that they are readily accessible the next time you teach the course.

Arrange to have one of your classes observed or videotaped so that an observer can help you evaluate what went well and what you can do to improve student learning.

Lectures are the major teaching method employed in many academic departments and schools.

Advantages of Lectures

- **Audience focus**: The lecturer can be aware and responsive to a specific audience so that each student feels that he or she is being talked to as an individual.
- **Versatile and flexible**: There are many variants of lectures, and other teaching methods can be included within the lecture format.
- **Easily updated**: Unlike some other teaching methods, changing lectures is easy and inexpensive. Material which is not otherwise available can easily be included in a lecture.
- **Low technology**: Little can go wrong other than the lecturer becoming ill.
- **Acceptable and familiar**: Some students like lectures because they are usually nonthreatening and they can hide in the multitudes.
- These can incorporate learning principles.
- **Live contact:** Rapport and immediate feedback to the student are possible.
- **Professor-efficient**: Preparation time can be kept within reasonable limits.
- **Time-efficient**: These can be presented to a large number of students which is an efficient use of the professor's time.
- **Instructor control**: Many professors prefer a teaching style which allows them to have direct control
- **Helps for motivation and for conveying information:** A professor can convey the interest and enthusiasm that he or she has in the topic. Information can be presented and rearranged in a variety of ways to help students learn.
- **Student learning can be high:** If clear objectives are given to students and good support materials are available, research shows that student learning in a lecture course as measured by a content examination is equal to that of other teaching methods (Taveggia and Hedley, 1972).

Disadvantages of Lectures

- **Audience ignored:** Poor lecturers push on despite the pain and suffering which is obvious
- to all but the lecturer.
- **Inappropriate lecture form may be used**: Many professors are unfamiliar with the many variants of lectures and try to force-fit one form onto all circumstances.
- **Stagnation**: Although lectures are easy to change and up-date every semester, many professors don't bother. This is obviously a teacher problem and not the fault of the technique.
- **Passivity**: Like stagnation of material, acceptability of the method may lead the professor to ignore looking for ways to improve.
- **Few learning principles may be satisfied:** This is often the case in lectures with lots of content and little professor-student interaction. The worst problem is usually the passivity of students in lectures unless special efforts are made to keep them active.
- **Boredom:** A "live" presentation where the professor is boring, speaks in a monotone, makes no eye contact, pays no attention to the students, receives no student feedback, gives no feedback to the students, and is impersonal is "dead."
- **Inadequate preparation or over preparation**: Inexperienced professors often spend too much time preparing for lectures, and experienced professors who no longer care, may not prepare. One of the problems of lecturing is that there is no mechanism which forces adequate preparation.
- **False economy:** The economic efficiency of large lectures is abused by many universities. Student learning of higher-level cognitive functions would be significantly enhanced in smaller classes with more interactions.

- **Lack of individualization**: Since the instructor controls the pace, it will necessarily be too fast for some students and too slow for others.
- **Anyone can lecture:** Unfortunately, the apparent ease of lecturing hides the fact that lecturing is one of the hardest teaching methods to truly master. In addition, what many professors have seen and are cloning are inferior lecture classes.
- **Not suited for higher level cognitive tasks**: Although lecturing is a good teaching method for conveying information, it is not as well suited for some higher-level cognitive tasks, such as analysis, synthesis, evaluation, and problem-solving.
- **Extremely stressful**: Lecturing can be an emotional trial for some professors. In extreme cases, these professors need to find alternate teaching methods which are less stressful for them.
- **Lack of supporting material**: If clear objectives are not given to students and good supporting material is not available, then student learning will be less than with an alternate teaching method which provides these.

DISCUSSION

Discussion is defined as two-way, spoken communication between the teacher and the students, and, more importantly, among the students themselves. Lowman (1995, p. 159) suggested: 'Useful classroom discussion consists of student comments separated by frequent probes and clarifications by the teacher that facilitate involvement and development of thinking by the whole group.'

Discussion engages students in what they are presented with in lectures or other class assignments. Discussion approaches are effective in developing students' thinking skills and higher-level learning, such as application, analysis, synthesis, and evaluation (Bloom et al, 1956), and also creativity (Anderson and Krathwohl, 2001; Bligh, 2000). As a teaching method, discussion permits students to be active in their own learning, which increases their motivation to learn and makes the process more interesting.

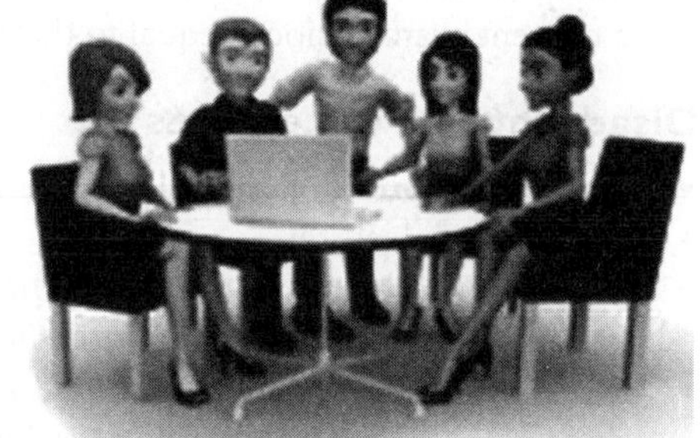

Effective Discussion Techniques

Group size: A successful discussion requires a relatively small number of participants—5 being an ideal number. (Schellenberg, (1959); Hare (1961). 'The five-participant rule' creates a problem for teacher who has more number of students in her classroom. There are two solutions to this problem. 1. Small group (5 in number) can be allowed to discuss by asking the others to observe. This is known as fishbowl strategy. 2. Break a class into small groups and allow for discussion in different occasions.

Seating Arrangements

The traditional seating arrangements: Students in rows facing the instructor—severely restricts participation in a discussion. Circular arrangement where a teacher and students can see each other is much more effective.

Stages of a Typical Classroom Discussion

- Define the question, topic, or problem to give the discussion focus.
- Have students suggest possible answers or solutions.

- Collect relevant information or data that might help answer the question(s) at issue.
- Evaluate positions argued by, or solutions proposed by, the students during the discussion.

Teacher's Role in Discussion

- **Get to know your students:** Particularly important for successful discussions. Develop rapport with your students.
- **Be prepared:** An effective discussion requires much more preparation than an effective lecture. In a lecture, you can decide what you will cover. In a discussion, you should be prepared to explore any issue reasonably related to the discussion topic. This means you must know the topic very well. Be ready to address potential issues or questions that the students might bring up. Outline your possible answers or responses.
- **Begin the discussion:** Many times, and certainly the first time, you as the instructor will begin the discussion. Svinicki and McKeachie (2011) discuss a number of ways to start the discussion with a question, a controversy, or a common experience. Choosing something from the students' 'real life' is one tactic. Providing a common experience by means of a reading, film, or similar example of mass media is another. Ensure that your students have sufficient information to make the discussion productive.
- **Facilitate the discussion.**
- Be patient, since discussions take time to get started. Allow for pauses and silence. Although silence may feel socially awkward, it gives both you and the students time to think. You may need to train your students (and yourself) to feel comfortable with silence.
- Listen to what each student says. Observe who is, and is not, participating.
- **Ask questions:** Ask a student for clarification, or to support his or her comment or opinion; use open-ended questions (that cannot simply be answered by a 'yes' or a 'no' or one word); ask divergent questions (where there can be more than one acceptable answer). However, do *not* question a single student too long.
- **Deal with conflicts:** It is important *not* to ignore conflicts. First, try to clarify what seems to be the disagreement; it might simply be a cognitive misunderstanding. Listing the pros and cons visually (e.g. whiteboard, handout, discussion board) can be helpful. If the conflict involves many students, let the group talk about their disagreement in some manner. (See also Kustra and Potter, 2008, pp. 59-65.).
- **Provide summaries:** Periodically during the discussion, and certainly at the end, provide a summary and perhaps some conclusions of the discussion. Verify group consensus and check to see whether *all* the students do actually agree: 'Does that statement reflect what all of you think?'
- **Reflect on what took place during the discussion:** After the discussion, think about what worked well and what you might do differently. Think about which student(s) did or did not participate in the discussion. Which of them contributed most? Did any student(s) dominate? What was the quality of the students' comments? And, especially, what did the students learn?

Students' Roles in Discussion

- **Students should be prepared:** In keeping with your expectations, students are to come to the discussion prepared. Typically, this means that not only are they to have read the assignment, but also thought about it in the context of the topic being studied.
- **Students should participate:** Assuming that discussions are a required part of the course, students must participate. Totally silent observers do not earn full credit in such a course. This does not mean that silent observers do not learn anything, but the students who participate learn more, which is the purpose of a discussion class.

- **Students should explain with clarity:** One purpose of discussions is to allow students test their ideas and conclusions. This requires not only that students develop ideas, but also that they explain their ideas or conclusions with clarity, and where possible, with reasonable brevity.
- **Students should listen:** Student participation involves not only speaking, but also listening to what other students are saying, and either indicating some level of understanding or asking for clarification.

Barriers to Good Discussion

Svinicki and McKeachie (2011, pp. 44–45) discuss five barriers to good discussion:

1. Habits of passive learning.
2. Fear of appearing stupid.
3. Trying too hard to find the answer the teacher is looking for.
4. Failing to see value in the discussion topic or process.
5. And wanting to settle on a solution before alternatives have been considered. Davis (2009, p. 107) outlines six faulty assumptions students often hold about discussions: one must argue for only one position; knowledge is really just opinion; personal experience is the real source of knowledge; issues should not be discussed unless there is agreement; individual rights are violated when ideas are challenged; and individuals in a discussion should never feel uncomfortable.

Enhancing Participation

- **Ask general (divergent) questions:** Questions that can have more than one acceptable answer (e.g. 'What is your opinion about...?') can lead to more discussion. In addition, give students your questions about the reading before you will be discussing them.
- **Avoid looking *only* at the student talking:** Although it may seem counterintuitive to look away, and eye contact does tell a student that you are paying attention, looking too long at one student can seem threatening. Also, you need to monitor how the other students in the group are reacting.
- **Control excessive talkers:** Even though the students who talk the most are sometimes the 'better' students, avoid automatically calling on them first, even after a seemingly long silence. Ask to hear from someone who hasn't said anything yet. If one student's excessive talking becomes a problem, you may want to talk with that student about it outside the class. Sometimes the excessive talker is you (or me) — the teacher! Videotaping a class and watching it later may provide useful information about this.
- **Ask for examples and illustrations:** This is particularly important when discussing complex ideas, or concepts students often have difficulty understanding.
- **Allow for pauses and silences:** Silence, even for a minute or more, allows the students, and you time to think. This 'wait time' is especially helpful to students who are more introverted and may not be getting an opportunity to participate (Davis, 2009).
- **Be sensitive to feelings and emotional reactions:** Some topics may generate strong negative, or positive, feelings, or you may notice that a student is becoming upset or angry as the discussion progresses, any of which may become obstacles to learning. You may simply wish to say, "You seem to have strong feelings about this." Or you may need to explore: "Would you say some more about that?" You may want to talk to the student after class.

Encourage and recognize students' contributions: Listen carefully to each student's comments, sometimes paraphrasing to show that you understand. Give students a chance to clarify what they meant, or link Student B's comment to something Student A said.

Advantages of Discussion Method

- Well suited to facilitate a number of course goals.
- Particularly effective at increasing student involvement and active learning in classes.
- Engages students in what they are presented with in lectures or other class assignments.
- Effective in developing students' thinking skills and higher-level learning.
- Help students acquire better communication skills as they learn to present their ideas clearly and briefly.
- Can contribute to students' affective development by increasing their interest in a variety of subjects, helping to clarify their values, and aiding in recognizing, and perhaps changing, some attitudes.
- Discussion permits students to be active in their own learning.
- Provides feedback.

Disadvantages of Discussion Method

- Discussions are *not* an effective way to cover a significant amount of content.
- Time-consuming, requiring more preparation and class time.
- Even when you are very well prepared, the discussion may not follow the direction you anticipated, resulting in less control. To some extent, you must go where the students' questions and interests take the group, which may not be consistent with your initial plan.
- Difficult to get students to participate in a discussion, particularly when some of them may not even know how to effectively participate.
- Finally, a topic may be very controversial or elicit excessive emotional reactions.
- Discussion is a complex teaching method that requires careful planning and preparation for both you and your students (Brookfield and Preskill, 2005).

DEMONSTRATION

Demonstration is an essential teaching approach in supporting the learning of a skill at any level or grade and is the most supportive of all teaching approaches (Cambourne 1988; Mooney 1990). Demonstration is a method by which the learner is shown by the teacher how to perform a particular skill. Return demonstration is the method by which the learner attempts to perform the skill with cues from the teacher as needed. These two methods require different abilities by both the teacher and the learner. Demonstration is of utmost importance in the teaching of nursing. Demonstration can be defined as the visualized explanation of facts, concepts and procedures. When using the demonstration model in the classroom, the teacher, or some other expert on the topic being taught, performs the tasks step-by-step so that the learner will eventually be able to complete the same task independently.

The eventual goal is for learners to not only duplicate the task, but also to recognize how to solve problems when unexpected obstacles or problems arise. After performing the demonstration, the teacher's role becomes supporting students in their attempts, providing guidance and feedback, and offering suggestions for alternative approaches. This method of teaching is based on the simple, yet sound, principle that we learn by doing. Students learn physical or mental skills by actually performing those skills under supervision. Demonstration method is otherwise known as performance method.

Every instructor should recognize the importance of student performance in the learning process. Early in a lesson, that is to include demonstration and performance, the instructor should identify the most important learning outcomes. Next, explain and demonstrate the steps involved in performing the skill being taught. Then, allow students time to practice each step so they can increase their ability to perform the skill.

Phases of Demonstration

Explanation Phase

Explanations must be clear, pertinent to the objectives of the particular lesson to be presented, and based on the known experience and knowledge of the students. In teaching a skill, the instructor must convey to the students the precise actions they are to perform. In addition to the necessary steps, the instructor should describe the end-result of these efforts. Before leaving this phase, the instructor should encourage students to ask questions about any step of the procedure that they do not understand.

Demonstration Phase

The instructor must show students the actions necessary to perform a skill. As little extraneous activity as possible should be included in the demonstration if students are to clearly understand that the instructor is accurately performing the actions previously explained. If due to some unanticipated circumstances the demonstration does not closely conform to the explanation, this deviation should be immediately acknowledged and explained.

Student Performance and Instructor Supervision Phases

Because these two phases, which involve separate actions, are performed concurrently, they are discussed here under a single heading. The first of these phases is the student's performance of the physical or mental skills that have been explained and demonstrated. The second activity is the instructor's supervision.

Student performance requires students to act and do. To learn skills, students must practice. The instructor must, therefore, allot enough time for meaningful student activity. Through doing, students learn to follow correct procedures and to reach established standards. It is important that students be given an opportunity to perform the skill as soon as possible after a demonstration that is called 'return demonstration.' Prior to terminating the performance phase, they should be allowed to independently complete the task at least once, with supervision and coaching as necessary.

Evaluation Phase

In this phase, the instructor judges a student's performance. The student displays whatever competence has been attained, and the instructor discovers just how well the skill has been learned. To test each student's ability to perform, the instructor requires students to work independently throughout this phase and makes some comment as to how each performed the skill relative to the way it was taught. From this measurement of student's achievement, the instructor determines the effectiveness of the instruction.

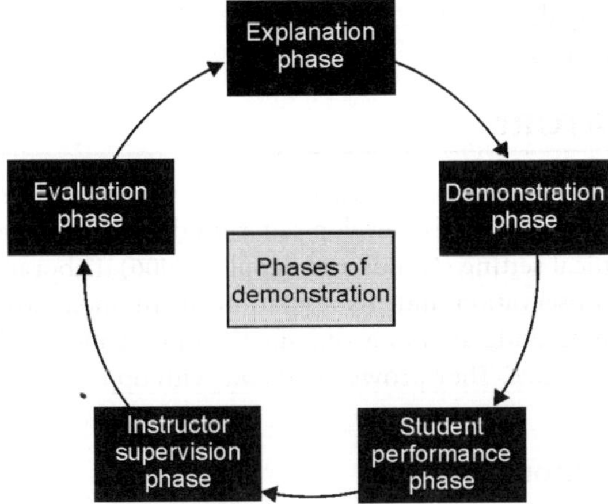

Advantages of Demonstration

- **Clarifies material:** Material presented by verbal methods alone may be misunderstood or misinterpreted. The demonstration method can eliminate misconception and improve understanding.
- **Supplement other method:** The demonstration method is rarely used by itself. It is usually preceded and accompanied by an explanation employing either lecture or conference method or both.
- **Appeals to senses:** A demonstration is an especially effective teaching method. It appeals to the sense of sight and many people learn more readily through the sense of sight than through any of other senses.
- Correlates theory and practice.
- Provides a base for concrete learning
- **Realistic:** The Demonstration stimulates interest because it is realistic.
- Helps in introducing new practices or procedures.
- **Saves time:** Students can observe in a few minutes what might take several hours to explain by lecture or discussion, demonstrations save time.
- **Sets performance standards:** Teaching performance standards by demonstration shows the student how a given procedure contributes.
- Provides direct experiences
- Reinforces learning
- Serves as a model laboratory instruction
- It is understood easily
- Permits teaching of theory with practice.

Disadvantages of Demonstration

- May fail
- May limit participation
- May limit audience/client input
- Requires large amount of preliminary preparation

- Danger of student being dishonest
- Good demonstrators are rare.

CLINICAL LABORATORY

During the course of their education, students are expected to acquire knowledge, incorporate critical thinking and psychomotor skills, develop self-confidence in their abilities, and then transfer this knowledge to the clinical setting (Childs and Sepples, 2006). Laboratory teaching assumes that first-hand experience in observation and manipulation of the materials of science is superior to other methods of developing understanding and appreciation. Laboratories are wonderful settings for teaching and learning science. They provide students with opportunities to think about, discuss, and solve real problems.

Significance of Laboratory Method

Infante (1985) describes laboratory as a workshop from the Latin word 'Laboratorium' where the laboratory method provides the students with real experience. The goal of laboratory experiences (labs) is to become practiced and confident in nursing psychomotor skills (skills that require varying levels of well-coordinated physical activity and precise procedures), in order to provide the basis for safe, competent care to patients and families in the clinical setting.

Boxer and Kluge (2000) identified those skills beginning registered nurses (RNs) perform most often: universal precautions for infection control, vital sign assessment, intravenous therapy management, medication administration, and patient hygiene. Patient care and safety can be compromised when such basic skills are deficient (Bloomfield, Roberts, and While, 2010). Patients have reported that the proficiency and efficiency with which the practitioner performs skills can produce or reduce patient anxiety (Bjork, 1995).

Laboratories are wonderful settings for teaching and learning science. They provide students with opportunities to think about, discuss, and solve real problems. Developing and teaching an effective laboratory requires as much skill, creativity, and hard work as proposing and executing a first-rate research project.

Shulman and Tamir, in the Second Handbook of Research on Teaching (Travers, ed. 1973), listed five types of objectives that may be achieved through the use of the laboratory in science classes:

- **Skills**: Manipulative, inquiry, investigative, organizational, communicative
- **Concepts**: For example, hypothesis, theoretical model, taxonomic category
- **Cognitive abilities**: Critical thinking, problem-solving, application, analysis, synthesis
- **Understanding of the nature of science**: Scientific enterprise, scientists and how they work, existence of a multiplicity of scientific methods, interrelationships between science and technology and among the various disciplines of science
- **Attitudes**: For example, curiosity, interest, risk taking, objectivity, precision, confidence, perseverance, satisfaction, responsibility, consensus, collaboration, and liking science.

Approaches to Teaching Labs

The approach one takes to laboratory instruction has important consequences for student motivation and learning. Domin (1999) distinguishes four different approaches to laboratory instruction, ranging from those in which students have little ownership over their own learning to those in which they have considerably more control, motivation, and incentive to work together to solve problems.

Purposes

- Teaching manuals and observational skills relevant to the subject
- Improving understanding of methods of scientific inquiry
- Developing problem-solving and doing by self-skills.

Ideal Methods of Teaching Laboratory

- Self-preparation
- Right-explanation
- Starting-experiments
- Handling instruments
- Explaining observations
- Writing reports
- Lab safety.

Advantages

- Students learn by doing and come in contact with raw data or materials object in teaching learning process
- Develops the power of observation and reasoning
- Develops the scientific attitudes on range of nursing procedures
- Gives an understanding of what research is and how to apply the scientific method of research
- Gives training in organizing data gathered from real materials object and how these objects are manipulated to attain the objectives
- Since students come in contact with real-life situations, it can be a preparation for solving real-life problems.

Disadvantages

- Uneconomical way of learning in time and material.
- Does give much training in verbal expression and when the time equipment is used, most of the time its use becomes mechanical, i.e. used without much thinking anymore.

PROJECT METHOD

A project is a list of real life that has been imparted into the school. It demands work from the pupils. The class may be divided into 4–6 groups and each group could be assigned one part of the project depending on their interest, ability and skill. In this strategy, students involve them in performing some constructive activities in natural condition. Kilpatrick (1918), influenced by Dewey's and Thorndike's theories, deduced that the 'psychology of the child' was crucial to the learning process and they needed to be able to decide what they wanted to do and this motivation would lead to learning success since they pursued their own purpose. Kilpatrick (1921) identified the term 'project' to refer to any unit of purposeful experience, any instance of purposeful activity where the dominating purpose, as an inner urges, fixes the aim of the action, guides its process, and furnishes its drive, its inner motivation.

Popular Definitions of Project Method

- According to Kilpatrick, 'A project is a whole-hearted purposeful activity proceeding in a social environment'.
- According to Stevenson (1908), 'A project is a problematic act carried to completion in its natural setting'.
- Charter (1923) viewed the project as 'a problematic act carried to completion in a natural setting'.
- L Arpin and L Capra (2001) give a large characterization to the project method, defining it as a 'pedagogical method which allows the pupil to imply himself into the building of his knowledge interrelating with the colleagues and with the environment, the role of teacher being of pedagogical mediator, privileged by pupils and knowledge that must be studied'.

Principles of Project Method

- **Principle of Purposefulness:** The project should be purposeful, and that should have some main objective. The objective should give the enthusiasm and work to the students, otherwise that will be a wastage of time and energy.
- **Principle of Utility:** The project should be useful to the students and the society. It will give some value to the students. From a good project, the students as well as the society get the benefit a lot.
- **Principle of Freedom:** The students are free to select the topic and execute the work according to their will and wish, interest, attitude and capacity. The teacher is just a guide and gives guidelines to execute that.
- **Principle of Activity:** Project means the purposeful activity. At the end of the project, the students gain knowledge through their activity. It is based on the principle of 'learning by doing'.
- **Principle of Reality:** Project should be real and related to the life situation of the students and the society. Only then they would be able to complete the project naturally and really. Imaginary problems are not taken up in the project.
- **Principle of Social Development:** A good project focuses health needs, social development and societal awareness. It is a good method to concentrate on the affective domain of the student which is many times a neglected learning domain. A single project solves the problem of thousands of people or the society. Nursing projects give solution for many day-to-day problems in the field of care and educational areas of nursing in the hospital and community.
- **Principle of Planning:** The student develops prior planning in advance about the project. They find solutions for— How? When? What? Where? Why? So, a good project develops the problem-solving capacity and prior planning for the execution.
- **Based on Pragmatic Thoughts:** Project method follows pragmatic principles.

Types of Project

Kilpatrick classified project method into four types. They are:

1. **Constructive:** When learners have to construct something related to social life, e.g. charts, models, maps, etc.
2. **Artistic:** Generally allotted in aesthetic field of life. e.g. Music, drawing, painting and culture.
3. **Problem-solving:** Projects are given to solve problems related to life situations or related to any subjects.
4. **Group work:** A team of students assigned to perform a group work.

Elements of Project Method

- Spontaneity
- Purpose
- Significance
- Interest

The project method assures a dynamic and continuous interaction of the three elements of the pedagogical structure: teacher, pupil and knowledge acquired by the pupil. The Project Method permits an 'ideal mode' of complete activities to be carried out in series of steps.

General Steps in Project Method

- **Informing:** The teacher becomes the ultimate motivator. Student chooses the project topic in consent with the teacher. Students must be given enough freedom to express their interest and suggestions in the topic chosen. Teacher must ensure that the project meets specific learning objective of the course or the subject.
- **Planning:** Students are helped to come out with a guiding plan individually or as a group based on the type of project planned. The entire 'go ahead' plan considering manpower, money, material and time should be in place to guide the project. The teacher advises and guides the student(s) adequately to run the project by keeping a watch on any upcoming errors.
- **Implementing:** This is the most important step where the project is given live track to run. All the energy and work are utilized in an appropriate way to achieve something useful that will enhance the students.
- **Evaluation:** The teacher evaluates the project work and gives the feedback to the student.

Specific Steps Involved in Carrying Out a Project

1. **Providing a set of problems:** The teacher provides a set of problems to the students and initiates discussion on them. The student(s), individually or in groups are asked to choose a particular problem that interests him/them.
2. **Selecting and defining a problem:** The students select a particular problem (individually or in groups) and define the problem precisely. The precise definition of the problem is very important because the student should be clear about the problem in which he/she works.
3. **Formulating hypotheses:** Hypotheses are probable solutions to the problems. The students at this point, after reflection and discussion, frame a hypothesis for the problem selected.
4. **Planning/Designing methods to test the hypotheses formulated:** The teacher then asks the students to plan or design methods to test the correctness of the hypothesis framed for the problem selected. The students reflect on the nature of the problem, the hypothesis framed, the data required to validate the hypothesis, the mode of collecting such data, etc. and plan/design a comprehensive method to test the hypothesis. The teacher, before the commencement of the execution stage, discusses the evaluation criteria with the students and briefs them on the format of the project report to be submitted.
5. **Collection of data:** The students move out of the classroom and as per their plan, begin to gather data from various sources. They have to carefully record the information collected and later organize the information in a way that would facilitate further study and interpretation.
6. **Interpretation of data:** At this point, the students carefully study the data collected and interpret information collected. The interpretations are noted down and the findings and conclusions are arrived at.

7. **Reviewing:** The students then critically examine the methods adopted to collect the data, the adequacy of the data collected, the interpretation of the data and the conclusions arrived at, which either support or reject the hypothesis formulated. After this, the teacher is consulted and a review of the entire project exercise is made. The suggestions and recommendations of the teacher are incorporated in the first draft of the project report.
8. **Reporting**: The students present their findings in the form of a project report after receiving the corrected first drafts submitted.
9. **Evaluating:** The teacher evaluates the work submitted, on the basis of the evaluation criteria discussed and decided upon with the students. The evaluation criteria should be clear, specific and comprehensive.

Advantages of Project Method

- It is a democratic way of learning. The students choose, plan and execute the project themselves
- It teaches dignity of labor and the pupils develop respect and taste for all types of work
- It affords opportunity to develop keenness and accuracy of observation and to experience the job of discovery
- It helps to widen the mental horizon of students and analyze the problems in their natural settings
- It sets up a challenge to solve a problem and this stimulates constructive and creative thinking.

Disadvantages of Project Method

- It absorbs a lot of time, with the result that the quantity of knowledge suffers
- The whole syllabus, especially for more advanced classes, cannot well be included in a collection of projects and it is difficult to finish the syllabus in the limited period of time
- It is expensive in the sense that a well-equipped library and a laboratory are required and, at the same time, the pupils have to bear the expenses on excursion and other visits, etc.
- The teacher will have to be exceptionally gifted, knowledgeable as well as alert and helpful.

WORKSHOP

A workshop is a single, short (although 'short' may mean anything from 45 minutes to two full days) educational program designed to teach or introduce to participants' practical skills, techniques, or ideas which they can then use in their work or their daily lives.

Size: An ideal size is 8–12. It is small enough so that everyone has an opportunity to have his questions answered and to get some individual attention from the presenter, but still large enough to generate some lively discussion. If the group is larger than 15, the voices of some people, usually those who are quieter, tend to get lost; if it is smaller than 6–8, there may not be enough opinions, questions, and ideas flying around.

Purposes of Workshop

- Teaching a skill which the participants then might have to use or will use in the future
- Giving participants a chance to practice and receive feedback on techniques and concepts they already know
- Enhancing participants' current knowledge of concepts, techniques, and methods (new research, improvement of techniques, etc.)

- Familiarizing people with material important for, but not directly connected to, their jobs.
- Providing, or helping to provide, a job-related credential for advancement or initial employment for instance, or for some certification or licensure.

Common Features of Workshop

- They are generally small, usually from 6 to 15 participants, allowing everyone some personal attention and the chance to be heard.
- Often designed for people who are working together, or working in the same field.
- Conducted by people who have real experience in the subject under discussion.
- They are often participatory, i.e. participants are active, both in that they influence the direction of the workshop and also in that they have a chance to practice the techniques, skills, etc. that are under discussion.
- They are informal; there is a good deal of discussion in addition to participation, rather than just a teacher presenting material to be absorbed by attentive students.
- They are time-limited, often to a single session, although some may involve multiple sessions over a period of time (e.g. once a week for four weeks, or two full-day sessions over a weekend).
- They are self-contained. Although a workshop may end with handouts and suggestions for further reading or study for those who are interested, the presentation is generally meant to stand on its own, unlike a course, which depends on large amounts of reading and other projects (papers, presentations) in addition to classroom activities.

Ideal Occasions for Workshop Method

- **The beginning of something new:** If your organization is adopting a new method, or your community initiative is taking a new track, there are often new pieces of information or ways of functioning that people must learn. A workshop, or series of workshops, is a way to introduce these in a short time and get people ready for the change.
- **The initial training of staff or volunteers:** Workshops are often a good way to train new staff members or volunteers in the philosophy, methods, and functioning of your organization, or in techniques they will need to do their jobs.
- **The in-service or ongoing training of staff or volunteers:** Workshops in different issues, techniques, etc. are a good way to keep staff and volunteers fresh and thinking about what they are doing.
- **Staff development:** Workshops are often used as a way of honing professional skills and learning about new developments in the field.
- **The demonstration of a new concept:** If someone in an organization has been exposed to a particularly exciting new idea or technique, he may want to conduct a workshop on it for his colleagues, or the organization may want to bring in someone to do so.
- **The explanation of something to the public:** An organization may conduct a public workshop on its issue, in order to make sure that people are informed about its cause or about what it is doing.
- **The availability of a knowledgeable presenter:** If you have particular expertise in a subject, you may be asked to present a workshop to staff or members of another organization, to the public, at a conference, etc. Well-known people in a given field are often invited (and paid) to travel long distances to present workshops.

Advantages of a Workshop

- A workshop provides a way to create an intensive educational experience in a short amount of time, when the time for a more comprehensive effort may not be available
- A workshop can introduce a new concept, spurring participants to investigate it further on their own, or can demonstrate and encourage the practice of actual methods
- It is a great way to teach hands-on skills because it offers participants a chance to try out new methods and fail in a safe situation
- Feedback, from both the presenter and peers in the group, helps a participant understand what she can do to avoid failure in a real situation
- A workshop is a way for someone to pass on to colleagues ideas and methods that he has developed or finds important
- Able to reach large numbers of people by conducting workshops in various situations
- A workshop can help to create a sense of community among its participants.

Preparation

- Find out about the space you will be using, if possible
- Carry everything you need to the spot
- Arrange well beforehand for any equipment you will need
- Make materials and handouts as attractive and interesting as possible so that participants will return to them
- Be overprepared
- Make up a pre- and postevaluation form and overall assessment form
- Get a good night's sleep the night before.

Implementation

Planning and preparation are done. You are incredibly organized; you have all your handouts color-coded and arranged in the order you want to distribute them; you have activities planned down to the second, with plenty of extras if they do not fill the time completely; you have the room arranged so it will welcome participants and work for the activities you have planned. Now IT IS SET TO GO.

Steps in Conducting a Workshop

- **Consider the time available:** Workshops can run from as little as an hour or less to as much as a day or even longer. Workshop goals should match with the time availability. Rehearse different parts to see how long they will take, or how long you want them to take.
- **Present with different activities:** Breaking up the time by involving participants in a number of different kinds of activities is far more conducive to their learning than asking them to sit still and do one thing for the whole time. (Studies have shown that most people start to lose concentration after 20 minutes to half-an-hour. By the end of an hour, their level of attention has fallen by more than 50%).
- **Level of seriousness of the material:** Mixing activities and ideas that are fun or humorous with others that are more serious can not only keep participants awake and on their toes, but can aid learning as well.
- **Small break is healthy:** This will speak to the attention-span issue and allow participants a chance to get coffee, go to the bathroom, etc. without disturbing the flow of the workshop. Breaks always take longer than what is planned.

- **Exclusive time participants—to know each other:** The opportunity to get to know others and to exchange ideas is one of the main values of a workshop for many people, and there should be provision for it.
- Concentrate on the purpose of the workshop and do not deviate.
- **Consider your presentation:** The style of your presentation, both your personal style and the actual methods of presentation you employ, will do much to determine the effectiveness of your workshop.

Tips to Keep the Audience into Your Track

- Include some sort of hands-on activity where people can be physically active
- Include both group and individual activities
- Activities should be entertaining, or at least involving. Avoid being a 'talking head' as much as possible
- Include various kinds of audiovisual material where appropriate videos, audiotapes, overheads, projected computer-screen images, etc.
- Include innovative ways of presenting material directly: a play, an interactive skit, a song, a cartoon, etc.
- Always include practice of a particular technique or method that is being presented, even if only for a short time, to give participants the chance to see what it feels like.

Closing the Workshop

- In the final phase of the workshop, you will need to wrap things up and give participants a chance to react to what they have just been through. You may want to go through some formal activity for this purpose, or you may want to just throw out some questions and listen to what people have to say.
- Sum up and review agenda
- Revisit expectations
- Give participants a chance to sum up
- Ask for feedback on the ideas, techniques, methods, etc. that you presented
- Collect evaluation forms
- Follow-up.

ROLE-PLAY

Role-play is a powerful and effective teaching method for children and adults and can be adapted to deliver any learning objectives from simple to complex concepts. It really lends well to practice communication skills, debate complex ethical issues or explore attitudes and beliefs. Role-playing is the spontaneous acting out of situations, without costumes or scripts. In acting, role-playing is a rehearsal tool, not a performance. It is a chance for the actor to 'try on' different aspects of his character and explore relationships with his scene partner—without judgment.

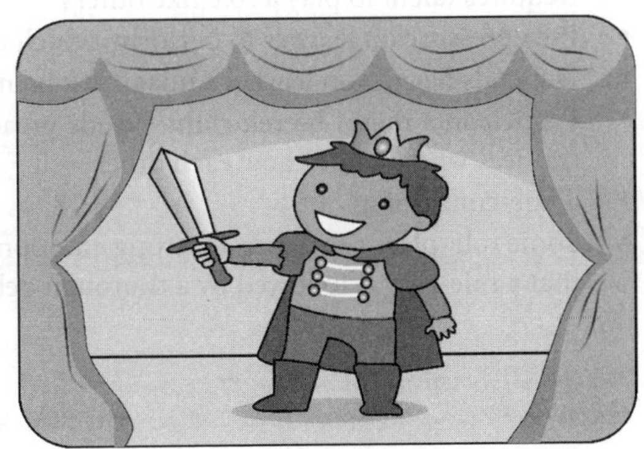

Good directors foster an environment of acceptance and experimentation during rehearsal. The context for the role-play is presented and roles are selected. Students have minimal planning time to discuss the situation, choose different alternatives or reactions and plan a basic scenario. The success lies in the construction and delivery with careful facilitation. This is deeply rooted in the principles of constructivist teaching. Role-playing differs from simulation, where learners are rehearsing behaviors or roles that they will need to master and apply in real life. Role-playing is best done in small groups so that all learners can actively take part as players or as observers. This provides students with opportunities to explore and practice new communication skills in a safe, nonthreatening environment, express feelings, and take on the role of another person by 'walking in another's shoes.'

Steps for Effective Role-playing

1. Be specific and know your goals.
2. Step into your client's shoes.
3. Forget what you know about your profession/service, be in your role.
4. Create a safe environment.

Advantages

- Actively involves participants
- Adds variety, reality, and specificity to the learning experience
- Develops problem-solving and verbal expression skills
- Provides practice to build skills before real-world application and when 'real' experiences are not readily available
- Enables learners to experiment in a safe environment with behaviors which strike them as potentially useful and to identify behaviors which are not
- Can provide an entirely new perspective on a situation and develop insights about feelings and relationships
- Provides the teacher immediate feedback about the learner's understanding and ability to apply concepts
- Improves the likelihood of transfer of learning from the classroom to the real world.

Disadvantages

- Requires talent to play a role like others
- Puts pressure on learner to perform, which can create embarrassment and even resistance
- Depends heavily on learner's imagination and willingness to participate
- Participants might be reluctant. Needs greater coordination among them; may not work with trainees who do not know each other well.
- Time-consuming
- Some role-plays can generate strong emotions amongst the participants. It is, therefore, essential that a role-play is followed by a thorough debriefing.

PANEL DISCUSSION

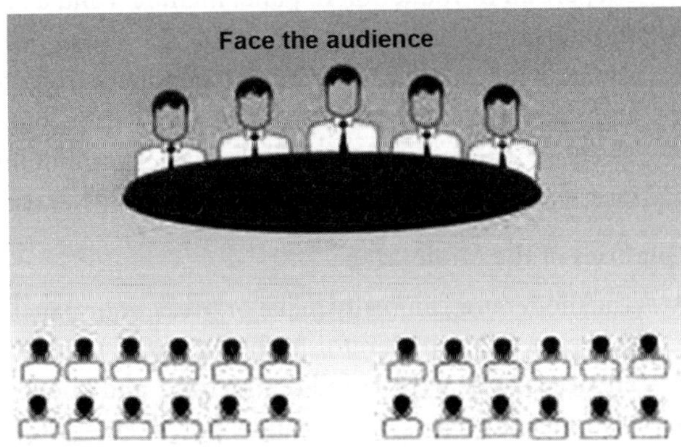

Discussion method could be conducted in any of the following modes:

- Small group discussion technique
- Socialized classroom discussion technique
- Panel discussion technique
- Direct instruction or classroom technique
- Recitation technique
- Interview technique.

Panel discussion is a form of discussion method. A panel is a group of four to six persons who have special knowledge about a topic and who present their viewpoints. The size of the panel is critical. The typical rule of thumb is between 5 and 6 panelists. Even if someone cancels at the last minute, you still have at least 4 panelists, to conduct the panel discussion. Several presenters can broaden the knowledge base and provide interest for mixed audiences. Panel discussions permit the presenters to focus on one specific issue of the problem; therefore, one person does not need to cover the entire problem.

Advantages

- Promotes learning by doing (Discussion provides for participation)
- Encourages good listening
- Stimulates thinking
- Makes use of peer groups and adds credibility to the topic
- Permits the presenters to focus on one specific major issue of the problem, and one individual does not need to cover the entire problem
- Allows experts to present different opinions
- Can provoke better discussion than a one-person presentation
- Frequent change of speakers holds participants' attention.

Disadvantages

- Experts may not be good
- Speakers may not hold participants attention
- Famous personalities may overshadow content
- Information may not be presented in a logical order.

Panelists in a panel discussion should:

- Define the problem and state it in question form
- Select a leader or moderator (The leader should be the quietest person on the panel)
- Be selected on the basis of their ability

- Prepare an introduction of panel members and a statement of the topic
- Arrange the room for good discussion
- Maintain a favorable environment conducive to good discussion at the conclusion of the panel
- Remind them of the other panelists who will be there and to limit their comments to 2–3 minutes
- Keep some time in their schedule to stick around for a few minutes after the panel discussion in case any audience members would like to speak with them on a one-on-one basis.

Qualities of the Moderator

- The moderator can really make or break your panel discussion. So select someone who has prior experience as a moderator in the panel discussion
- He needs to be well-versed on the topic and know something about each panelist
- A moderator needs to be a guide, not an entertainer
- The audience is not there to hear the moderator. The moderator needs to be able to move the conversation along
- The moderator must make sure that every panelist gets adequate time to speak
- A good moderator should always stay neutral
- The moderator is not there to be an expert or part of the panel. He is not there to show the audience how much knowledge he has. He is simply there to moderate
- A moderator should be firm and direct, yet personable.

Giving Structure to Panel Session

Session flow and sequence of the session should be decided in advance to allow panelists to prepare A brief presentation (not more than 5 minutes) from each panelist on the main question/topic, followed by questions from the chair and then from the audience. An introduction piece from the chair or someone not on the panel, should be ideally thought-provoking or inspiring followed by a response from each panelist and then followed by questions. It is a widely seen pattern launching the panel discussion, with the chair asking a few key questions around the topic, then opening it up to the audience for more questions.

Preparing the Session

Panelists are usually invited directly by session organizers. It is important to invite panelists with a wide range of views and approaches. In addition, inviting panelists with a range of backgrounds, e.g. academia, policy, practice, end-user will provide a strong starting platform for different viewpoints. Consider inviting panelists for whom the topic is not their specialism, but whose background might offer a new view.

Organizers should prepare a brief title and abstract for their session, as panelists need to understand the format and goals of the session in order to prepare their contribution. Before the conference, the session organizers might ask the panelists to provide a short summary of their thoughts on the session's topic or challenge, but even better would be a short conference call (e.g. via Skype) that allows panelists to meet each other, chat and understand the main goals of the panel sessions from the organizers.

Implementation

- Seat the panelists in such a way that they can see the audience and each other. Eye contact makes for good discussion
- Do not spend much time on introducing the topic or the panelists
- Make the session audible to everyone. Microphone can be used
- There need to be very good interactions among the panelists through thought-provoking questions to each other
- Moderator must be a well-experienced person who knows when and how to cut some people off, and when to encourage more from others.

CONFERENCE

The Latin roots of the word 'conference' mean, literally, 'bring together.' A conference brings together people and ideas. The structure and contents of conferences can vary greatly, but a typical framework would include one or more presentations of work and/or ideas about a given topic. Conference may be conducted using different teaching strategies, like lectures, slideshows or films, workshops, panel discussions, etc. Most conference-organizers encourage and invite posters and paper presentations as part of the conference. A conference may last a few hours or several days. It may be a one-time event, or a regular (usually annual) fixture on participants' schedules.

A conference refers to a formal meeting of people (with shared interest) to discuss some issue (and the issue may not be highly academic or about specialized academic subject; it is more of a general nature). It typically takes place over several days and a relatively larger group meets here (which may not be the case in seminars or symposia).

Types of Conferences

- **Academic conferences:** Most academic conferences are centered around a single subject, and sometimes on a single topic within that subject. A major focus of academic conferences, besides the exchange of ideas, is networking, which, in academia as elsewhere, is a key to collaboration, funding, employment, and other professional benefits.
- **Professional association conferences**: These are similar to academic conferences in some ways, but presentations tend to be focused more on practical issues, both having to do what the actual work participants do, and with regulations, funding, and other forces that affect the profession. For example, Trained Nurses Association of India conducting a conference.
- **Training conferences:** A training conference may be run by a professional association. Its purpose is training, and so it might include workshops on methods and techniques, information on new regulations, or simply an exchange of experience and methods among people from a number of different organizations.
- **Issue- or problem-related conferences:** These might be convened by almost any association, organization, institution, or citizens' group to focus on a particular concern.

Reasons for Organizing Conference

- Issue that needs to be examined
- The field needs a conference. There are several possible reasons for this:
  - The field may be a new one, and still lack a clear identity.
  - The field may not be cohesive to bring people together.

  - New concepts and research to be shared.
  - People may need to be energized, and to know they are not alone.
- Get together by organization
- Crisis that to be addressed
- When you want to establish the legitimacy of the field
- Feedback from the field
- It is a part of your job
- Steps in organizing the workshop
- Decide on the purpose of the conference
- There are many reasons for conducting a conference. Mostly organizers combine more than one reason: passing on information, new practice orientation, training, networking, decision-making.

Find Your Target Audience

Many conference organizers are interested in attracting more than just their 'normal' participants.

- **Fix the length and date for the conference:** How long the conference will be depends on what needs to get done; what most potential participants can afford, in time and money; and what the sponsoring organization can do and what the institution can afford. The conference date should be set in order to avoid conflict with other events that affect the intended audience, or with the realities of their work.
- **Set the overall theme and structure of the conference:** An often-used general format for a large conference, and one that many smaller conferences follow as well, begins with a keynote address – a speech or presentation, usually by a well-known or inspirational speaker, that is meant to introduce the theme of the conference, kindle attendees' enthusiasm, and/or make them think. Two to six short sessions continue after the key speaker. Each day's session includes lunch if it is charged already. Many conferences end with a wrap-up of final speaker, in order to send people home thinking about the issue, and feeling that they had a coherent experience.
- **Address conference logistics:** This is the part where the conference organizers earn their keep.
  - *Geographical location:* Consider what people can afford, how far they may be willing to travel, and where they are willing to go.
  - *Conference site:* A conference that keeps all participants together can do with one large or not-so-large, depending on the number of participants – hall or auditorium.
  - *Food:* An informal, one-day conference might be brown-bag (i.e. bring your own lunch) or provide a simple meal (pizza or sandwiches). Another possibility is a mid-morning and/or mid-afternoon beverage and snack break.
  - *Lodging*: If attendees, speakers, or presenters are coming from a distance, they may need a place to stay.
  - *Fees:* If the conference is local, and has few or no expenses, then it might be free to participants. Most large, multi-day conferences charge fees to cover costs, which include materials, mailings, space and equipment rental, catering, expenses and/or payments for keynote speakers and other presenters, copying and printing, etc.
  - *Signage:* You will need sign-boards pointing the way to various conference rooms, exhibitors, meals, rest rooms, and other points of interest in the conference site, as well as to official conference tables or booths – for registration, information, advocacy, etc.

- *Identification:* Conference staff, volunteers, technical assistants, and other 'officials' should have name badges that stand out (a different color, perhaps) and that identify them as people to approach with questions.
- *Safety and security:* A hotel or other conference site will usually employ on-site security and people with emergency medical training.

- **Publicity and recruitment**
  - Print advertising, particularly in journals, newsletters, and other print media read by your intended audience
  - Posters and/or other announcements sent to organizations and institutions
  - General communication to an e-mail list
  - Blogs
  - Word of mouth
  - Preconference registration.

This gives the organizers an estimate of how many people will attend. If the conference has a fee, participants are generally expected to send it in with their registration. Registration forms should be sent out early – several months before the conference.

- **Inviting the speakers :** Potential keynote speakers, will be contacted personally and request made to receive information about him or her.

Logistics just before and during the conference. This must be taken care.

- **Conference registration/check-in:** People who preregistered should have conference packets waiting ready for them. There should also be a clear procedure for walk-in registrations—what to do with conference fees, when to stop accepting walk-ins, etc.

Care of Speakers

Someone should be assigned to make sure that they have what they need, get to the right places at the right time.

Evaluation forms: Administered at the end of the session to all the participants.

SYMPOSIUM

Meeting or conference for the public discussion of some topic, especially one in which the participants form an audience and make presentations. Symposium originally refers to a drinking party (the Greek word 'sympotein' means 'to drink together') but has since come to refer to any academic conference, whether or not drinking takes place.

'Symposium is a technique in which two or more persons under the direction of a chairman present several speeches, which give several aspects of one question'.

'Symposium consists of a set of program of prepared speeches followed by audience discussion'.

Features of Symposium

- It provides the broad understandings of a topic or a problem
- The opportunity is provided to the listeners to take decision about the problem
- It is used for higher classes to specific theme and problem

- It develops the feeling of co-operation and adjustment. The objectives as synthesis and evaluation are achieved by employing the symposium
- It provides the different views on the topic of symposium.

Advantages

- It is suited to a large group or classes
- This method can be frequently used to present broad topics for discussion
- Organization is good because of the set speeches prepared beforehand
- Gives deeper insight into the topic
- Hands itself to the teaching of clinical subjects
- This method is useful in political meetings.

Disadvantages

- Inadequate opportunity for all the students to participate actively
- The speeches are limited to 15–20 minutes
- Limited audience participation.
- Question-and-answer session limited to 3 or 4 minutes
- Possibility of overlapping the subjects.

Procedure on the Day of Symposium

Record Attendance: Have participants sign in and give you their contact information for follow-up opportunities. Have several people assigned to greet participants as they arrive. We asked for names, e-mail addresses, majors, intended year of graduation and how they heard about the event. Guiding the Conversation.

Guiding the Conversation:

- ***Conversation Leader:*** This person helps the group stay on topic, guides discussion and keeps the event on schedule. Make sure to let participants know about any ground rules. Usually most institutes like the rules to those for a 'kitchen table conversation.' Everyone participates, no one dominates.
- ***The Discussion:*** It is important to start the symposium with an explanation for the event, along with what is expected of participants. Visual aids help spark conversation and keep people interested. Small-group moderators and the overall conversation leader should remember to summarize themes that develop.
- Find a way to give participants some kind of 'take-away' thoughts: conclusions from the discussion, ideas about how the key-points might come up in the future.
- Engage in follow-up activities.

SEMINAR

Seminar is, generally, a form of academic instruction, either at a university or offered by a commercial or professional organization. It has the function of bringing together small groups for recurring meetings, focusing each time on some particular subject, in which everyone present is requested to actively participate. A seminar is an advanced group technique which is usually used in higher education. It is an instructional technique. It involves generating a situation for a group to have a guided interaction among themselves on a theme. This seminar method is employed to realize the higher objectives of cognitive and affective domains. The seminar method applies such technique of human interaction intervention with the learning and teaching experience.

Types of Seminars

Seminars are conducted in various stages. Based on the size and organizational aspects, the seminars can be classified into four types, viz.:

1. Mini seminar
2. Major seminar
3. National seminar
4. International seminar.

Mini Seminar

Its coverage and scope are small and simple. A small population is enough to hold this seminar. A discussion held over the topic taught or to be taught with the students is known as Group discussion. Such group discussions held in an organized way within a classroom, are called mini seminars.

Major Seminar

The seminar conducted at an institutional or departmental level for a specific topic or subject is known as major seminar. Usually, students and teachers participate in this type of seminar. This major seminar can be organized at departmental level every month. A specific topic or subject is selected for the theme of the seminar.

National Seminar

An association of any kind particularly with academic or professional interest or an organization (government, firm, etc.) conducting the seminar at national level is called national seminar. The subject experts are invited to the seminar for discussion. The secretary of the seminar prepares the schedule and functionaries for the seminar.

International Seminar

Usually the seminar conducted by an international organization or agency is known as international seminar. The theme of this seminar has wider aspects. A nation or its body can conduct or organize the international seminar.

Seminar Committee

Seminar is conducted or organized by the committee proposed for this purpose only. This committee constitutes a chairperson, organizing secretary and subject experts, who are expertise in the theme proposed for seminar. The organizing committee guides and helps with the functions of chairperson and organizing secretary.

Usually, a seminar has been conducted with the following team of organizing body:

- ***Chairperson or President/Convener of Seminar:*** Naturally, she may be the apex person of the Institution/Department/Government/Firm/Policy maker of the concerned body or agency.

- ***Organizing Secretary of Seminar:*** Usually, he is nominated by the chairperson or president of the seminar committee. S/he must be a good administrator and subject expert in the field proposed theme of the seminar. He must be the person of tolerance and capable of doing things in right time with right persons.
- ***Chairperson of the Technical Session of Seminar:*** S/he must be the person with expertise in the theme proposed for the seminar. S/he would have a good experience to perform all the activities of technical session which is vital to the seminar
- ***Speaker of Seminar:*** S/he is the active participant of seminar presenting his/her paper among the other participants in the presence of Chairperson of technical session of seminar.
- ***Participants/Paper Presenters of Seminar:*** The people who are presenting papers and observing the paper presentation by participating in the seminar are termed as paper presenters and participants of the seminar.

Merits of Seminar Method

- Naturally, the spontaneous learning can be achieved effectively in this method
- Seminar is usually learner-centered
- Information seeking and retrieval behavior is encouraged very much in this method
- The learner himself prepares and compiles his own paper for the seminar, gives readiness of mind and learning becomes structured
- Learning by doing is encouraged in this method
- The paper presenter/participant receives a reinforced learning experience from the group discussion
- Learning experience is highly structured by the learner himself
- The teacher or chairperson of technical session only plays the guidance and instructional role
- Develops cognitive, affective domain-based learning
- Norms of behavior are developed and reinforced
- Develops open-mindedness, suppress the subjective ideas from the learners
- The interactions and interrogations develop the spirit of information seeking behaviors (norms of behavior)
- The data-processing skills, compilation skills, communication skills are easily inculcated in this method
- Learner gets in-depth knowledge of the subject he presented
- This method builds better social values and fault tolerance levels in the minds of learners.

Limitations of Seminar Method

- Setting up of a seminar for every topic in the text is not feasible
- The subject area to be taught must be relevant to the theme of the seminar
- The seminar themes must conform the learning experiences to be inculcated to the students
- This method is found fit for higher learning only
- Implementation of this method for lower classes is cumbersome
- Only matured and balance-minded teachers can make this method successful
- The teacher must be resourceful (both academically and administratively) in nature.

Be an Effective Presenter

- **Preparing an Effective Presentation:** An effective presentation is more than just standing up and giving information. A presenter must consider how best to communicate his/her information to the audience. Use these tips to create a presentation that is both informative and interesting.
- **Organize your thoughts:** Start with an outline and develop good transitions between sections. Emphasize the real-world significance of your research.
- **Have a strong opening**: Why should the audience listen to you? One good way to get their attention is to start with a question, whether or not you expect an answer. Define terms early. If you are using terms that may be new to the audience, introduce them early in your presentation. Once an audience gets lost in unfamiliar terminology, it is extremely difficult to get them back on track.
- **Finish with a bang:** Find one or two sentences that sum up the importance of your research. How is the world better off as a result of what you have done?
- **Design PowerPoint slides** to introduce important information. Consider doing a presentation without slides. Then consider which points you cannot make without them. Create only those slides that are necessary to improve your communication with the audience.
- **Time yourself:** Do not wait until the last minute to time your presentation. You only have 15 minutes to speak, so you want to know, as soon as possible, if you are close to that limit. Create effective notes for yourself. Have notes that you can read. Do not write out your entire talk; use an outline or other brief reminders of what you want to say. Make sure the text is large enough that you can read it from a distance.
- **Practice, practice, practice:** The more you practice your presentation, the more comfortable you will be in front of an audience. Practice in front of a friend or two and ask for their feedback. Record yourself and listen to it critically.
  Make it better and do it again.
- **PowerPoint Tips:** Microsoft PowerPoint is a tremendous tool for presentations. It is also a tool that is sometimes not used effectively. If you are using PowerPoint, use these tips to enhance your presentation.
- **Use a large font:** As a general rule, avoid text smaller than 24 points.
- **Use a clean typeface:** Sans serif typefaces, such as Arial, are generally easier to read on a screen than serifed typefaces, such as Times New Roman.
- **Use minimal text:** Use bullet points, not complete sentences. The text on your slide provides an outline to what you are saying. If the entire text of your presentation is on your slides, there is no reason for the audience to listen to you. A common standard is the 6/7 rule: no more than six bulleted items per slide and no more than seven words per item.
- **Use contrasting colors:** Use a dark text on a light background or a light text on a dark background. Avoid combinations of colors that look similar. Avoid red/green combinations, as this is the most common form of color-blindness.
- **Use special effects sparingly:** Using animations, cool transition effects, sounds and other special effects is an effective way to make sure the audience notices your slides. Unfortunately, that means that they are not listening to what you are saying. Use special effects only when they are necessary to make a point.

- **Presenting effectively:** When you start your presentation, the audience will be interested in what you say. Use these tips to help keep them interested throughout your presentation.
- **Be excited:** You are talking about something you find exciting. If you remember to be excited, your audience will feel it and automatically become more interested.
- **Speak with confidence:** When you are speaking, you are the authority on your topic, but do not pretend that you know everything. If you do not know the answer to a question, admit it. Consider deferring the question to your mentor or offer to look into the matter further.
- **Make eye contact with the audience:** Your purpose is to communicate with your audience, and people listen more if they feel you are talking directly to them. As you speak, let your eyes settle on one person for several seconds before moving on to somebody else. You do not have to make eye contact with everybody, but make sure you connect with all areas of the audience equally.
- **Avoid reading from the screen:** First, if you are reading from the screen, you are not making eye contact with your audience. Second, if you put it on your slide, it is because you wanted them to read it, not you.
- **Blank the screen when a slide is unnecessary**: A slide that is not related to what you are speaking about can distract the audience. Pressing the letter B or the period key displays a black screen, which lets the audience concentrate solely on your words. Press the same key to restore the display.
- **Use a pointer only when necessary**: If you are using a laser pointer, remember to keep it off unless you need to highlight something on the screen.
- **Explain your equations and graphs**: When you display equations, explain them fully. Point out all constants and dependent and independent variables. With graphs, tell how they support your point. Explain the x- and y-axes and show how the graph progresses from left to right.
- **Pause**: Pauses add audible structure to your presentation. They emphasize important information, make transitions obvious, and give the audience time to catch up between points and to read new slides. Pauses always feel much longer to speakers than to listeners. Practice counting silently to three (slowly) between points.
- **Avoid filler words:** Um, like, you know, and many others.

To an audience, these are indications that you do not know what to say; you sound uncomfortable, so they start to feel uncomfortable as well. Speak slowly enough that you can collect your thoughts before moving ahead. If you really do not know what to say, pause silently until you do.

- **Relax:** It is hard to relax when you are nervous, but your audience will be much more comfortable if you are too.
- **Breathe:** It is fine to be nervous. In fact, you should be—all good presenters are nervous every time they are in front of an audience. The most effective way to keep your nerves in check—beside a lot of practice beforehand—is to remember to breathe deeply throughout your presentation.
- **Acknowledge the people who supported your research:** Be sure to thank the people who made your research possible, including your mentor, research team, collaborators, and other sources of funding and support.

PROGRAMMED INSTRUCTION

Programmed instruction, one of the earliest teaching methods derived from behavior analysis, involves analyzing comprehensive concepts into small, sequential tasks that teach, test, and self-correct in units referred to as 'frames'. Programmed Instruction (PI) has evolved from the rudimentary teaching machines of the 1920s to present-day computer programs and Internet activities. First ideas on 'instruction automation' can be tracked to even earlier years, first notable steps in programmed instruction were taken by Sidney Pressey in the 1920s and further developed by BF Skinner in the mid-1950s. In Pressey's words, the teacher is:

'*... burdened by such routine of drill and information-fixing...*', but a mechanical device could be used to '*lift from her shoulders as much as possible of this burden and make her free for those inspirational and thought-stimulating activities which are, presumably, the real function of the teacher*'.

The components of Skinner's Programmed Instruction include:
- Behavioral objectives
- Small frames of instruction
- Self-pacing
- Active learner response to inserted question
- Immediate feedback.

Styles/Types of Programming

There are three types of programming:
1. Linear Programming.
2. Branching Programming.
3. Mathetics.

Linear Programming

The founder of this programming is BF Skinner. It is based on the theory of operant conditioning. It tells that 'A certain direction can be given to human behavior'. For this purpose, activities are needed to be divided in small parts and to make their analysis.

Linear programming is based on five fundamental principles:
- Principle of small step.
- Principle of active responding.
- Principle of immediate confirmation.
- Principle of self-pacing.
- Principle of student testing.

The assumption behind the linear programming is that student learns better if content is presented in small units. Student response if immediately confirmed, results in better learning. Student's errors create hindrance in learning. Student learns better in Laissez Faire environment.

Frame size in small steps; include only one element of topic at a time. Each step is complete in itself. It can be taught independently and can be measured independently. Frame structure is based on stimulus-response-reinforcement. There are four types of frames—introductory frames, Teaching frames, practice frames and testing frames. Responses in linear programming are structured responses and are controlled by programmer and not by learners. Immediate confirmation of correct responses provides reinforcement. Wrong responses are ignored.

It is used for secondary level students, is used for achieving lower objectives of learning, especially for recall and recognition, is useful for students of average and below average intelligence, and it can be used in distance education program.

Limitations of Linear Programming

- No freedom for student to response.
- Based on learning theories which were formulated by experience conducted on animals. A human being is more intelligent, than animals. He has got an intelligent brain.
- Every learner has to follow the same path; therefore, students may cheat one another.
- Wrong responses are avoided in the program. No remedy is provided for them.

Branching Programming

The founder of Branching programming is Norman A Crowder. It is based on configuration theory of learning. It is a problem-solving approach. It is a stimulus-centered approach of learning. It is based on three basic principles: 1. Principle of Exposition, 2. Principle of Diagnosis, 3. Principle of Remediation.

Assumptions behind this programming are:

- Student learns better if he is exposed to whole situation or content.
- Student errors help in diagnosis.
- Student learns better if remediation is provided side by side.
- Student learns better in democratic environment.

Frame size is large. There may be a para or page in the frame. Frame structure is Exposition-Diagnosis-Remediation types. There are two types of frames: Home page (for teaching and diagnosis) and Wrong pages (for remediation). Responses are not rigidly structured and are selected by the learner and not by the programmer. Confirmation of correct responses provides reinforcement.

The purpose of Branching programming is to draw out weak points of learner and provide remedy for recovering those weaknesses.

Branching programming is used for secondary as well as higher classes. Higher objectives can be achieved, such as multiple discrimination, etc. It is useful for students of above average and high intelligence. It can also be used in distance education programs.

Limitations of branching Programming

- It does not consider learning process, whether learning is taking place or not. Main emphasis is on diagnosing the weakness of learners and providing remedy to them.
- There is no sequencing of pages. Student finds it difficult to follow the steps. He does not find it exciting or motivating. Therefore, he does not want to go through these pages.
- More emphasis on remediation rather than teaching. Hence, it is only a tutorial approach.

Mathetics Programming

The founder of Mathetics is Thomas F Gilbert. 'Mathetics is defined as a systematic application of reinforcement theory to the analysis and construction of complex repertoires which represent the mastery in subject matter.' It is based on connectivist theory of learning. It is a reverse chaining approach. It is based on principle of chaining, discrimination and generalization. Mathetics programming is based on following assumptions.

- Chaining of responses helps in learning to reach up to mastery level.
- Reverse chaining of stimuli helps in learning, i.e. from whole to part, from complex to simple.
- Completion of task provides motivation to students.

Frame size is organized in small step but in a reverse chain, i.e. from complex content to its small, simple units to attain mastery level. Frame structure is based on demonstration-prompts-release. There are two types of frames: 1. Demonstration frames; 2. Prescription frames.

Responses are structured responses and responses determined by the programmer. Completion of task provides reinforcement. Wrong responses are ignored. Error helps in discrimination but not in learning. Its main purpose is to develop mastery of the content. Main focus is on Mathematics and grammar. It is used for higher classes for complex and difficult task. It can be used in distance education.

Limitations of mathetics programming

1. Main emphasis is on mastery of the content rather than changes in behavior of the learner.
2. Retrogressive chaining of stimuli if not effective for terminal behavior.
3. It is very difficult to develop retrogressive learning package.

QUESTIONING

A question is any sentence which has an interrogative form or function. In classroom settings, teacher questions are defined as instructional cues or stimuli that convey to students the content elements to be learned and directions for what they are to do and how they are to do it.

Purposes of Teachers' Classroom Questions

- To develop interest and motivate students to become actively involved in lessons
- To evaluate students' preparation and check on homework or seat-work completion
- To develop critical thinking skills and inquiring attitudes
- To review and summarize previous lessons
- To nurture insights by exposing new relationships
- To assess achievement of instructional goals and objectives
- To stimulate students to pursue knowledge on their own.

Guidelines for Questioning

- Ask questions which focus on the salient elements in the lesson; avoid questioning students about extraneous matters
- When teaching students factual material, keep up a brisk instructional pace, frequently posing lower cognitive questions
- With older and higher ability students, ask questions before (as well as after) material is read and studied
- Question younger and lower ability students only after material has been read and studied
- Ask a majority of lower cognitive questions when instructing younger and lower ability students. Structure these questions so that most of them will elicit correct responses
- Ask a majority of higher cognitive questions when instructing older and higher ability students
- In settings where higher cognitive questions are appropriate, teach students strategies for drawing inferences
- Keep wait-time to about three seconds when conducting recitations involving a majority of lower cognitive questions

- Increase wait-time beyond three seconds when asking higher cognitive questions
- Be particularly careful to allow generous amounts of wait-time to students perceived as having lower ability
- Use redirection and probing as part of classroom questioning and keep these focused on salient elements of students' responses
- Avoid vague or critical responses to student answers during recitations
- During recitations, use praise sparingly and make certain it is sincere, credible, and directly connected to the students' responses.

Audiovisual Aids

Chapter Highlights

- Learning Experience-Actual, Vicarious and Symbolic
- Importance of Instructional Aids
- Types of Instructional Aids
- Definitions of Audio-Visual Aids
- Chalkboard
- Whiteboards
- Display Board
- Flannel Board
- Flip Chart
- Charts
- Posters
- Cartoons
- Flash-Cards
- Graphs
- Maps
- Models
- Print Media
- Books
- Audiotapes
- Radio
- Projected Aids
- Slide Projector
- Film Strips
- Overhead Projector (OHP)
- Compact Disk (CD)
- Videotapes

Learning Objectives

Upon completion of this chapter, the students will be able to:

- Describe the actual, vicarious and symbolic
- Identify the importance of instructional aids in teaching
- Classify the instructional aids
- Define the terms audio, visual and audiovisual aids
- Explain the different instructional aids used in day-to-day practice of teaching

LEARNING EXPERIENCE

All the individuals do not act in the same way when they go through the process of learning. Psychologists and educationalists believe that the knowledge has few sources. They are:

- Transcendental experience
- Actual experience
- Vicarious experience
- Symbolic experience.

The first 'source' that just pops into your head. This 'source' of information or knowledge can be dismissed out of hand. Transcendental knowledge has no consistent relationship with truth. In fact it is typically thought to be true regardless of the facts. The acceptability of transcendental knowledge is best understood when it cuts against you rather than for you. Knowledge which is not provable it is foisted off as transcendental has no place in science. All knowledge comes from experience, either your personal experience, or from other people who communicate their experiences to you. Therefore any knowledge can always be examined for its truthfulness. The next three sources are considered here for discussion:

Knowledge Gained Through Actual Experience (Empirical Research)

The first credible source of information is what a person comes to know by direct personal experience. These empirical sources can be categorized into several general classes. These classes could be seen as lying on a rough continuum which varies from a relatively passive observation to the active manipulation of abstract variables in a completely controlled environment.

It occurs through direct firsthand experience which provides immediate sensory contact with reality. Hospitals provide firsthand experience to nursing students. There are may things which the nursing students wants to know which they cannot experience directly. Consequently vicarious experience becomes a necessity.

Knowledge Gained Through Vicarious Experience

The second source of knowledge is gained through some means other than your own direct experience. Each person cannot directly experience for themselves all possible events. Varied activities and situations which people come across provide them the additional experience. It acts like direct experience in its relevant aspects. It makes it possible to predict what would happen (i.e., respond correctly) in a new situation which has never been personally or directly experienced. Audiovisual materials maybe considered as second level of experiencing and learning. Audiovisual materials include chalkboard, flannel, and magnetic boards, models, specimens, radio, etc.

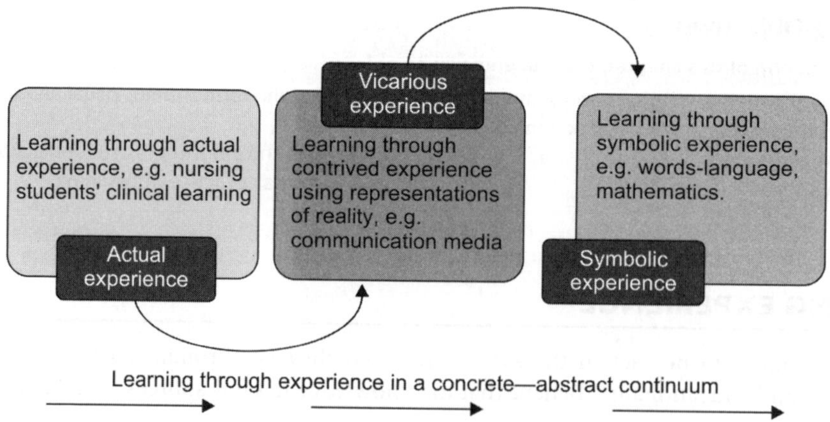

Knowledge Gained Through Symbolic Experience

This is most abstract experience that comes through the use of words, written oral and other symbols. We rely on language, logic, and mathematics to provide us with information indirectly. A synonym would be symbolic experience. This maybe called as symbolized experiencing and learning.

Instructional aids help you reach your objectives by providing emphasis in a different way than speaking. Psychologists have long recognized the importance of concrete illustration in teaching. Devices whether visual or audiovisual materials, are valuable in the learning-teaching process because they stimulate interest and make possible the enrichment of the pupil's experience. Clear pictures, graphs, or models multiply your students level of understanding of the material presented, and they can be used to reinforce your message, clarify points, and create interest. They enable you to appeal to more than one sense at the same time, thereby increasing your student's understanding and retention level. With drawings, posters, transparencies and other visuals, the concepts or ideas you present are no longer simply words—but words plus images. A device is an incentive introduced into the method of teaching for the purpose of stimulating the pupil and developing understanding through experiencing. The basis for all learning is experience, and usually the most effective type of learning is gained by concrete, direct, first-hand experience.

The word instructional aid refers to any material or device used to assist the instructor in:

- Preparation of the lesson(s)
- Presentation (teaching) of the lesson(s)
- Facilitation of learning.

IMPORTANCE OF INSTRUCTIONAL AIDS

Instructional aids assist to reinforce and supplement the instructor's communication during the presentation of the lesson. This is done by:

- Clarifying the concept or idea
- Making the communication channel more explicit
- Helping the learners to develop a good conceptual understanding of the content or skill taught.

For example an idea which would be difficult (abstract) can easily be simplified when an instructional aid is used to present it. Therefore learners are able to relate an idea to their common reality or environment with the use of aids.

Types of Instructional Aids

There are many types of instructional aids. Each instructional aid, however, may have inherent advantages and disadvantages (or limitations). Instructional aids can be grouped in four main categories:

- **Visual aids: Visual** implies relating to the sense of seeing. They include the blackboard, posters, charts, displays, models, pictures, etc.
- **Auditory aids: Audio** refers to sound waves that can normally be heard by the human ear. This type of instructional aids appeal to learners' sense of hearing. They include radio and many types of audio recording.

  Aids implies those instructional devices or teaching aids which make teaching more effective.
- **Audiovisual Aids: Audiovisual aids** are those instructional devices that maybe used by a teacher or a communicator in order to facilitate better understanding on the part of learners by involving their many senses, particularly those relating to seeing and hearing. They include sound motion pictures, slides on sound and television.

Value of instructional aid:

- Their appeal to learners' senses and perceptions
- Their ability to attract and hold learners' attention and interest
- The ability in developing understanding of the material to be learned
- Helps the trainees to learn faster and save instructional time
- Helps trainees to understand the relationships between different concepts or ideas
- They guide learners/students to learn well and reduce the stress involved in the process of teaching and learning
- Ability to improves students' comprehension.

Definitions of Audiovisual Aids

- Audiovisual aids are those aids, which help in completing the triangular process of learning, i.e. Motivation, classification and stimulation. —*Carter V. Goo*
- Audiovisual aids are any device, which can be used to make the learning experience more concentrate, more realistic and more dynamic. —*Kinder S. James*
- Audiovisual aids are anything by means of which learning process maybe encouraged or carried on through the sense of hearing or sense of sight. —*Good's dictionary of education.*

VISUAL AIDS

Nonprojected aids are those which require no projection material or any electric power. There is much sense in the Chinese saying that 'a thousand hearing are not as effective as one seeing'. Wordsworth has also realized this fact and he put it in his own poetic way, saying: 'Things seen are mightier than things heard'.

Advantages

- Strengthen the clarity of the speaker's message
- Increase the interest of the speaker's information
- Make a speaker's message easier for listeners to retain
- Enhance the speaker's credibility
- Can improve the speaker's persuasion
- Helps combat stage fright.

Nonprojected aids are those which require no projection material or any electric power.

CHALKBOARD

The term 'blackboard' dates from around 1815 to 1825 while the newer and predominantly American term, 'chalkboard' dates from 1935 to 1940 is a reusable writing surface on which text or drawings are made with sticks of calcium sulfate or calcium carbonate, known, when used for this purpose, as chalk. Chalkboards were originally made of smooth, thin sheets of black or dark gray slate stone. Modern versions are often green or brown and are thus sometimes called a green board or brown board instead.

Uses of Chalkboard

Chalkboards are often used in teaching, although in wealthier countries their use has diminished. Chalkboards are also used in many establishments (typically public houses) as a form of advertising often for upcoming events and menus and to record the score in dart matches. Also in homes, specifically in the kitchen, for writing messages, shopping lists and things to remember, as well as sometimes serving a decorative purpose.

Tips for Effective use of Chalkboard

- Plan the layout of the chalkboard. Before you begin your lesson session, draw exactly what you are going to write-draw on the chalkboard in your notebook.
- Draw two vertical lines from the top of the board to the bottom. The board is now divided into three separate areas
- Draw a large H on the chalkboard. You have divided the chalkboard into four separate areas
- Organize your stuff while writing on the board
- Do not speak to the board; speak to your students.

The Advantages of Using Chalkboards in Teaching

- Most areas assigned for instruction are equipped with chalkboards. Also, if more board space is needed, portable boards of various types and styles are handy
- The chalkboard is inexpensive, especially when the usable life of the board is considered. (Zeitlyn, 1992)
- It is flexible in use in the sense that instructors may use it, learners may use it and changes can be easily made through erasure
- Space: Lots of writing space is usually provided
- The chalkboard can be used to present more formally prepared lessons, or for informal, spontaneous sessions
- Ideas can be dealt with at all levels from facts to concepts, from cognitive to affective learning
- Various coloured chalk or pens can be used to develop the topic, show parts or build associations
- A point-by-point outline of a presentation can be made on the spot with diagrams, charts, and other accentuation drawn at the appropriate moment
- The visual communication of the chalkboard directs attention of the class to the purposes of the lecture or discussion
- Ideas or topics suggested in discussion can be listed on the board, reorganized, deleted, added to, and put in final form
- Test or discussion questions can be put on the board and covered up before the class assembles, then revealed at the appropriate time. This can save on time and cost of duplication materials
- A number of learners can do practice or drill work on the board at one time, allowing the instructor to give feedback immediately.

Disadvantages or Limitations

According to Jones et al. (1994) the following are the disadvantages of using a chalkboard:

- The chalkboard carries with it a 'temporariness.' Material put on the board cannot be saved or made permanent

- Chalkboards are often fixed in such a way that they are not always at a comfortable height for all potential users
- Being fixed, chalkboards can put restrictions on the use of classroom space and classroom activities as learners need to be placed where they can see the boards
- Problems can arise for learners who have vision impairments
- With age, use of certain types of chalk, and/or improper cleaning practices, boards can become 'cloudy' as they retain chalk dust
- Some instructors are psyched-out of using the board because they feel a lack of artistic ability.
- Motion cannot be easily shown
- A teacher's handwriting or spelling deficiencies are most obvious when using the chalkboard.
- Chalkboard work can be messy
- Writing on the board can be 'down time' and may break the class's train of thought and/or discussion.

WHITEBOARDS

For almost 20 years, many schools have chosen to replace the familiar chalkboard with high-tech and advanced whiteboards. These particular whiteboards, whose surfaces are smooth polypropylene, use dry-erase markers and, sometimes, colored pencils. Teachers and students like the option of using whiteboards because they do not require chalk and there is no dust.

Advantages

- Whiteboards offer a clean, modern and business like look
- More appealing than darker chalkboards
- White surface is very attention getting
- Also offers preprinted lines and lettering to help in certain classes, such as music and geometry
- Whiteboards can also perform double-duty as effective projection screens in a room
- With its colorful dry-erase markers, the whiteboard can engage an entire class to become actively involved in a lesson.

Disadvantages

- It will, age soon
- They are so slick that students end up writing faster than their brains can think, making handwriting not as clear
- Whiteboards far outnumber chalkboards in classrooms today, but they face competition from the next step in the evolutionary chain, the interactive whiteboard.

DISPLAY BOARD

A display board is any kind of board on which visual and written materials can be pinned or glued. It can be used to display students' work, give information about a new development activity or perhaps display instructions for operating machinery (for example, a photocopier).

It is especially appropriate for use in teaching or training situations where there are no solid walls to display material, in mud houses classrooms for example. It can be free-standing, mounted on a or hung from a ceiling or tree. It can be made of wood, line, cork cardboard, woven mats or other materials.

FLANNEL BOARD

It is a board that is usually covered in either felt or flannel and propped up on a easel. It is usually used in preschool classes as a storytelling device. This teaching tool is called by different names like Visual Board, Frick Board, Slap Board, Felt Board, Choreograph, Videograph. The tool consists of only two Parts—a board covered with flannel and objects having fluzzy and napped backing. The principle involved is the interlooking of fibers of two rough or bairy surfaces, so that the pieces pressed on to a background which is hard and vertical will stay. It can be illustrated on a larger scale by proooing two tooth bruohoo or hair bruohoo togcthcr, oo thc briotlc intcr 1ook. In caoc of flannol graph similar principle of friction helps an object to cling to the surface of the board.

Uses of Flannel Board

Teachers often use flannel boards to enhance storytelling.

- They may use pictures of the characters and other important parts of the story to illustrate it as they read
- Flannel boards are also used for 'acting out' songs and poems
- They can be used to demonstrate science and math concepts to young children, like the life cycle of a frog or butterfly or addition
- They are also commonly used in Sunday school to tell Bible stories
- Flannel boards can also be used in students' centers so that the students can manipulate the pieces, providing hands-on learning
- Useful to health educate the community.

Benefits

There are many benefits to using flannel boards in the classroom. They make learning more visual for young students, and the students remember what they have learned better. Flannel boards are more cost-effective than some other classroom aids. They can be used over and over again for a wide variety of activities, and you can easily switch the pieces from activity to activity. It is also easy to make your own flannel board and story pieces.

Principles of teaching while using flannel board

- Outline what you want to say
- Plan the lay-out keeping in view the principles of teaching
- Arrange the materials in such a way that they lend themselves best to illustrate what you want to say
- Try the lay-out to see that it fits the space on the flannel board
- Place the flannel board at eye level and at a slightly inclined angle. Lighting should also be checked
- Use a minimum number of objects to let the students focus their eyes on a few items at a time
- Talk to the class as much as possible but not to the board
- Remove the cut-outs from the board as soon as you have finished talking about them and place the next cut-outs in position. It is better to have the interest focused on one or two cut-outs than to have the attention wandering back to the illustrations already discussed. In case of story telling or developing a chart, however, the characters might be left on the board.

Advantages

- Permits numerous and varied arrangements of visua1 materials
- It is appealing, because the audience is fascinated in watching the steps in the presentation
- Permits the development of a complete story
- Permits the use of either chart or small pieces of material
- Promotes conscientious planning, which must precede the development of the material in the first place
- Challenges one to develop symbols to portray such things as abstractions
- Materials can be packed and transported
- Permits use of various colors, which may be used for specific purposes
- Materials can be left on board after meeting closes for those who wish more complete notes
- It is effective because it permits two techniques for delivering a message, word of mouth-sound and symbols or pictures-sight
- Easier to construct materials for flannel board than to make slides or movies
- Speaker works in front of his audience in well-lighted surroundings
- Chronological development of ideas on board promotes ease in note taking
- After symbols are developed they can quite easily be used in constructing attractive designs.

Disadvantages

- Transportation and storing of boards and materials is a problem
- Suitable tables to support boards must be available
- Time and cost of making material for presentation present a problem
- Cost of boards themselves can not be overlooked
- Presentation is limited a new idea involves a lapse of time before the new material can be added
- Might tend to deter one from using other more effective methods and techniques when it is evident that other methods might be more appropriate
- To tell a complete story it often takes either too much board space Or smaller designs and materials some of which cannot be seen well
- Requires considerable ingenuity and imagination to construct effective varied materials
- Materials must be attractively prepared.

FLIP CHART

Flip chart is a stationery item resembling a whiteboard, typically supported on a tripod or four-legged easel. A pad of paper sheets is typically fixed to the upper edge. Such charts are commonly used for presentations. The flip chart is thought to have been invented by Peter Kent who built one to help him in a presentation.

Types of Flip Charts

- Stand-alone flip chart: Resembles a big isosceles triangle box that usually sits on a table. Imagine a book that you would open at 270° angle and then lay on a table. The paper is flipped from one side of the top of the triangle box to the other.

- Metallic tripod (or easel) stand: Usually has 3 or 4 metallic legs that are linked together at one extremity. A support board is attached to two of these legs to support the large paper pad. This is the most common type of flip chart stand.
- Metallic mount on wheels: usually has a flat base to support the paper pad and is mounted on one or two legs that then have a set of wheels. The advantage of these more recent forms of stands is that it is easier to transport the flip chart from one location to another.

Flip Charts are Used in

- Presentations where the papers pads are prefilled with information on a given topic
- For capturing information in meetings and brainstorming sessions
- In classrooms and teaching institutions of any kind
- As a creative drawing board for art students
- A palette for artists in 'life-drawing' classes
- For strategy coaching for sports teams.

Advantages of Using a Flip Chart

- Do not need electricity
- Flip charts are economical
- Color can be added very easily
- An inexpensive box of flip chart markers allows you all the creativity you want
- Flip charts allow spontaneity
- Any last minute changes can be easily made.

Ten Tips for the Effective Use of a Flip Chart

1. Arrive early and be sure that the flip chart is positioned so that you can get to it easily when you need it.
2. Ensure that the flip chart is positioned so that you can stand next to it and write while still facing your audience. Do not turn your back on your audience.
3. Make sure you have to hand several markers pens that work. Throw away any pens that do not work.
4. Only use blue or black marker pens: It will be difficult for those at the back of the room to see any other colors. You can however use the color red to accentuate things already written in blue or black.
5. When writing on the flip chart, make your letters at least 2–3 inches tall so that everybody can clearly see what you have written.
6. Draw lines in pencil on blank pages before your presentation—to help you keep your writing legible and straight.
7. Plan out your pages as you are writing the outline for your presentation. They will be the support for your public speaking presentation.
8. Write notes to yourself, in pencil, on the flip chart to help remind yourself of all the important points to be included. Your audience will not see the pencil notes.
9. If you have something that you want to present and then accentuate during the presentation or discussion, write out the flip chart page beforehand so that you can just flip the page to it.

10. If you need to refer to something that you wrote on a page at a later point in your presentation, rip off the page and affix it to the wall.

CHARTS

A chart is a combination of pictorial, graphic, numerical or vertical material which presents a clear visual summary. Edgar Dale defines charts as, 'a visual symbol summarizing or comparing or contrasting or performing other helpful services in explaining subject-matter'. The main function of the chart is always to show relationships such as comparisons, relative amounts, developments, processes, classification and organization.

Characteristics of Charts

- Charts can be carefully stored and preserved for use in the future
- They have an educational value
- Usually the charts are teacher made
- Charts can be of any size
- Charts display specific information
- Easy to carry.

Types of charts

- Picture charts
- Time charts
- Table charts
- Graphic charts
- Flow or organization charts
- Tree charts
- Pie charts.

Uses of Charts

- Motivates the students
- Shows continuity in the process
- Shows relationships by means of facts, figures and statistics
- Presents matter symbolically
- Presents abstract ideas in visual form
- Summarizes information
- Shows the development of structures
- Creates problems and stimulates thinking
- Encourages utilization of other media of communication.

Limitations of Charts

- If the selection of material for preparing the charts is not good they will not last long
- Takes up the time of the teacher if she has to prepare the chart
- Charts only emphasize the key points. This leaves the students in doubt, if the clarification is not clear

- Charts lose their charm, if it contains too much matter on it
- Poor use of color combination, improper spacing and margins creates confusion in the minds of the students.

POSTERS

According to SL Ahluwalia 'A poster is a pictorial device designed to attract attention and communicate a story, a fact, an idea, or an image rapidly and clearly.'

Good's Dictionary of Education says, 'A poster is a placard, usually pictorial or decorative, utilizing an emotional appeal to convey a message aimed at reinforcing an attitude or urging a course of action'. The poster can be defined as a graphic representation of some strong emotional appeal that is carried through a combination of graphic aids, like pictures, cartoons, lettering and other visual arts on a placard. It aims at conveying the specific message, teaching a particular thing, giving a general idea, etc. Posters exert a great influence on the observer.

Characteristics of a Good Poster

- *Brevity:* Use of minimum words, i.e. four or five
- *Idea:* Idea or a feeling should be put in original form
- *Simplicity of layout:* It refers to the arrangement of the elements of the poster
- *Efficient use of colors:* (i) Use bold illustrations, (ii) Avoid fancy lettering style, (iii) Proper use of color.

Uses of Posters

- Present a single idea or a subject forcefully
- Publicize important school and community events and projects
- Add atmosphere to the classroom
- Capture attention by some attractive features and thus convey the message attractively and quickly
- Motivate the class
- Strong lasting impression
- Satisfy the viewer emotionally and aesthetically.

Limitations of Posters

- Convey a single theme
- The lettering if not attractive and accurate, makes the poster illegible
- Smudge marks make the posters unattractive and futile.

Suggestions for preparing posters

- Decide the theme
- Decide the most suitable words to provide a title or a slogan
- Sketch some layouts and decide on the best
- Gather all the needed material to prepare the poster
- Prepare the lettering.

- Add desired objectives
- Give the finishing touches and erase the smudge marks.

CARTOONS

Using humor in class is a 'valuable teaching tool for establishing a classroom climate conducive to learning' (Kher, 1999). One way of introducing humor into our classes is by using cartoons.

There are a number of benefits to using cartoons in teaching because they can motivate students and arouse interest in a particular idea or topic, grab and maintain attention.

- Motivate students to engage with the lesson's teaching point
- Arouse interest in a particular idea or topic
- Grab and maintain attention
- Strengthen analytical and critical thinking skills
- Give an insight into the world around us and help students think 'outside the box'
- Encourage students to use their imagination
- Help interpret meaning that is otherwise difficult to explain
- Make students laugh and smile which can relieve their stress and anxiety
- Help teachers build a closer rapport with their students by being able to laugh together
- Help students retain information through a visual and memorable stimulus.

FLASHCARDS

Flashcards are used for the presentation of an idea in the form of posters, pictures, words and sentences. A single card or a whole series may be flashed in front of the class. They aim to develop the power of observation, identification, quick comprehension and retention.

Characteristics of Flashcards

- Small compact cards
- Made out of cardboard or any other thick material
- Simplest of all aids.

Uses of Flashcards

- The pictorial contents presented in a series are easily recognized by the group
- These are flashed before the class one by one to bring home an idea
- Communication of new ideas requires repetitive study methods, drill-work and review of the discussion
- Provides pupils with a systematic approach to drill
- Helpful to teach recognition by sight
- Easy to carry.

Limitations of Flashcards

- If used for a prolonged period, it becomes boring for the students
- The students cannot get the complete view of the concept, as the points are flashed one by one.

GRAPHS

Graph is defined as a visual representation of numerical data. Graph is fundamentally a tool for expressing number relationships, which is much easier to visualize than can be done if the statement were made only in words and figures. It offers a judicious technique for analyzing, comparing and prophesying of facts which are vital to an intelligent study of a problem.

Characteristics of Graphs

- Graphs are by nature a summarizing device
- Effective tool for comparisons and contrast or for presenting complicated facts
- Made according to exact specifications and depict specifically quantitative data for analysis, interpretation or comparison
- Graphs, being symbolic, are abstract in character
- Self-explanatory and simple
- Regarded as flat pictures which employ dots, lines or pictures to visualize numerical and statistical data to show statistics or relationships.

Types of Graphs

- Line graph
- Bar graph
- Circle or pie graph
- Pictorial graph
- Flannel graph.

Steps in Presenting Graphs, Maps, Diagrams

They are repotent spark plugs because they can be ignited at the crucial moments.

To ensure success

- Prepare students
- Present the aid
- Apply information
- Test students after the aid has been presented
- Review or reshow the illustration if the previous step reveals misunderstanding.

Uses of Graphs

- *Awareness:* The teacher should be well aware of the method of drawing of graph in a neat and accurate manner
- *Neatness:* The graph should be neat, clean and artistic. It should be of good quality
- *Accuracy:* The scales and the measurement of the graph should be accurate and intelligible to the students
- *Drawing and paper:* The graph should be properly drawn. The graph paper should be good. The pencil that is used should also be good
- *Hints:* The hints should be properly explained. The marks on the graph should be such that the students may know them by themselves
- *Blackboard:* The teacher may draw a graph on the blackboard.

Limitations of Graphs

- If the graph is not drawn neatly, it loses it purpose
- The teacher should be adept at drawing the graphs and presenting it properly to the students
- Graphs cannot be preserved for a long time if the quality of the paper is not good
- Graphs will not be self-explanatory, if proper hints and scale are not given.

MAPS

Maps easily orient us to the location and boundaries of any place in the world. These constitute an indispensable aid in teaching many subjects, like geography, history, economics and social studies. The learning of these subjects becomes unreal, inadequate and incomplete without map media. A resourceful teacher will turn the fear of map into the genuine love by motivating the students. Maps are the part and parcel of community health nursing services.

Meaning

Maps are called 'Encyclopedia of Man's Existence'. The map as a record of spatial concepts tells a story as nothing else can. A map is an accurate representation plane surface in the form of a diagram drawn to scale, the details of boundaries of whole of earth's surface, continents, countries, etc. Geographical details like location of mountains, rivers, altitude of a place, contours of the earth's surface and important locations can also be represented, taught and learnt accurately. Maps depict the climatic conditions, natural conditions, location, etc. of certain countries and continents.

Purpose or Uses of Maps

- To depict geographical features of earth's surface and to understand the position of earth in the universe
- To show relationship between places
- To furnish information concerning distances, directions, shapes and sizes
- To clarify descriptive materials
- To reduce the scale of areas and distances and thus bring the abstract concepts of size, distance and directions into the region of reality
- To understand the lines, such as boundary lines, lines of communication, lines indicating the rivers, contours, meridians and parallels
- To understand the colors, tints, shadows, symbols in a map or globe
- To understand the distinction between various types of maps, such as relief, political, distribution maps
- To make epidemiological investigations on any disease-specific epidemic, pandemic, etc.

  Richard E Servey states that maps can be used in a wide variety of ways to express many different statements:

  - With color as a basic symbol
  - Through the use of conventional or invented symbols
  - Re-arranged maps
  - Three-dimensional maps
  - Globe.

Limitations of Maps

- Maps should be accurate, well-planned, well-printed, wall-mounted and durable
- Many of the maps are not visible to all the students in the class
- The teacher often does not take effort to teach map reading to the students
- Each type of map should have the relevant details
- If the lettering is not taken care of, it will prove futile.

Models

Models are three-dimensional instructional tools that allow the learner to immediately apply knowledge and psychomotor skills by observing, examining, manipulating, handling, assembling, and disassembling objects while the teacher provides feedback (Rankin & Stallings, 2001). Whenever possible, the use of real objects and actual equipment is preferred, but a model is the next best thing when the real object is not available, accessible, or feasible, or is too complex to use.

The three specific types of models used for teaching and learning are replicas, analogues, and symbols. To differentiate the three types of models, Babcock and Miller (1994) suggest associating a replica with the word *resemble*, an analogue with the terms *act like*, and a symbol with the words *stands for*.

A ***replica*** is a facsimile constructed to scale that resembles the features or substance of the original object, e.g. 1. Resuscitation dolls are a common type of replica used to teach the skills of cardiopulmonary resuscitation. 2. Human skulls in teaching anatomy.

An ***analogue*** performs like the real object because it has the same properties as the dynamic system under consideration. Mechanical devices such as, extracorporeal and dialysis machines are good examples of analogues. Popular analogue is the use of a computer model to see how the human brain functions (Babcock & Miller, 1994).

Advantages

- Useful when the real object is too small, too large, too expensive, too complex, unavailable, or a potential source of difficulty for learners
- Help learners to practice acquiring new skills
- Learners become more actively involved
- Application of knowledge and skills is immediate
- These tools are especially attractive and useful for the kinesthetic learner who prefers the hands-on approach to learning
- A vast array of models can be purchased from commercial vendors at varying prices (some for free) or improvised by the teacher
- Models do not need to be expensive or elaborate to get concepts and ideas across (Rankin and Stallings, 2001).

Disadvantages

- Some models may not be suitable for the learner with poor abstraction abilities
- Some models are fragile
- Some are very expensive
- Many are bulky to store and difficult to transport
- Unless models are very large, they cannot be observed and manipulated by more than a few learners at any one time.

Print Media

Printed materials are one of the oldest and most widely used forms of educational resources. They include books, pamphlets, magazines and newspapers. Printed material can be distinguished from other forms of media by the fact that they are composed of leaves or sheets on which information is displayed in rows of characters or symbols. Printed materials are frequently combined with other forms of media to form multimedia packages, which may be either locally or commercially produced.

Advantages

- As a medium of communication
- As a medium of instruction
- Permits a reader to skim their contents and to react spontaneously to them by making marginal comments or underlining
- Can be produced in multiple copies, and can thus be used for independent study
- A reader can stop, put the material away, and return later to the pint of termination. Because they allow a reader to return again and again to the same point, print materials facilitate the study of difficult, complicated concepts
- They are easily portable, and do not require expensive or complicated procedure to carry
- They can be quickly and easily revised and updated
- They are familiar format to teachers and students alike.

Limitations

- They cannot present motion materials effectively. As a result, their ability to engage all our senses for a total learning experience is quite limited
- They are difficult to revise and update if produced in a hardbound format.

Types of Printed Material

Books

- Picture book
- Textbooks
- Workbooks
- Paperback books
- Reference books, newspaper and magazines.

Books

A book is a written or printed work, produced and used as an independent unit, and generally more than 50 pages in length. It may be composed solely of printed material, or it may contain a mixture of visual and textual elements. If the visual material functions merely to decorate or enhance the text, the book is called an illustrated book. If the illustrations carry the essence of the book's meaning, however, it is termed as a picture book.

Reference books are the forms of book designed to be consulted for a specific piece of information rather than to be read through form cover to cover. They contain large number of facts organized for use, and may be arranged alphabetically, chronologically or topically. There are two types of reference books: those which contain the needed information and those which tell the user as to where information can be found.

Teachers are obligated to see whether the students receive instruction in the effective use of reference books. Effective utilization of reference books also entails study of the characteristics of a reference book, as its purpose and objectives, how it is arranged, the nature of its entries, the types of study aids it provides, the cross-reference and index structure, the type of bibliographies provided, and any special features it may possess. Nursing students should be taught how to use the databases for any kind of assignment or research work.

Audiotapes

It is a plastic tape covered in ferrous oxide or chromium oxide, it is pulled at a constant speed past two electromagnetic heads. This tape is capable of being magnetized. Then when it passes over the 'record head' the magnetic impulses from the sound sources are recorded on it, following which it is played back through the loudspeaker by converting the magnetic impulses into sound. The audiotape recorder can be a powerful tool to augment other teaching methods by providing the listener with the opportunity to review previously heard information, to receive taped feedback from instructors, or to hear information available from no other source (Haggard, 1989).

Advantages

- Learner can use them at his free time
- Repeated listening possible
- They can be used almost anywhere
- Instructor can record the instructions/health programs
- Low cost and easy storage
- Pictures, diagrams, and printed handouts can accompany to fit the needs of a variety of learners.
- Captures the interest of the patients.

Disadvantages

- Audiotapes address only one sense—hearing
- Learners may become easily distracted from the information being presented unless they have visuals to accompany with the tapes
- To be effective, with it has to be used with various other methods of instructions
- One-way communication.

RADIO

Radio is the oldest form of audio technology. In developing countries, however, radio has been used extensively as a vehicle for health, nutrition, and agricultural education. Because of its commercial nature and appeal to mass audiences, it has typically been used more for pleasure than for education.

Advantages

- It helps the students to keep up with the current information about the world
- Easily reaches all people
- Its widespread use makes it versatile
- Portable
- Major source of information to public.

Disadvantages

- Announcers or radio-jockeys are essential to grab the attention of public.
- Radio does not allow the opportunity for repetition of information.
- One-way communication.
- Scheduled programs, those stick on to time.
- Only few schools have their own system of broadcasting to educate students.

PROJECTED AIDS

Projected aids are those aids where a bright light is passed through a transparent picture, and by means of a lens, an enlarged picture is thrown or projected on the screen. Projected aids mainly fall into three groups, viz. opaque projections, transparent still projections and cine projections.

SLIDE PROJECTOR

Among the various types of materials available for still projection, slides and film strips are the foremost visual aids. Slide projector popularly known as magic lantern, is an optical aid to the process of teaching. It is used for projecting pictures from a transparent slide on a wall or screen. It helps in showing the magnified image of the slide. When the figure or illustration is very small and it is required that the whole class should see it clearly, a transparent slide of this small figure is prepared. The slide is placed inverted into the slide carrier part of the magic lantern (slide projector). The slide projector projects its erect image on the wall or screen by enlarging its dimension and making the vision more sharp and clear. If he slide or film strip is colored, then it would be more attractive. The slide projector is useful for small as well as large groups.

Advantages

- *Educational information:* The slide projector has immense educational value because a variety of information may be given using maps, drawings, diagrams, photographs, etc. The subject can be taught with detail and clarity. To make it more effective, a tape-recorder can also be used along with the slide projector. The teacher records the narration in a tape-recorder and the latter is hooked up with the slide projector in such a way as to give the necessary commentary about the slide without the help of the teacher.
- *Motivational force:* It arouses attention and interest of the students. A projected image has great power to hold attention of the audience for a long time. They can easily motivate the students for better learning.
- *Easy to transport:* Slide projector is light and easy to transport.
- *Easy to use:* It is very easy to use. It is a simple device of showing the magnified objects on the screen. It can be operated and focused by a remote control.
- *Picture on the screen:* The picture on the screen can be allowed to remain there as long as the students wish.
- *Interesting:* The whole activity is interesting.
- *Economical in time:* There is no wastage of time and energy.
- *Not costly:* Slide projector is not costly. Any school can afford to have it.

- *Nonfragile:* It is not easily broken.
- *Noninflammable:* It is noninflammable.

Limitations

- All types of material cannot be projected by the slide projector. The glass slides are becoming costlier now
- It may not be put to excessive use
- Slides have proved very useful for teaching various subjects. It helps the teacher to demonstrate different types of figures, diagrams, and pictures through the slides.

FILM STRIPS

It is an improvement upon slide projector (magic lantern). The device may be used as a slide projector or as a film strip projector. Instead of using different slides for different topics or more slides for one topic, one strip or piece of still film is prepared. Slides produced on films are called film strips. A film strip consists of a strip of cellulose acetate film 16 mm or 35 mm wide and 2 to 5 feet long. It usually consists of 40 to 100 separate pictures related to a particular subject, topic or theme. Such strip or a piece of still film serves the same purpose as served by a number of slides. There is not much difference between a slide projector and a film strip projector. In a slide projector, we use separate slides while in a film strip, a strip of film (having long strip of many slides) is exhibited. Various commercial firms sell such film strips readymade for different topics.

Advantages

- It is easy to operate
- A frame may be held on screen as long as it is required
- Strips of educative value according to special needs are available
- By reversing the operating knob, previously exhibited frames can be illustrated again for reference
- It draws the attention of the students
- Varieties of information may be given
- Now film strips with commentary recorded on tapes are available
- The teacher can also tape his comments and play the tape synchronizing it with the frame of the film strip
- Film strips are light-weight and easy to carry
- Even a low-voltage lamp can serve the purpose while using film strips
- With every film strip projector, a 2" × 2" slide attachment is also provided and the same projector can be used for projection slides also
- Its use does not restrict the normal flow of conversation between the teacher and the class
- The numbered film strips prove advantageous to the learner, especially when one or two students use them in independent work. Numbering makes it possible to locate a frame to be reshown
- Since film strips present the pictures in a fixed sequence, they provide a structure for the subject
- Film strips provide an economical means of presenting information.

Limitations

Film strips lack audition. Teacher has to do the work of a commentator. Just showing a film strip is not enough.

OVERHEAD PROJECTOR (OHP)

The overhead projector has opened a new avenue for communication. It represents a lot of improvement over magic lantern, slide and film projectors. The name 'overhead projector' comes from the fact that the projected image is behind and over the head of the speaker/teacher. In an overhead projection, a transparent visual is placed on a horizontal stage on top of light source. The light passes through this transparency and then is reflected at 90° angle on the screen at the back of the speaker.

Characteristics

- *Vertical projection:* It contains an area of vertical projection besides the straight horizontal path of the light available with the usual projectors
- *Horizontal path:* The path of the light rays is again changed to a horizontal one by mirror placed at 45° angle and continues over the shoulder of the teacher to the screen
- *Large aperture:* It contains a large aperture of the size of 20 × 20 cms or 25 × 25 cms for placing the slides and other visual materials
- *Focusing of the image:* It provides for the focusing of the image on the screen by vertical movements of the projection head containing the objective lens and mirror
- *Flow of air:* There is a provision of a constant flow of air passing the lamp by a cooling fan in the base of the projector.

Advantages

- *Large image:* It projects a very large image on the screen form a minimum of projection distance.
- *Face the class:* In this projector, the image is projected over the shoulder of the teacher. Therefore, he can face the class at all times. He can maintain eye contact with the students. It helps the teacher to keep watch on the class or indicate points of importance on transparency.

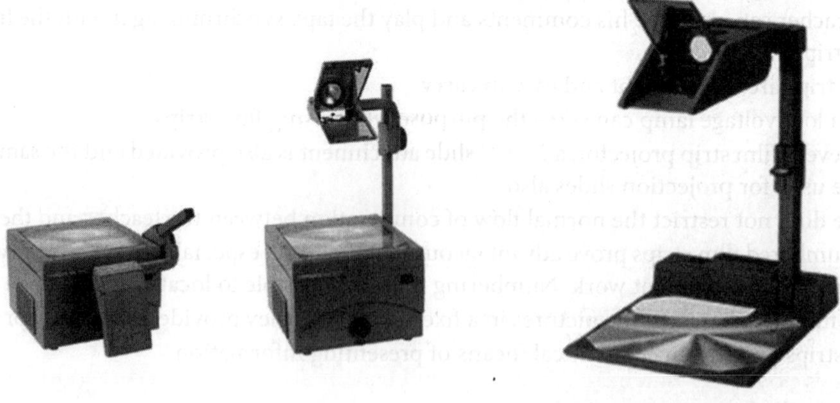

- *Lighted room:* OHP can operate in an illuminated room. There is no need of darkening the room. It enables the teacher to develop a 'circuit of understanding' by watching expression of others.
- *Bright image:* The lens and mirror arrangement in over-head projector makes it possible to have a bright image even in a well-lighted room.
- *Simple operation:* It is simple, easy and convenient to operate the overhead projector. It does not need separate projector operator or the instructor. It permits the teacher to face the class and, at the same time, operate the machine. Slides can be changed quite easily.
- *Light weight:* The light weight of the equipment makes it portable.
- *Class control:* The teacher can maintain complete class control and interest in a lesson by turning a switch on or off. He, while sitting on his desk, can indicate specific items on the screen by locating them with his pencil on the slides.
- *Process on the screen:* By putting a piece of ground glass over the slide space, the teacher can draw a sketch with pencil or wax pencil and the class can watch the process on the screen. He can also place sheets of transparent plastic over the slides for writing on them. Thus, the overhead projector permits the teacher to use the screen as a blackboard.
- *Large slide:* Due to largeness of its aperture, it may allow the use of slides of the size 20 × 20 cms or 25 × 25 cms. It may facilitate the preparation of art work for slides.
- *Use of pointer:* The teacher can use a pointer or pencil to point out important details of a slide. He has not to run about the machine to the wall to explain things to the students.
- *Preparation and presentation of transparencies:* Transparencies can be prepared ahead of time, presented exactly when required and quickly remove when they serve their purpose.
- *Low cost:* Effective visuals can be made in a minimum of time and at low cost. Once a transparency is made, it is permanent. It need not be erased as in a blackboard. It can be stored for recall at any later time.
- Easier to write on horizontal surface.
- Permits the use of color.

Limitations

- Cannot be used for long time
- Writing by some types of writing pens get blotted out on plastic
- Transparencies create a storage problem.

COMPACT DISK (CD)

A compact disk is an optical storage medium that can store over 500 megabytes of information. The disk is of 120 mm in diameter with a 15 mm hole in its center. The disk is made of a polycarbonate plastic and coated with a reflective material. Data is stored by etching small holes in the reflective material called pits. The non-etched areas that reflect light are called lands.

Advantages

- Capability to store large amounts of information
- Ability to store data, graphics, audio, and video on the same disk
- There is no danger of a head crash, wear and tear, or accidental data corruption that magnetic media suffer.

Disadvantages

- High initial cost to produce a single disk
- Slow access and data transfer times compared with high performance of fixed disk systems.

There are different types of CDs:

- *Writable disks (or CD Recordable):* This means that you can only burn data a single time on it, or multiple times when using multisession mode until the capacity is exhausted. You cannot physically delete data (unless you damage the disk and the like).
- *Rewritable disks (CD Rewritable):* You can not only add data, but you can also erase the whole data on disk in order to put different contents on it. Usually you can erase it a few hundred times. If you want to use this type of disk like a floppy disk, you have to use programs like Nero in CD.

VIDEOTAPES

Advantages

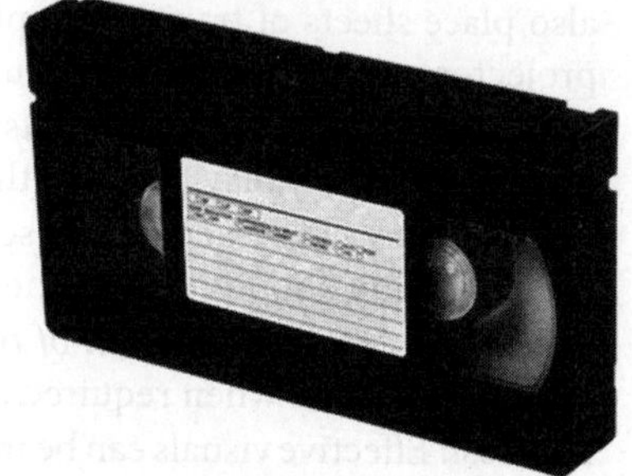

- Teacher can maintain eye contact
- Motion enhances the realism
- Learners are exposed to same teaching
- Can be used by individual learner in his own place.

Disadvantage

One-way communication

DVD (DIGITAL VIDEO DISK OR DIGITAL VERSATILE DISKS)

Advantages

- Replaces videotapes.
- More portable, durable and easier to store.
- Have higher quality audio-video.
- DVDs can be played on desktop or laptop computers with a DVD drive or televisions with a DVD player.
- Old video tapes can be converted as DVD.
- Digital Versatile Disk (or DVD Read Only Memory). Basically the same as CD-ROM, however, a DVD typically has a 6 times greater capacity than a CD.
- Writable DVDs (or DVD Recordable). Basically the same as CD-R with greater capacity. Note that DVD–R (say, DVD minus R) and DVD+R (say, DVD plus R) are different kinds of disks. There is virtually no difference between those types, but it might be the case that your DVD burning device can only burn DVD–R or only burn DVD+R. Most modern devices support both formats equally though.
- Rewritable DVDs (DVD Rewritable). Basically the same as CD-RW with greater capacity.

21

Measurement and Evaluation

Chapter Highlights

- Measurement
- Meaning and Definitions of Evaluation
- The Purposes of Educational Evaluation
- Formative Evaluation
- Summative Evaluation
- Assessment
- Types and Approaches to Assessment
- Formative vs Summative Assessment
- Informal vs Formal Assessment
- Process vs Product Assessment
- Divergent Assessments vs Convergent Assessment
- Continuous vs Final Assessment
- Continuous Assessment
- Features of Continuous Assessment
- Advantages of Continuous Assessment
- Disadvantages of Continuous Assessment
- Teachers' Quality to Run Good Continuous Assessment
- Test
- Qualities of a Good Test
- Base for Writing Test Items
- Objective Tests
- Multiple Choice Item Construction
- Myths Related to Multiple Choice Items (MCIs)
- Functions of the Parts of Multiple Choice Item
- Types of Multiple Choice Items
- Using Cognitive Levels of Learning (Bloom's Modified Version) In Multiple Choice Items (MCIs)
- Item Analysis
- True or False Questions
- Matching Items Questions
- Completion Questions
- Subjective Tests
- Essay Questions
- Short-answer Questions

Learning Objectives

Upon completion of this chapter, the students will be able to:

- Define measurement and evaluation
- Describe the types and approaches to assessment
- List qualities of a good test
- Describe various types of objective tests
- Describe the types of subjective tests
- List the purposes of educational evaluation
- Differentiate between various types of assessment
- Provide the base for writing test items
- Demonstrate skill in performing item analysis
- Demonstrate skill in test construction

The concepts of test, measurement, assessment and evaluation in education are often used interchangeably by practitioners. Actually these concepts carry different meanings. As educators and teachers we must understand the meaning of these terms clearly.

Measurement is a process of assigning numerals to objects, quantities or events in other to give quantitative meaning to such qualities. Measurement stops at ascribing the quantity but not making value judgment on the child's performance. It implies involves carrying out actual measurement in order to assign a quantitative meaning to a quality. In the classroom, to determine a student's performance, you need to obtain quantitative measures on the individual scores of the student.

MEANING AND DEFINITIONS OF EVALUATION

Evaluation has the potential to be beneficial or harmful. In other words, it might be easily misleading. It might lead to excellent or poor outcomes and decisions. It is for that reason that all elements underlying an evaluation should be carefully examined.

Evaluation is defined as an effort involving collection, analysis and interpretation of data in order to judge the achievement of a program's objectives. Rossi and Freeman define evaluation as: 'the systematic application of social research procedures for assessing the conceptualization, design, implementation and utility of social intervention program's.'

Patton uses the term evaluation as 'any effort to increase human effectiveness through systematic data-based inquiry' and defines evaluation research as: 'the systematic examination of accomplishment and effectiveness in program and services'.

Evaluation is a qualitative measure of the prevailing situation. It calls for evidence of effectiveness, suitability, or goodness of the program. It is the estimation of the worth of a thing, process or program in order to reach meaningful decisions about that thing, process or program. It is the process of delineating, obtaining and providing useful information for judging decision alternatives (Stufflebeam et al 1971).

The Purposes of Educational Evaluation

According to Oguniyi (1984), educational evaluation is carried out from time to time for the following purposes:

- To determine the relative effectiveness of the program in terms of students' behavioral output; to make reliable decisions about educational planning
- To ascertain the worth of time, energy and resources invested in a program
- To identify students' growth or lack of growth in acquiring desirable knowledge, skills, attitudes and societal values
- To help teachers determine the effectiveness of their teaching techniques and learning materials
- To help motivate students to want to learn more as they discover their progress or lack of progress in given tasks
- To encourage students to develop a sense of discipline and systematic study habits
- To provide educational administrators with adequate information about teachers' effectiveness and school need
- To acquaint parents or guardians about students' performances
- To identify problems that might hinder or prevent the achievement of set goals
- To predict the general trend in the development of the teaching-learning process
- To ensure an economical and efficient management of scarce resources
- To provide an objective basis for determining the promotion of students from one class to another as well as the award of certificates
- To provide a just basis for determining at what level of education the possessor of a certificate should enter a career.

There are two main levels of evaluation. Program evaluation has to do with the determination of whether a program has been successfully implemented or not. Student evaluation determines how well a student is performing in a program of study. Each of the two levels can involve either of the two main types of evaluation–formative and summative at various stages.

Formative Evaluation

The purpose of formative evaluation is to find out whether after a learning experience, students are able to do what they were previously unable to do.

Uses of formative evaluation

- Draw more reliable inference about his/her students than an external assessor, although he may not be as objective as the latter.
- Identify the levels of cognitive process of his students.
- Choose the most suitable teaching techniques and materials.
- Determine the feasibility of a program within the classroom setting.
- Determine areas needing modifications or improvement in the teaching-learning process
- Determine to a great extent the outcome of summative evaluation.

Summative evaluation is judgmental in nature and often carries threat with it in that the student may have no knowledge of the evaluator and failure has a far reaching effect on the students. However, it is more objective than formative evaluation. Some of the underlying assumptions of summative evaluation are that:

- The program's objectives are achievable
- The teaching-learning process has been conducted efficiently
- The teacher-student-material interactions have been conducive to learning
- The teaching techniques, learning materials and audio-visual aids are adequate and have been judiciously dispensed
- There is uniformity in classroom conditions for all learners.

Assessment

In the most general sense, *assessment* is the process of making a judgment or measurement of worth of an entity (e.g. person, process, or program). *Educational assessment* involves gathering and evaluating data evolving from planned learning activities or programs. This form of assessment is often referred to as *evaluation. Learner assessment* represents a particular type of educational assessment normally conducted by teachers and designed to serve several related purpose (Brissenden and Slater).

Assessment is a fact finding activity that describes conditions that exists at a particular time.

Assessment often involves measurement to gather data. However, it is the domain of assessment to organize the measurement data into interpretable forms on a number of variables.

Assessment in educational setting may describe the progress students have made towards a given educational goal at a point in time. However, it is not concerned with the explanation of the underlying reasons and does not proffer recommendations for action. Assessment is used generally for measuring or determining personal attributes (totality of the student, the environment of learning and the student's accomplishments).

A number of instrument are often used to get measurement data from various sources. These include tests, aptitude tests, inventories, questionnaires, observation schedules, etc. All these sources give data which are organized to show evidence of change and the direction of that change. A test is thus one of the assessment instruments. It is used in getting quantitative data.

These purposes include:

- Motivating and directing learning
- Providing feedback to student on their performance
- Providing feedback on instruction and/or the curriculum
- Ensuring standards of progression are met.

TYPES AND APPROACHES TO ASSESSMENT

Numerous terms are used to describe different types and approaches to learner assessment. Although somewhat arbitrary, it is useful to these various terms as representing dichotomous poles (McAlpine, 2002).

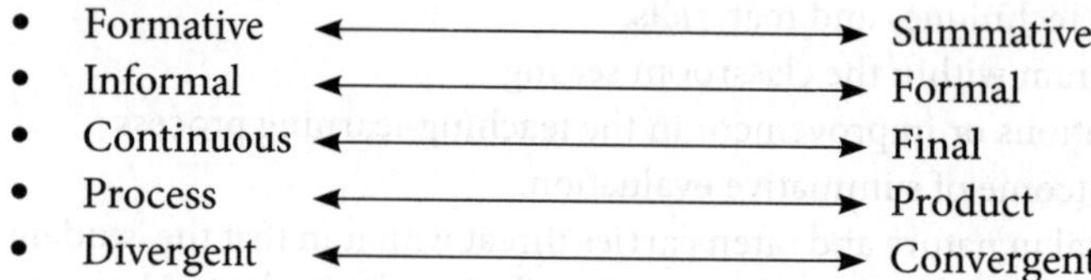

Formative vs Summative Assessment

Formative assessment is designed to assist the learning process by providing feedback to the learner, which can be used to identify strengths and weakness and hence improve future performance. Summative assessment is used primarily to make decisions for grading or determine readiness for progression. Typically summative assessment occurs at the end of an educational activity and is designed to judge the learner's overall performance.

Informal vs Formal Assessment

With informal assessment, the judgments are integrated with other tasks, e.g. lecturer feedback on the answer to a question or preceptor feedback provided while performing a bedside procedure.

Formal assessment occurs when students are aware that the task that they are doing is for assessment purposes.

Process vs Product Assessment

Focuses on steps or procedures, e.g. giving injection, improving performance, different concepts.

Divergent Assessments vs Convergent Assessment

Divergent assessments tend to be more authentic and most appropriate in evaluating higher cognitive skills. However, these types of assessment are often time consuming to evaluate and the resulting judgments often exhibit poor reliability.

A convergent assessment has only one correct response (per item). Objective test items are the best example.

For any form of assessment to be able to serve the above functions, it cannot be a one shot kind of assessment. It has to be an on-going exercise throughout the teaching and learning processes. This is why continuations assessment is advocated in the classroom.

Continuous vs Final Assessment

Continuous assessment occurs throughout a learning experience Continuous assessment is most appropriate when student and/or instructor knowledge of progress or achievement is needed to determine the subsequent progression or sequence of activities.

Final (or terminal) assessment is that which takes place only at the end of a learning activity.

It is most appropriate when learning can only be assessed as a complete whole rather than as constituent parts.

Continuous Assessment

Continuous assessment is defined in the Federal Ministry of Education handbook as:

'A mechanism whereby the final grading of a student in the cognitive, affective and psychomotor domains of behavior takes account in a systematic way, of all his performances during a given period of schooling. Such an assessment involves the use of a great variety of models of evaluation for the purpose of finding and improving the learning and performance of the students.'

Continuous assessment tests are used to evaluate the progress of students periodically. Continuous assessment tests can be done daily, weekly, monthly, depending on the goals of teaching and learning. The continuous assessment equalizes the term internal assessment.

Features of continuous assessment

- Periodical, systematic and well planned
- Continuous assessment tests can be in any form (oral, written, practical, announced, or unannounced, multiple choice objective, essay, or subjective, assignment, etc.)
- Often based on what has been learnt within a particular period. It should be a series of tests or others
- Continuous assessment tests are part of the scores used to compute the overall performance of students
- Designed and produced by the subject teacher.

Advantages of a continuous assessment

- It provides useful information about the academic progress of the learner
- It makes the learner to keep on working in a progressive manner
- It informs the teacher about the teaching-learning effectiveness achieved
- It gives a true picture of the student academic performance since it is a continuous process rather than one duration type of test which may be affected by many variables, such as sickness, fatigue, stress, etc.
- It makes learning an active rather than a passive process.

Disadvantages of continuous assessment

- Constructing the test extremely easy so that undeserving students can pass. Inflating the marks of the continuous assessment tests so that undeserving students can pass the final examinations and be given certificates not worked for
- Conducting few (less than appropriate) continuous assessment tests and thus making the process not a continuous or progressive one

- Reducing the quality of the tests simply because the classes are too large for a teacher to examine thoroughly
- Chances for examination malpractices, e.g. giving the test to favored students before-hand, inflating marks, or recording marks for continuous.

Teachers' quality to run good continuous assessment

- Honest and firm
- Be fair and just in their assessments
- Dedicated and disciplined
- Shun all acts of favoritism, corruption, and other malpractice activities.

Test

A test item is the basic unit of observation in any test. A test item is intended to measure some aspect of human ability generally related to learning or training. A test is a measuring device intended to describe numerically the amount of learning under uniform, standardized conditions. Typically, a set of items are intended to measure a domain of knowledge or skills or cognitive ability.

Tests are detailed or small scale task carried out to identify the candidate's level of performance and to find out how far the person has learnt what was taught or be able to do what he/she is expected to do after teaching. Tests are carried out in order to measure the efforts of the candidate and characterize the performance. Test is therefore an instrument for assessment. Types of tests can be determined from different perspectives. Discrete point tests are expected to test one item or skills at a time, while integrative tests combine various items, structures, skills into one single test.

Qualities of a good test

- *Purposeful:* A good test serves a purpose, either formative, to help learners improve their performance or knowledge, or summative, to certify that learners have indeed learned what they should have learned.
- *Valid:* A good test is valid because the test conditions, behavior and standards are the same as in the objective.
- *Reliable:* A good test is reliable, because it provides sufficient evidence of the desired knowledge or skill.
- *Objective:* A good test is objective, meaning that two trained evaluators would obtain the same result with the test.
- *Comprehensive:* A good test tests on samples of all the course requirements.
- *Differentiating:* A good test differentiates between those who know and those who do not know. This means that competent learners score high on the test and incompetent learners score low.
- *Expected:* A good test tests what is expected. Tell learners the objectives so they can practice what is on the test.
- *Instructive:* A good test is instructive, because it tells the test-taker what was well done or what is in need of improvement. Good feedback is one of the qualities of good learner assessment.
- *Useful:* A good test is useful if it can be implemented with available resources. Objective structured clinical exams, in which simulated patients and trained observers are used to help assess students' clinical skills, can be very valid, objective, instructive, differentiating, and comprehensive.

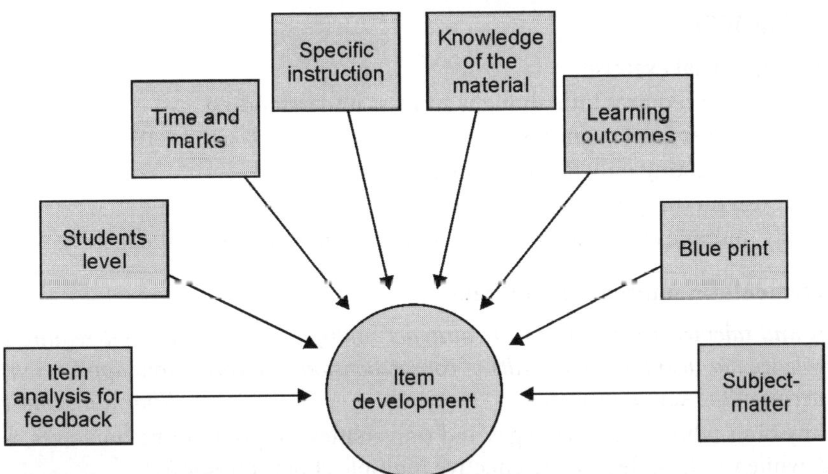

Base for writing test items

- Subject-matter content to be tested
- Learning outcomes to be measured by the test
- Clear table of specifications/blue print
- Time and marks
- Specific instructions
- Knowledge and understanding of the material being tested
- Understanding of the students for whom the items are intended. Item analysis for feedback.

There are two major categories of tests. They are objective tests and subjective tests.

Objective Tests

Multiple Choice Item Construction

Nurse academicians who sought to study MCQs found that neither test bank questions (Masters, Hulsmeyer, Pike, Leichty, Miller, & Verst, 2001) nor instructor-developed test questions (Tarrant, Knierim, Hayes, & Ware, 2006) yielded quality items. Masters et al (2001) examined 2,913 textbook test bank questions and found 76.7% violated test-writing guidelines.

Almost half (46.2%) of the questions contained violations of item-writing guidelines and over 90% were written at low cognitive levels. Only a small proportion of questions were teacher generated (14.1%), while 36.2% were taken from test banks and almost half (49.4%) had no source identified. MCQs written at a lower cognitive level were significantly more likely to contain item-writing flaws (Tarrant et al, 2007).

Multiple choice items are widely used in higher education. Many universities, teaching institutions and various firms usc it as a testing tool.

Purposes vary:

- Enroll students and trainees, recruit employees
- Appraisal and promotion
- Regular examinations, continuous assessment, professional examination

Myths Related to MCI

- It is only a superficial exercise
- Multiple guess that requires little thought and less understanding
- MCI tests only lower level cognition
- MCI is meant for testing only factual information
- Any teacher can do this job.

So, obviously multiple choice items have a mixed reputation among the faculty.

Scholars' statements on multiple choice items

An ingenious and talented item writer can construct multiple choice items that require not only the recall of knowledge but also the use of skills of comprehension, interpretation, application, analysis or synthesis to arrive at the keyed answer. —*Thorndike and Hegen, 1969*

How many of us who teach at colleges and universities would describe ourselves as 'ingenious and talented' while we struggle to write effective multiple choice questions?

—*Wilbert J. Mckeachie, 1986*

'... the greater your experience in their construction, the longer it takes per [multiple-choice] item to construct a reasonably fair, accurate, and inclusive question.' —*Wilbert J. McKeachie*

Parts of multiple choice item

Each item has:

- Item stem
- Correct or keyed option/response
- Several distracters

Functions of the parts of multiple choice item

1. *Stem:* presents the problem
2. *Keyed response:* correct or the best answer
3. *Distracters:* appear to be reasonable answers to the examinee who does not know the content
4. *Options:* include the distracters and the keyed response.

Types of multiple choice items based on stem

- Complete question
- Incomplete sentence

Types of multiple choice items based on options

- **Correct Answer**
  - Only one correct response
- **Best Answer**
  - Requires examinee to select alternative closest to being correct
- **Multiple Answers**
  - More than one correct or best answer.

Complex multiple-choice format. (e.g., A and D, A and C, A, B and C, etc.)

General guidelines

- Include four or five alternatives
- List possible responses one below the other
- The item should test only one idea
- Omit responses that are obviously wrong
- Alignment on the paper should show stem and options separately
- Give appropriate instructions
- Scoring instructions.

Writing the stem

- The stem should clearly formulate a problem
- Eliminate excessive wording and irrelevant information
- Include in the stem any word(s) that might otherwise be repeated in each alternative
- When using incomplete statements avoid beginning with the blank space
- Avoid teaching in the stem
- Ensure that the directions in the stem are very clear
- Include the central idea in the stem instead of the choices
- Avoid window dressing (excessive verbiage)
- Word the stem positively, avoid negatives, such as NOT or EXCEPT
- When a negative item is used emphasize the negative word or phrase. It can be ***underlined, capitalized, and italicized.***

Writing Item Alternatives

- Develop effective choices of four and above
- Make sure that only one of these choices is the right answer or the best answer
- Keep choices independent; choices should not be overlapping
- Keep choices homogeneous in content and grammatical structure
- Keep the length of the choices about equal
- Make all distracters plausible
- Use typical errors of students to write your distracters
- When possible, present alternatives in some logical order (e.g. most to least and chronological)
- Word all responses in such a manner that the student must know the subject matter to select the correct answer
- Many testing authorities do not agree including 'all of the above' and 'none of the above' as options
- Scatter position of the correct answer
- Avoid ambiguity
- Avoid overlapping
- Two sets of opposites are better than one set
- Avoid writing repetitive options in combinations
- Go for succinct options.

Time

Allow 1 minute each for simple multiple choice and 1½ minutes each for multiple-multiple choice items.

Advantages of MCI

- Versatility in measuring all levels of cognitive ability
- Highly reliable test scores
- Scoring efficiency and accuracy
- Objective measurement of achievement or ability
- A wide sampling of content or objectives
- Different response alternatives which can provide diagnostic feedback
- They deemphasize writing skills.

Limitations

Multiple choice items:

- Are difficult and time-consuming to construct
- Lead an instructor to favor simple recall of facts
- Place a high degree of dependence on the student's reading ability and instructor's writing ability
- Are particularly subject to clueing (students can often deduce the correct response by elimination)
- They limit creativity.

Example-(incomplete stem-type)

While learning about the culture of her patient the nurse needs to show

a. respect and patience
b. judgment and command
c. intimacy and priority
d. Kindness and sympathy.

Best response

Which of the following clients should the nurse attend first? A client who is in need of

a. a dressing change
b. a suctioning
c. pain medications
d. incontinence sheet

Best response (case scenario)

Case Scenario: A patient who is visibly upset says to the nurse, 'I want to talk with the head nurse, no, get me the supervisor and the director of nursing and the owner of the hospital. I am mad.'

Stem: The best initial response for the nurse to make is:

Distracters: A. 'Whom do you wish to see first?'
B. 'Don not be angry.'
C. 'Why do you want to talk to them when I can help'

Correct Answer D. 'You seem upset.

Writing flaws-Examples

Vitamin B_{12}

a. Contains iron
b. Is absorbed by mouth
c. Is stored in liver
d. Is given for hemolytic anemia.

The stem does not contain the problem. The learner has to examine each option to decide what is required.

Wrong

The name of the nursing diagnosis is linked to the etiology with the phrase:

a. 'As manifested by'.
b. 'related to'
c. 'evidenced by'
d. 'due to'

Corrected version

While formulating a nursing diagnosis, which of the following phrases should an educator recommend to link the problem with the etiology?

a. As manifested by
b. Related to
c. As evidenced by
d. Due to.

Wrong

The secretion of the sebaceous gland is called:

a. cerumen
b. sebum
c. semen*
d. sweat.

Distracter: (c) not plausible. Easy to identify.

Negative form

Which of the following does normal urine not contain?

a. Urea
b. Albumin
c. Phosphate
d. Chloride.

Corrected version: Would be better stated in a positive form.

Which of the following is an abnormal constituent of urine?

a. Urea
b. Albumin
c. Phosphate
d. Chloride.

In objective testing, the term 'objective' refers to the method of:

a. method of identifying the learning outcomes
b. method of selecting the test content
c. method of presenting the problem
d. method of scoring the answers*

Words are repeated unnecessarily in the above options

Corrected version

In objective testing, the term 'objective' refers to the method of:

a. identifying the outcomes
b. selecting the test content
c. presenting the problem
d. scoring the answers*

Using cognitive levels of learning (Bloom's modified version) in MCIs:

Remembering

Furosemide (Lasix) is a:

- stimulant laxative
- beta blocker
- diuretic*
- cholinergic.

Understanding

Furosemide (Lasix) acts to:

- prevent reabsorption of water.
- increase peristalsis
- block the reuptake of serotonin.
- inhibit beta receptor activity.

Applying

Before helping a patient receiving furosemide (Lasix) get out of bed, the nurse would:

a. put slippers on the patient
b. dangle the patient at bedside*
c. check blood pressure while supine
d. calculate intake and output chart.

Analyzing

The nurse is administering furosemide (Lasix) to the patient. Which of the following complications is the patient at risk for?

a. Hypertension
b. Arrhythmias*
c. Crackles
d. Tachypnea

Which of the following would be the most accurate in evaluating the effectiveness of furosemide (Lasix)?

- Decreased weight*
- Degree of shortness of breath
- Diastolic blood pressure
- Intake and output chart

There are varieties of test items available to test the learners. 1. There are questions where the learner recognizes the answer (true/false, multiple-choice, matching); and 2. Questions where the learner supplies the answer (completion, short-answer, essay, production, procedure: criterion checklists).

Item Analysis

Item analysis is the systematic evaluation of the effectiveness of each item of a test.

Benefits of item analysis

- The difficulty of the item
- The discriminating power of the item
- The effectiveness of each alternative.

All the above three help the test constructor to review the questions and strengthen the items to test the students effectively. This also helps to make valid contribution to the evaluation of students' achievement that would assure quality in teaching.

Item-Analysis-Procedure

There are a number of different item-analysis procedures that might be applied (Downie, 1967).

For informal achievement tests used in teaching, only the simplest of procedures seems warranted. The following steps outline a simple but effective procedure. We shall use 32 test papers to illustrate the steps.

- Arrange the test papers (all 32 papers) in order from the highest score to the lowest score. Select approximately one-third of the papers with the highest scores and call this the upper group (10 papers). Select the same number of papers with the lowest scores and call this the lower group (10 papers). Set the middle group of papers aside (12 papers). Although these could be included in the analysis, using only the upper and lower groups simplifies the procedure.
- For each item, count the number of students in the upper groups who selected each alternative. Make the same count for the lower group.
- Record the count, from step 3, on a copy of the test, in columns to the left of the alternatives to which each count refers. The count may also be recorded on the item card or on a separate sheet, as follows:

Item 1	Alternatives	A	B*	C	D	E
	Upper 10	0	6	3	1	0
	Lower 10	3	2	2	3	0

*Correct answer

- Estimate item difficulty by determining the percentage of students who got the item right. The simplest procedure is to base this estimate on only those students who are included in the item-analysis groups. Thus, sum the total number in the upper and lower groups (10 + 10 = 20); sum the number selecting the correct answer. For item 1 above, 6 + 2 = 8; divide the first sum into the second and multiply by 100 as follows:

Index of Difficulty = 8/20 × 100 = 40%

Although our computation is based on the upper and lower groups only, this provides a close approximation to the estimate that would be obtained with the total group. Thus, it is proper to say that the index of difficulty for this item is 40 per cent (for this particular group). Note that since difficulty refers to the percentage getting the item right, the smaller the percentage figure, the more difficult the item.

- Estimate item-discriminating power by comparing the number of students in the upper and lower groups who got the item right. Note in our sample item above that six students in the upper group and two students in the lower group selected the correct answer. This indicates positive discrimination, since the item differentiates between students in the same way that the total test score does. That is, students with high scores on the test (upper group) got the item right more frequently than students with low scores on the test (lower group).

Index of Discrimination

Index of discrimination can be easily computed. Simply subtract the number in the lower group who got the item right from the number in the upper group who got the item right and divide by the number in each group.

Thus, for our sample item, the computation would be as follows:

Index of Discrimination = (6 – 2) ÷ 10 = 0.4

Note that the discriminating power of an item is reported as a decimal fraction. Maximum positive discriminating power is indicated by an index of 1.00. This is obtained only when all students in the upper group select the correct answer and no one in the lower group does.

For our illustrative upper and lower groups of 10, the computation for an item with maximum discriminating power would be as follows: Index of Discrimination = (10 – 0) ÷ 10 = 1.0

Note that this item is at the 50 per cent level of difficulty (upper 10 got it right, lower 10 missed it). This explains why test makers are encouraged to prepare items at the 50 per cent level of difficulty. It is only at this level that maximum discrimination is possible. Zero discriminating power (.00) is obtained when an equal number of students in both groups get the item right, and negative discriminating power when more students in the lower group than in the upper group get it right. Both types of items should be removed from general achievement tests and be discarded or improved.

- Determine the effectiveness of the distracters by comparing the number of students in the upper and lower groups who selected each incorrect alternative. A good distracter will attract more students from the lower group than the upper group. Thus, for our illustrative item-analysis data, in step 4, alternatives A and D are functioning effectively, alternative C is poor since it attracted more students from the upper group and alternative E is completely ineffective since it attracted no one. An analysis such as this one is useful in evaluating a test item, and, when combined with an inspection of the item itself, it provides helpful information for improving the item.

True or False Questions

A true or false question is essentially a statement called a proposition. The learner judges whether the proposition is true or false.

Specifications for writing a true or false item:

- There should be about an equal number of true and false statements

- Both true and false statements should be about equal length
- False items should be plausible.

Good Example

The MDR of vitamin D for a normal 160-pound male adult is 4,000 units *(assuming the correct response is 400 units).*

Bad Example

The MDR of vitamin D for a normal 160-pound male adult is 4 pounds

- The proposition should be clearly true or false.

Good Example

A fracture of the femur protruding through the skin is an example of a compound fracture.

Bad Example

A simple fracture of the femur protruding through the skin is an example of a compound fracture. *('Simple' and 'compound' as technical terms are mutually exclusive.)*

- The proposition should be simple
- The proposition should be specific.

Good Example

Fifteen percent of all American males aged 55 and over suffer from cardiac arrhythmia.

Bad Example

About 25–35% of Americans suffer from some sort of heart condition.

- The proposition should contain one idea.

Good Examples

Vitamin C is useful in the prevention of scurvy. Vitamin D is useful in the prevention of scurvy.

Bad Example

Vitamin C and Vitamin D are useful in the prevention of scurvy.

- The proposition should include sources if needed.

Good Example

According to Street, 42.3 out of 127 people will tell the truth on a survey.

Bad Example

42.3 out of 127 people will tell the truth on a survey.

- Avoid broad statements. Statements with too broad a scope are usually false.

Good Example

High levels of LDL (>180 mg/dl) is a risk factor for heart disease in men over 40.

Bad Example

Cholesterol is bad for men over 40.

- Avoid trivia.

Good Example

The incidence of tuberculosis among all people living in Greenville, NC is .05%.

Bad Example

The incidence of Crumbler's Syndrome among blue-eyed Caucasians from Greenville, NC is .0000000005%.

- Avoid qualifiers. Adjectives that qualify the meaning of a noun, such as 'always' and 'never,' usually make the statement false.

Good Example

AIDS is characterized by the co-occurrence of opportunistic infections.

Bad Example

AIDS is always accompanied by opportunistic infection.

- Avoid indefinites.

Good Example

AIDS is characterized by the co-occurrence of opportunistic infections.

Bad Example

Some AIDS patients suffer from opportunistic infections.

- Avoid negative statements.

Good Example

One can use a summative evaluation design for formative evaluation purposes.

Bad Example

One should not use a formative evaluation design for summative evaluation purposes.

Matching Items Questions

A matching item question is the one that requires the test taker to match an item in one column with an item from a second column. In general, the items that have a blank space next to them are called the 'questions' and the items that you choose from to fill in the blank are called the 'answers'.

Guidelines for writing matching items

- Instructions indicate the basis for matching
- Questions and responses are all from the same category
- Questions and responses include 5 to 8 items
- There should not be an equal number of test items; 2 to 3 more possible responses should be available
- Questions and responses should be grammatically consistent; they should not contain any grammatical cues
- Questions and responses should all be on the same page

- Reponses are short phrases
- All the responses are plausible for the questions
- Responses are listed to the right of the questions
- Responses are in a systematic order: alphabetic for lists of names; numeric for dates and numbers.

Completion Questions

A completion item is a form of short-answer question in which the learner completes a sentence by supplying a keyword or phrase. A completion item is comprised of two parts, the 'cue' and the 'blank'. Completion questions are the simplest types of test items in which the learner is required to supply the correct answer, rather than to choose the correct answer. As such, it requires a higher level of learning—recall learning—rather than simple recognition. Every completion question should follow these specifications.

Example

- The causative organism of tetanus is ___________. *(Answer: clostridium tetanic)*

Guidelines for constructing completion items

- The sentence describes the blank(s).
- Blank(s) are at the end of the sentence. The point of the item can be lost if the blank occurs earlier in the item. Also, learners may have to return to the beginning of the item to recall what is being asked of them.
- Blank(s) should be equal in length. Blanks of unequal length may be misread as an additional cue to learners. All blanks should be of sufficient length to accommodate any correct answer for all completion questions.
- There should be few blanks per question.
- Each blank should be worth one point. Assigning differential point values to different blanks is an invitation to charges of unfairness in grading.

Subjective Tests

Essay Questions

An essay question calls for an extended response from the learner. The response can be extended, with virtually no restrictions on the answer, or it can be restricted according to length.

Essay questions challenge students to create a response rather than to simply select a response. Essay questions allow the learner maximum freedom to respond. Higher order mental processes can be tested using essay questions, such as description, comparison, evaluation and prediction. All essay questions should follow these specifications.

There are many definitions found in literature on 'essay questions'. A definition given a long time ago by Stalnaker (1951, p.495) is perhaps the most helpful. An essay question is '…a test item which requires a response composed by the examinee, usually in the form of one or more sentences, of a nature that no single response or pattern of responses can be listed as correct, and the accuracy and quality of which can be judged subjectively only by one skilled or informed in the subject.'

Advantages

- Essay questions provide an effective way of assessing complex learning outcomes that cannot be assessed by other commonly used paper-and-pencil assessment procedures

- Essay questions allow students to demonstrate their reasoning
- Essay questions provide authentic experience. Constructed responses are closer to real life than selected responses.

Limitations

- Essay questions necessitate testing a limited sample of the subject matter, thereby reducing content validity
- Essay questions have limitations in reliability
- Essay questions require more time for scoring student responses
- Essay questions provide practice in poor or unpolished writing.

Common Misconceptions

- By their very nature, essay questions assess higher-order thinking
- Essay questions are easy to construct
- The use of essay questions eliminates the problem of guessing
- Essay questions benefit all students by placing emphasis on the importance of written communication skills
- Essay questions encourage students to prepare more thoroughly.

Guidelines for constructing essay questions

- Essay question is used for an appropriate objective
- Establish a framework to guide the student. To establish a framework, limit the area covered by the question
- Use descriptive words, such as *define, outline, classify, summarize.* Avoid the use of the word *discuss*
- The question is realistic in terms of difficulty, time allotted, and complexity
- A model response is prepared for each question. Preparation of model responses will result in more reliable and objective scoring of essay questions. Preparation of model answers as questions are being written will help reduce question ambiguity, unrealistic expectations and other problems
- Always tell the time allotted and point value of each question. These indications on a test will give students a basis for pacing themselves.

Evaluating Essay Questions

Subjective nature of essay exams makes it difficult to grade. The following guidelines are helpful for grading essay exams in a consistent and meaningful way.

- Construct a model answer for each item and award a point for each essential element of the model answer. This should help minimize the subjective effects of grading.
- Essay items must be graded anonymously, if at all possible, in order to reduce the subjectivity of the graders. That is, graders should not be informed as to the identity of the examinees whose papers they are grading.
- Grade a single essay item at a time. This helps the grader maintain a single set of criteria for awarding points to the response. In addition, it tends to reduce the influence of the examinee's previous performance on other items.

- Evaluate all the students' answers to one question before proceeding to the next question.
- Unless it is a test of language mechanics, do not take off credit for poor handwriting, spelling errors, poor grammar, failure to punctuate properly, etc.
- Ideally, there should be two graders for each item. Any disagreements between these two graders must be resolved by a third grader.

Short-answer Questions

Short-answer questions are open-ended questions that require students to create an answer. They are commonly used in examinations to assess the basic knowledge and understanding (low cognitive levels) of a topic before more in-depth assessment questions are asked on the topic.

These do not have a generic structure. Questions may require answers, such as complete the sentence, supply the missing word, short descriptive or qualitative answers, diagrams with explanations, etc. The answer is usually short, from one word to a few lines.

Guidelines for setting and marking

- Make the questions precise
- Direct questions are better than incomplete statements
- If a numerical answer is required, indicate the units and degree of precision required
- Prepare a structured marking sheet
- Allocate marks or part-marks for acceptable answer(s)
- Be prepared to accept other equally acceptable answers, some of which you may not have predicted.

Advantages

- Relatively fast to mark and can be marked by different assessors, as long as the questions are set in such a way that all alternative answers can be considered by the assessors
- Relatively easy to set compared with many assessment methods
- Used as part of a formative and summative assessment. As the structure of short-answer questions are very similar to examination questions, students are more familiar with the practice and feel less anxious
- There is no guessing on answers, students must supply an answer.

Disadvantages

- May overemphasize memorization of facts
- Take care—questions may have more than one correct answer
- Scoring is laborious
- Inexperienced teachers may not follow the guidelines. It will be difficult for the assessors to score
- Since it falls between subjective and objective tests, paper-setter must show careful evaluation on objectives to be placed under short-answer questions.

22

Guidance and Counseling

Chapter Highlights

- Definitions and Meaning of Guidance
- Characteristics of Guidance
- Need for the Guidance Service in Schools
- Principles to Disseminate Guidance
- Types of Guidance
- Counseling
- Types of Counseling
- Phases of Counseling
- Difference between Counseling and Guidance
- Benefits of Counseling Service to Student

Learning Objectives

Upon completion of this chapter, the students will be able to:

- Define the terms guidance and counseling
- Identify the importance of guidance service to students in the schools
- List the types of guidance
- Describe the phases of counseling
- List the benefits of counseling in schools
- List the characteristics of guidance
- List the principles to disseminate guidance
- State the types of counseling
- State the difference between guidance and counseling

Guidance is the process of helping people makes important choices that affect their lives, such as choosing a preferred lifestyle. While the decision-making aspect of guidance has long played an important role in the counseling process, the concept itself, as an often-used word in counseling, 'has gone the way of 'consumption' in medicine' (Tyler, 1986, p. 153).

Shartzer and Stone (1976) defined guidance to mean, 'to direct, pilot or guide.' Bakare (1996) refers to guidance as a more directive or prescriptive form of assistance. Idowu (1998) sees it as a family name for all the helping service within the general educational and community systems. To make the meaning to be more explicit, Akinade (2002) remarked that some specialists assert that guidance is a broad term used to cover a number of specialist services available in schools.

Guidance can be defined as a cognitive educational services that help people understand themselves, provided the client reveals accurate, reliable and valid information about himself and his environment.

DEFINITIONS AND MEANING OF GUIDANCE

'Guidance seeks to help each individual become familiar with a wide range of information about himself, his abilities, this pervious development in the various areas of living and his plans or ambitions for the future.'

—*Chisholm*

'Guidance is an assistance given to the individual in making intelligence choices and adjustments.'

—*AJ Jones*

'Guidance is a means of helping individuals to understand and use wisely the educational. Vocational and personal opportunities they have or can develop and as a form of systematic assistance whereby students are aided in achieving satisfactory adjustment to school and to life.' —*Dunsmoor & Miller*

Both Guidance and counseling are process used to solve problems of life. The basic difference is in the approach. In the process of guidance, the client's problems are listened carefully and readymade solutions are provided by the expert whereas in the process of counseling the client's problems are discussed and relevant information are provided in-between. In the end of the counseling process, the client himself/herself have a insight to the problem and he/she become empowered to take own decision. Since readymade solutions (taking decision for others) were provided in guidance, the client may or may not follow it but most often decision taken in the process of counseling are followed sincerely. The set of decisions comes out from guidance and counseling process may be same but in the first process the decision is taken by the guide whereas the client take own his/her own decisions in the later process.

Characteristics of Guidance

- Guidance is a continuous process
- Concerned with problem and choice
- An assistance to the individuals in the process of development
- It is both a generalized and specialized service
- It is a service meant for all.

Need for the Guidance Service in Schools

- To help in the total development of the student
- To help in making proper choice at various stages of their educational career
- To help the students in vocational development
- To help students make the best possible adjustments to the situations in the schools as well as in the homes
- To minimize the mismatch between education and unemployment
- To identify and motivate the students from weaker sections of society
- To identify and help students in need of special help
- To minimize the incidence of indiscipline
- To make the idea inclusive education successful.

Principles to Disseminate Guidance

- The dignity of the individual is supreme
- Each individual is different from every other individual
- The primary concern of guidance is the individual in his own social settings
- The attitude and personal perceptions of the individuals are the bases on which he acts
- The individual generally acts to enhance his perceived self
- The individual has the innate ability to learn and can be helped to make choices that will lead to self-direction consistent with social improvement.
- Each individual may at times need the information and personalized assistance best given by competent professional personnel.

Types of Guidance

'Paterson' has suggested five types of Guidance.

1. Educational Guidance
2. Vocational Guidance
3. Personal Guidance
4. Economic Guidance
5. Health Guidance.

Counseling

There is no single individual live in this world without seeking a help or advice from another individual. The only difference exist is whether the individual is adequately qualified to function as a counselor in the given context. Counseling is defined by many scholars. It is simply a process of helping individuals or people to gain self-understanding in order to be themselves. Burker and Steffler (1979) sees counseling as a professional relationship between a trained Counselor and a client. Olayinka (1972) defined it to be a process whereby a person is helped in a face-to-face relationship while Makinde (1983) explained counseling as an enlightened process whereby people help others by encouraging their growth.

'Counseling is an interaction process which facilitates meaningful understanding of self and environment and result in the establishment and or clarification of goals and values for future behavior'

—*Shertzer and Stone*

'Counseling is a process by which a troubled person (client) is helped to tell and behave in a more personally satisfying manner through interaction with an uninvolved person (counselor) who provides information and reactions which stimulate the client to develop behavior which enable him to deal more effectively with himself and his environment.'

—*Edwin Lewis*

Jones calls counseling the intimate and vital part of entire guidance. Webster's Dictionary defines counseling as 'consultation, mutual interchange of opinions, deliberating together'. Wren says, 'counseling is a dynamic and purposeful relationship between two people who approach a mutually defined problem with mutual consideration for each other to the end that the younger or less mature, or more troubled of the two is aided to a self-determined resolution of his problem.

Types of Counseling

There are two major types of Counseling, namely: individual counseling and group counseling.

Individual counseling: This is referred to as one-to-one counseling. It occurs between the professionally trained Counselor (Therapist) and his client (Counselee). The goal of this is to help the client to understand himself, clarify and direct his thought, in order to make a worthwhile decision.

Group counseling: This is a counseling session that takes place between the professionally trained counselor and a group of people. Number of this group should not be more than seven, or at least ten, in order to have a cohesive group and an effective well controlled counseling session.

Phases of Counseling

Interview Stage/Phase

Any counseling process starts with the interviewing. This stage could also be referred to as the familiarization, orientation or introductory stage. This stage is the base and the counselor needs to approach this stage in a carefully using 'go smooth and get more' approach. This stage is the one that decides the fait of the other stages as well the success of the other stages.

- The counselor makes deliberate effort to get acquainted with the client by establishing rapport. This is done by asking the client to sit down, so that he or she would be emotionally relaxed.
- The counselor inquires about the client's name, class, parents, friends, progress in school and his mission to the counselor's office. This should be done with caution so that the client does not feel as if he or she is being interrogated.
- The counselor further assures the client that whatever is discussed will be kept confidential. This is to win the client's confidence and make him or her open up to say his purpose for coming to the counselors' office. The client may or may not present his problem during this stage.

How does the counselor conduct and maintain him at this point?

- The counselor should not be in a hurry to make him/her disclose his mission
- Be patient and listen carefully
- Show empathy
- Show unconditional positive regards that is treating his clients with respect, warmth, irrespective of his age, sex, race, color, religion and socioeconomic status. This is very important as counselors are not expected to be discriminative.

Working Stage/Phase

In this stage the counselor fully engages the client in discussion about what to do and how it will be done concerning the problem of the client. If the client has not disclosed his/her mission in the first stage, the counselor now asks the client. He uses questioning techniques to make the client open up. Questions such as: Are you okay? Can I help you? What is the matter? What has brought you to my office? The client now responds. The counselor having listened to the client will suggest different techniques depending on the nature of the problem presented on how the problem can be handled.

The counselor uses techniques such as responding, exploring, restatement, interpretation, confrontation, unconditional positive regards, empathy, silence and catharsis to diagnose the problem. Also it is during this stage that the goals for counseling are set by the client and counselor.

Termination Stage/Phase

This stage is the third stage in the counseling process. Termination means bringing an end to the counseling relationship between the counselor and client. Different reasons have been given by many authors on why a counseling relationship may end or terminate. Some of these reasons are given below for you to understand.

It is important to stress here that termination of counseling relationship may be a temporary or permanent one. The following reasons are given by different authors.

Counseling goals are achieved: When the goals have been realized to the satisfaction of the client and counselor, the relationship can be called off temporarily or permanently. Temporarily because the counselor may want to follow-up the client to see if he is doing well or putting into practice what has been discussed and suggested. If the client's problem is solved permanently he may not need to see the counselor again. The client should be told that if he has problem in future, he should be free to see the counselor.

Uncooperative attitude from the client: If after several attempt nothing good is coming out of the relationship, the counselor can terminate the relationship temporarily and ask the client to think over his behavior and may decide to come back if convinced to continue.

Client may decide not to continue: After some time of counseling, the client may decide not to continue for reasons best known to him. Sometimes it may be due to the fact that the client is not honest in the relationship with the counselor and when his attention is drawn to this fact he may decide to stay away and remain with his problem.

Referral to an expert/specialist: The counselor may discover that the client has problem that is beyond his competence, area and experience, when this happens the client should be referred to the appropriate quarters for specialized treatment.

Death of counselor or client: Counseling relationship may be terminated permanently when the counselor or client dies. If it is the counselor that dies, the client may seek for counsel from another counselor.

Follow-up Phase

The follow-up aims at finding out whether the client is carrying out the decisions arrived at before you ended the session and what problems are being experienced. All the clients do not need this stage.

Benefits of counseling service to students

- Understand what she can do and should do, about her progress
- Understand the choices she faces, the opportunities available and the qualification required to choose a particular goal in life
- Understand the difficulties, handle them in a rational mannered strengthen her best qualities and abilities
- Make decisions and plans on the basis of self-understanding
- Acceptance of responsibilities and formulate the future action-plan, in that direction.

Difference between counseling and guidance

Guidance	Counseling
Broader and comprehensive	Counseling is in-depth, narrowing down the problem until the advise understands his/her own problem
More external	Help people to understand themselves, it is an inward analysis
Focus is on finding solution	Focus on counseling is not on solution but on understanding the problem
The guidance may bring attitude change on the advise	Adviser may be able to bring emotional change or change in feeling
Guidance is generally education and career related, it can be on personal problems too	Counseling mostly on personal and social issues

It is always essential school and nursing colleges appoint an educational psychologist to help the students on day-to-day basis. Faculty members take an active role in guidance and counseling programs of the students. This would aid the timely interventions.

Section IV

Quality Assurance

23. Quality Concepts
24. Assuring Quality in Nursing Colleges
25. Mission, Vision, Goals and Student Learning Outcomes
26. Quality Assurance System in Nursing Education

23

Quality Concepts

Chapter Highlights

- Need for Quality Assurance
- Origin and Meaning of Quality Assurance in Education
- Meaning of Quality
- Meaning of Quality—Juran and Crosby
- Dimensions of Quality
- Elaborate Definitions of the Terms Used by Boyce et al
  - Quality Assurance and Related Terminologies

Learning Objectives

Upon completion of this chapter, the students will be able to:

- Describe the importance and need for quality assurance
- State the meaning and origin of quality assurance
- Describe the various dimensions of quality
- Provide various definitions on quality
- Define the terminologies related to quality assurance

'An examination of a knife would reveal that its distinctive quality is to cut, and from this we can conclude that a good knife would be a knife that cuts well'.

—Aristotle

NEED FOR QUALITY ASSURANCE

We tend to look for quality whenever we buy a product. Ultimately, the manufacturers/producers/product owners are bound to assure quality in their products. If the said product does not meet the required standards, the consumers say 'no' to it. Nursing care at the hospital and nursing education in the college/school are equally responsible in assuring quality to its consumers. Quality assurance 'in' education is part of the day-to-day work. Over the past two decades, quality assurance processes in higher education have become increasingly common in most of the countries.

The profession's interest in quality assurance and nursing standards began with the publication of Florence Nightingale's Notes on Nursing: What it is and what it is not. In 1859, Ms. Nightingale outlined aspects of good practice and noted the types of behavior and actions expected of nurses to achieve high levels of performance. She actually developed a standard for good nursing practice and showed how a professional group evaluates its own performance.

It is a well-known fact that the nursing education given in the nursing schools and colleges is the base for the quality of nursing care provided in the hospitals. The primary responsibility for the quality of education delivered rests with the organization that provides those services. Quality assurance focuses on the quality of learning outcomes recognized through qualifications as a whole. It also examines the systems and processes that support delivery of quality by providers. Quality assurance helps to support faculty and build expertise and capacity in the education system to deliver positive outcomes. Quality assurance helps to raise standards and expectations, and levels of consistency across faculty and colleges.

Rigorous and robust quality assurance gives confidence in judgments and provides assurance to stakeholders and others that all learners receive appropriate recognition for their achievements in line with agreed national standards and are progressing in line with expectations.

ORIGIN AND MEANING OF QUALITY ASSURANCE IN EDUCATION

The phrase 'quality assurance' found to be popular and familiar in business/industries. The concept of Quality Assurance emerged as a principal business methodology in the Western world throughout the 1950s and in the early 1960s. Now this had taken a giant tide in education as well as in nursing education all over the world. Quality assurance has implicitly taken its journey of life from industry, service centers and hospitals to education. Education seeming to be the most essential basic need of the man, he has no second thought to spend money for getting a good education.

What is good education? The rating goes on as 'good,' 'better' and 'the best'. These are considered the measurement criteria. The best equals the superior quality. Whether a doctor or a nurse, it is a routine practice to ask where he or she was qualified. This question indirectly seeks to assess the quality of the candidate by knowing the name of the institution. Quality remains the most important attribute that creates value about the product/service for the receiver. In educational institutions, the word 'product' means the candidate who passes out from the institution. The products of the nursing colleges are the nursing graduates who pass out from the institution. These nursing graduates represent their parent college or school, their goodness and competencies reflect on the institution.

Organizations that provide quality and value in the provision of their educational services are likely to grow and prosper. Such organizations gain benefits, like stronger student and staff loyalty, less staff turnover, good admission status and lower vulnerability to economic changes and forthcoming challenges of the profession.

MEANING OF QUALITY

Harvey and Knight (1996) identify the following meanings attributed to quality:

- Quality as exceptional, i.e. exceptionally high standards of academic achievement
- Quality as perfection (or consistency), which focuses on processes and their specifications and is related to zero defects and quality culture
- Quality as fitness for purpose, which judges the quality of a product or service in terms of the extent to which its stated purpose—defined either as meeting customer specifications or conformity with the institutional mission—is met
- Quality as value for money, which assesses quality in terms of return on investment or expenditure and is related to accountability
- Quality as transformation, which defines quality as a process of qualitative change with emphasis on adding value to students and empowering them.

MEANING OF QUALITY—JURAN AND CROSBY

- 'Fitness for purpose'—Juran (industrialist)
- 'Conformance to requirements'—Crosby (industrialist)

An educational definition is that of an ongoing process ensuring the delivery of agreed standards. These agreed standards should ensure that every educational institution where quality is assured has the potential to achieve a high quality of content and results.

DIMENSIONS OF QUALITY

Boyce et al (1997) suggest that **quality** encompasses the following dimensions:

- **Effectiveness:** achieving increases in survival or improved quality of life
- **Efficiency:** maximizing benefits for a given cost
- **Access:** the capacity of individuals to obtain the same quality of care
- **Safety:** the extent to which potential risks are avoided
- **Acceptability:** the degree to which expectations of informed consumers are met
- **Continuity:** the extent to which episodes of care are co-ordinated and integrated into overall care provision
- **Technical proficiency:** (the extent to which care is consistent with contemporary standards and knowledge
- **Appropriateness:** the extent to which potential benefits of an intervention exceed the risk involved.

ELABORATE DEFINITIONS OF THE TERMS USED BY BOYCE ET AL

- **Effectiveness:** The degree to which an intervention produces measurable increases in survival or improved quality of life (or improved outcomes) when applied in routine practice. An indicator might be a measure of provider-assessed or patient-assessed outcome.
- **Efficiency:** Maximizing benefits (or outcomes) for a given cost. Technical efficiency refers to the degree to which the least cost combination of resource inputs occurs in production of a particular service, and an indicator might involve cost/activity ratios, such as cost per case mix-adjusted separation. Allocative efficiency refers to the degree to which maximum benefits are obtained from available resources, and an indicator might draw from frameworks for priority setting, such as program budgeting with marginal analysis.
- **Access:** The capacity of individuals to obtain the same quality of care. An indicator might involve waiting times, preventable admission/avoidable deaths, condition-specific utilization rates, etc.
- **Safety:** The extent to which potential risks were avoided and inadvertent harm minimized in care delivery processes. An indicator might involve adverse event monitoring.
- **Acceptability:** The degree to which the service meets or exceeds the expectations of informed consumers. An indicator might be a suitable patient satisfaction survey.
- **Continuity:** The extent to which an individual episode of care is co-ordinated and integrated into overall care provision. An indicator might involve a suitable patient survey, or an index of the numbers of service providers involved in the care of an individual.
- **Technical proficiency:** The extent to which the performance of interventions by service providers is consistent with contemporary standards and knowledge of skills relevant to that intervention. An indicator might involve compliance with guidelines for care.

- **Appropriateness:** The extent to which potential benefits of an intervention exceed the risk involved. An indicator might involve case-by-case comparison with expert clinician inferences based on variation in utilization.

Quality Assurance and Related Terminologies

Quality is the distinguishing characteristic guiding students and higher education institutions when receiving and providing higher education. Quality assurance is still a much-debated concept in many countries. The concept of quality assurance is not a new one, but the range of the terminology and methodologies, which are now used to define, develop and apply it, are relatively recent.

Quality assurance is the maintenance of a desired level of quality in a service or education or product, especially by means of attention to every stage of the process of delivery or production. Quality assurance is the systematic review of educational programs to ensure that acceptable standards of education, scholarship and infrastructure are being maintained.

Quality assurance is the means by which an institution can guarantee with confidence and certainty, that the standards and quality of its educational provision are being maintained and enhanced.

Quality control refers to the verification procedures (both formal and informal) used by institutions in order to monitor quality and standards to a satisfactory standard and as intended.

Quality enhancement is the process of positively changing activities in order to provide for a continuous improvement in the quality of institutional provision.

Quality assessment is the process of external evaluation undertaken by an external body of the quality of educational provisions in institutions, in particular, the quality of the student experience.

Quality audit is the process of examining institutional procedures for assuring quality and standards and whether the arrangements are implemented effectively and achieve stated objectives. The underlying purpose of Continuation Audit is 'to establish the extent to which institutions are discharging effectively their responsibilities for the standards of awards granted in their name and for the quality of education provided to enable students to attain standards'.

Standards describe levels of attainment against which performance may be measured. Attainment of a standard usually implies a measure of fitness for a defined purpose.

Quality culture is the creation of a high level of internal institutional quality assessment mechanisms and the ongoing implementation of the results. Quality culture can be seen as the ability of the institution, program, etc. to develop quality assurance implicitly in the day-to-day work of the institution and marks a move away from periodic assessment to ingrained quality assurance.

Quality chain series of relationships between customers and suppliers involving quality considerations can involve an individual being both supplier and consumer.

Quality circle is a group of people sharing responsibility for quality initiatives. It can involve people working in different organizational locations or in the same location.

Accreditation is the result of a review of an education program or institution following certain quality standards agreed on beforehand. It is a kind of recognition that a program or institution fulfills certain standards.

We will be learning in depth about assuring quality nursing education in nursing colleges in the forthcoming chapters.

24

Assuring Quality in Nursing Colleges

Chapter Highlights

- Need for Quality Assurance
- Permission from Statutory Bodies—India
- Quality Assurance Agencies—International Perspectives
- Standards for Accreditation—Common Areas of Concern
- Types of Accreditation
- National Qualifications Framework
- Elements Considered for Qualifications Framework

Learning Objectives

Upon completion of this chapter, the students will be able to:

- Describe the statutory process to start nursing colleges in India
- Identify the common sections or areas of concern under quality assurance process
- Explain the process of quality assurance in higher education in most countries

NEED FOR QUALITY ASSURANCE

Quality assurance plan should walk parallel to the other works even before starting a college. Earlier, the nursing colleges in India were very few in numbers; that too, most were government-owned with few religion-based. From the year 1990 onwards, new private nursing colleges started to appear at greater numbers. Currently, India has 1506 nursing colleges offering BSc nursing program, 465 colleges offer PG program in nursing, 648 colleges offering post-basic BSc nursing, 2450 DGNM schools offering diploma in nursing (Indian Nursing Council statistics).This statistics equals only the recognized nursing institutions of India by the apex body Indian Nursing Council. In addition, many colleges are offering postgraduate programs (MSc Nursing) in nursing. After schooling, students have too many career options to choose from, one among them is nursing career. Once decided to choose nursing as the career, students look for an ideal nursing school or college. Ideal means the quality. To opine, nursing college/school is not just a building constructed with bricks and cement, but a place of noble profession that dreams to create nurses with intellectual brains, skilled hands, merciful eyes and service mind to the mankind. In addition, nurses need to walk with technological advancements, but work with human courtesy and kindness, assuring 'quality' in each single step of the caring journey.

PERMISSION FROM STATUTORY BODIES—INDIA

To initiate any program in nursing discipline, the concerned institution needs to send a letter of interest to the government (in most countries, it is state government/Ministry of higher education).

In India, the experts assigned by the 'Directorate of Medical Education' of the concerned state examine the institution for suitability (like land area, faculty strength to start the college), following which the government order is issued to start the college. After obtaining the government order, the institution proposes the intent to Indian Nursing Council. Then the nursing college is inspected by the inspection team (one convener and a member) appointed by the Indian Nursing Council. After receiving the permission from Indian Nursing Council, the inspectors appointed by the state nursing council inspect the college. After getting permission from all the three statutory bodies, the university assesses the suitability of the institution to start the nursing program. When all the four steps are cleared, the name of the college is included in the single window system where the nursing applicants are given opportunities to choose their colleges that are available as per their academic merit and communities denomination. Once chosen the particular nursing college, students undergo the 4 years' nursing program (that includes integrated internship) in the same college.

QUALITY ASSURANCE AGENCIES—INTERNATIONAL PERSPECTIVES

In most countries, the Commission that assesses the quality assurance system of higher education is an independent authority reporting directly to the Higher Council of Education. Its role is separate from that of the Ministries and other government agencies to which institutions are administratively accountable and which may establish regulations and reporting requirements for the institutions for which they are responsible. The Commission's responsibilities relate to quality issues, which include the resources available, processes followed, the quality of services provided and the quality of students learning. The accreditation commissions of different countries have established the required standards in broad areas of activity, and have developed a national qualifications framework that specifies generic standards of learning outcomes for each level of qualifications. These accrediting commissions expect that institutions establish internal quality assurance systems that ensure high levels of quality in all of the required areas.

STANDARDS FOR ACCREDITATION—COMMON AREAS OF CONCERN

Most countries set standards for quality assurance and accreditation of higher education institutions in eleven general areas of activity and nursing education is no exception:

- Mission goals and objectives
- Governance and administration
- Management of quality assurance and improvement
- Learning and teaching
- Student administration and support services
- Learning resources
- Facilities and equipment
- Financial planning and management
- Employment processes
- Research
- Institutional relationships with the community.

These standards are what is generally accepted as good practice in higher education throughout the world. These general standards are broken into substandards. There are many substandards falling under each individual standard and within substandards, there are many good practices carried out by the institution.

TYPES OF ACCREDITATION

There are two types of accreditation assessment carried out. They are:

- Institutional assessment and accreditation
- Program assessment and accreditation

However, all the above standards are being utilized to assess both institution and program.

Institutional assessment

It means the critical evaluation of the entire institution and all the programs offered by the institution. Program assessment means the critical evaluation of a single program offered in the institution. Course evaluation/assessment means the specific course (subject) taught within the program in a particular institution.

Program assessment

It is defined as the systematic and ongoing method of gathering, analyzing and using information from various sources about a program and measuring program outcomes in order to improve student learning.

In India, we usually address the program as a course. Whereas in other countries, each individual subject is a course and all subjects (courses) put together are considered as the program. For example, fundamentals of nursing, pediatric nursing, mental health nursing, all these are separately called the courses and all these courses put together are a program; for example, BSc nursing program.

NATIONAL QUALIFICATIONS FRAMEWORK

The learning expectations for qualifications do not stop with simple acquisition of knowledge. The learning expectations go beyond this. Strong demand for a much wider range of learning outcomes is expected throughout the world. Internationalization has increased the need for common understanding of expectations from different levels of qualifications. Increasingly, graduates travel overseas for further study or work in an international environment in research and development projects. These pressures have led to the widespread introduction of qualifications frameworks in many parts of the world.

A commitment to lifelong learning is to make it likely that graduates will keep pace with the extremely rapid and accelerating development of new knowledge in their field.

Every country must develop a national qualification framework to assure the students and public that the nursing education provided in the country is equivalent to high international standards. It is intended to ensure consistency within the country of the standards of student learning outcomes regardless of institution attended, and to make clear the equivalence of those standards with those for equivalent awards granted by higher education institutions in other parts of the world.

Expectations on learners:

- Personal characteristics, such as honesty and reliability, capacity to work effectively in groups and provide leadership.
- A wide range of thinking and problem-solving skills:
- Ability to communicate effectively with different types of audience, the ability to investigate new and unexpected problems using a wide range of information sources.
- A commitment to lifelong learning to make it likely that graduates will keep pace with the extremely rapid and accelerating development of new knowledge in their field.

- Every country must develop a national qualification framework to assure the students and public that the nursing education provided in the country is equivalent to high international standards.
- It is intended to ensure consistency within the country of the standards of student learning outcomes regardless of institution attended, and to make clear the equivalence of those standards with those for equivalent awards granted by higher education institutions in other parts of the world.

Levels
Levels are numbered and linked to qualification titles to describe the increasing intellectual demand and complexity of learning expected as students progress to higher academic awards.
Credits
Points are allocated to describe the amount of work or volume of learning expected for an academic award or units or other components of a program.
Learning Domains
These are the broad categories of types of learning outcomes that a program is intended to develop.

ELEMENTS CONSIDERED FOR QUALIFICATIONS FRAMEWORK

Levels

The qualifications framework begins at an entry level, which is the successful completion of secondary education, and culminates with the degree of doctor. Levels in our Indian context include:

Entry	Completion of secondary education
Level 1	Diploma
Level 2	Bachelor
Level 3	Higher Diploma
Level 4	Master
Level 5	Doctor

Credit Hours

Credit hours mean the amount of learning expected to complete the program. In India, in nursing so far assigning credit hours for subjects/programmes are not in practice. In India, we allot specific number of hours for each subject (theory and practice); All the subjects put together make the total required hours to complete the nursing program. Practice in defining credit requirements for academic study varies in different countries.

25

Mission, Vision, Goals and Student Learning Outcomes

Chapter Highlights

- Importance of a Mission Statement
- Writing a Mission
- Defining the Program's Vision Statement
- Defining the Program's Values and Guiding Principles
- Defining Program Goals
- Writing Program Goals
- Reviewing Your Program Goals

Learning Objectives

Upon completion of this chapter, the students will be able to:

- Recognize the importance of a mission statement
- List down the guidelines for writing a mission statement
- Define mission statement
- Demonstrate skill in writing mission, vision statements and program goals

IMPORTANCE OF A MISSION STATEMENT

Mission statement of an institution takes the first place in assuring quality in nursing schools and colleges since this is going to be guiding the entire work. Mission statement functions as a backbone and guide of the organization. An effective mission statement describes the firm's fundamental, unique purpose. An important part of this description indicates how a firm is unique in its scope of operations and its product or service offerings. In simple, yet powerful, terms, a mission statement proclaims corporate purpose. This proclamation indicates what the organization intends to accomplish.

Guidelines to Write a Mission Statement

The mission statement should establish priorities for development and quality improvement and be a key element in the quality assurance process.

- Consequently, it should be prepared in a way that generates a sense of ownership across the institution, be periodically reviewed as a major policy issue by the institution's governing body, and consistently referred to as a basis for planning, evaluation and resource allocation.

The mission of *(name of your program or unit)* is to *(your primary aim)* by providing *(your primary functions or activities)* to *(your stakeholders)*. *Additional clarifying statements.*

- It should be consistent with the charter establishing the institution, and realistic in relation to the capacity of the institution in the environment within which it is operating, but at the same time, present challenges for development and improvement.
  The program mission statement is a concise one.

Definitions of Mission Statement

- 'Setting a clear, realistic mission and then working tirelessly to make sure everyone—from the chairman to the middle manager to the hourly employee—understands it.' (Henkoff 1990).
- The program mission is a *broad statement* of *what the program is, what it does, and for whom it does it.* It should provide a clear description of the *purpose of the program* and the *learning environment.* For a given program, the mission statement, in specific terms, should reflect *how the program contributes to the education and careers of students* graduating from the program. In addition, the mission should be *distinctive* for your program.
- To assure quality in nursing education, the mission statement of the institution should be:
  - Appropriate
  - Useful and guiding
  - Developed considering purpose, primary activity of the institution and it should include the beneficiaries/stakeholders

  Maintains relationship between mission, goals and objectives.

WRITING A MISSION

State the purpose of the nursing program. State the primary purpose of your program—the primary reason(s) why you perform your major activities or operations (e.g. teaching, research, and service). For example, this might include educating nursing students to function as a graduate nurse/instructor. You need to explain why you do what you do.

Check your mission statement

- Is your mission statement brief and memorable?
- Is it distinctive?
- Does it clearly state the purpose of the program
- Does it indicate the primary functions or activities of the program?
- Does it indicate who the stakeholders are?
- Does it clearly support the department's, college's and institution's missions?

- **Mention the primary functions of the program.**
  Highlight the most important functions, operations, outcomes, and/or offerings of the program.
- **Indicate who the stakeholders are.**
  Include the primary groups of individuals for whom we are providing the program and those who will benefit from the program and its graduates (e.g. students, faculty, staff, parents, employers, community etc.).
- **Ensure that the mission statement clearly supports the institution's mission.**
  Make sure that the programme mission is aligned with the mission of the University, college, and the department.
- **The mission should be distinctive.**
  Mission statement must distinguish it from other programs.

Structure of a program mission statement:

The mission of (***name of your program or unit***) is to (***your primary aim***) by providing (***your primary functions or activities***) to (***your stakeholders***)***. Additional clarifying statements, e.g. The mission of 'X' College of Nursing is to prepare excellent dependable graduate nurses by providing world class value-added nursing education to serve the individual, family and community at national and international levels.***

DEFINING THE PROGRAM'S VISION STATEMENT

A vision statement is a short and memorable description of what a program will look like if it succeeds in implementing its strategies and if it achieves its full potential.

Ask the following questions to write vision statement:

Your vision statement must answer these questions:

What would you like the program to become?

- In what direction(s) would you like the program to move?
- What program outcomes would you like to see in the future?

The above questions will be reminding you about the destination, competition, growth and achievements. Definitely, the program outcomes will be giving us the feedback to recheck, assess and act accordingly.

Check your vision statement

- What would you like to become?
- The best
- A leader
- Regionally or nationally recognized
- Other

What would you like to strive for?

- Reputation
- Excellence
- Other

What would you like your program to look like in the future?

DEFINING THE PROGRAM'S VALUES AND GUIDING PRINCIPLES

Values and guiding principles are short statements describing the code of behavior to which an organization or program adheres or aspires. **Value statements** indicate what your program holds and represents. Guiding principles indicate how you would like your program to operate.

Some examples of values include:

- Integrity
- Respect
- Community
- Excellence
- Trust
- Inclusiveness

Example of a value statement

Integrity, respect, community, and excellence are the core values that hold together our program and guide our conduct, performance, and decisions.

Example of a guiding principle

Our program strives to develop partnerships and work in teams to achieve our mission, build community among our students, and innovate to achieve excellence.

When developing your values and guiding principles, answer the following questions: What values would you like your program or students to uphold? How would you like your program or students to operate or behave?

DEFINING PROGRAM GOALS

Goals are broad statements that describe the long-term program targets or directions of development. They state in broad terms what the program wants to accomplish (in terms of student outcomes) or to become over the next several years. Goals relating to functions and administrative units throughout the institution should be thought of as applications of the mission to specific activities. They establish directions for detailed planning though they are usually expressed in general terms.

Goals provide the basis for decisions about the nature, scope, and relative priorities of various activities in a program. They are used in planning and should help move the program to attain its vision.

The general process for writing goals should start with the vision statement for the program (e.g. become the best in the nation). Think about what that program would look like and how it should operate (refer to your mission) to reach that vision and write down these characteristics. This may require improving student outcomes, maximizing employment rates, and minimizing time to degree. Generate a list of potential 'goals' and then prioritize them. Write these more formally as goal statements.

WRITING PROGRAM GOALS

Once you have reached an understanding of the mission of the program on what the program is trying to accomplish, you can start writing the program goals. The following are some guidelines for writing program goals:

- Identify **three or more goals** that are important (i.e. strongly related to the mission and that will help to achieve the vision)
- Goal statements should describe the expected performance of the student or specific behaviors expected from graduates of the program
- Do not identify too many goals, particularly when first starting out.

REVIEWING YOUR PROGRAM GOALS

After generating a list of program goals, the following questions can help to determine whether the list is complete and will be of value to your program:

- Do your goals describe the desired aspects of a successful program?
- Are your goals consistent with your mission?

- If you achieve your goals, have you reached your vision?
- Are your goals aligned with your values?

Student Learning Outcomes are specific statements that describe the required learning achievement that must be met on the way to attaining the degree and meeting ***the goals*** of the program. The outcome statements should be derived from the ***goal statements***, which, in turn, should be aligned with the mission. Goals are broad statements, while learning outcomes are precise, specific and clear statements about the intended outcomes of a program.

Student learning outcomes describe ***specific behaviors*** that a student of your program should demonstrate after having completed the program. Student learning outcome statements should focus on the *expected knowledge, abilities, values and attitudes* of a student after the completion of your program.

Objectives should be linked through ***strategic planning*** processes to the mission and goals of the institution. They should be more specific and include intended levels of performance to be achieved within a stated time period. A well-stated ***mission, vision, values, goals, student learning outcomes*** would provide a quality monitoring platform for the given program. All these statements need to be periodically assessed and reviewed by concerned higher head and faculty members of the organization.

26

Quality Assurance System in Nursing Education

Chapter Highlights

- Need for Quality Assurance in Nursing Education
- Main Tenets of Quality Assurance in Nursing Education
- Various Sections of Quality Standards
- Student Learning Outcomes
- Student Assessment
- Quality of Teaching
- Support for Improvements in Quality of Teaching
- Qualifications and Experience of Teaching Staff
- Quality and Adequacy of Facilities and Equipment
- Resources for Learning
- Relationships with the Community
- Research
- Measurements and Surveys

Learning Objectives

Upon completion of this chapter, the students will be able to:

- Recognize the need for quality assurance in nursing education
- Identify the main tenets of quality assurance in nursing education
- Identify various sections of standards of quality assurance in nursing education
- Describe the process of quality assurance in all the standards related to nursing education

Defining quality is difficult but the expanse of quality is an interaction process between customers and providers. Quality can be defined as the extent of resemblance between the purpose of education and the truly granted care as an outcome of education. In an economic dimension, quality is the extent of accomplished relief case with justified use of means and services (Williamson, 1999). Quality assurance is a dynamic process through which nurses in both academic and clinical practice assume accountability for quality of care they provide (George, Veigas and Isaac, 1984). It is a guarantee to the society that members of the nursing profession are regulating services provided by nurses. Kozier et al. (2004) define quality assurance as the defining of nursing practice through well-written nursing standards and the use of those standards as a basis for evaluation on improvement of client care.

NEED FOR QUALITY ASSURANCE IN NURSING EDUCATION

All over the world, nurses represent the largest group of health care professionals. They are constantly in touch with all the hospital staff and they stay longest with patients performing dependent, interdependent and independent functions (Badru, 2006). Quality assurance has also been reported to assist nurse educators to define educational and clinical guidelines and standards, operating procedures to assess performance compared with selected performance standards as well as take tangible steps towards improving program (English National Board for Nursing, Midwifery and Health Visiting, 1997).

Quality assurance had been found to be cost-effective in nursing education since it promotes confidence, improves communication and fosters clearer understanding of educational and practice needs and expectations (Peterson, Kovel-Jarboe). Quality assurance also provides the nurse education institutions with tools that gauge current performance levels and facilitate continuous improvement. It is found to assist the nurses' satisfaction and motivation (Quinn, 2001). Quality assurance can also be seen as a logical approach for conveying the importance of excellence to individuals who are nursing care recipients. (Schwartz, 1997)

The field of quality assurance is as old as modern nursing. Florence Nightingale in 1860 introduced the concept of quality in nursing when she started a school of nursing to train those who were to give care to the public although within the hospital setting. (Koziers et al, 2004)

Structure/Input

Structure evaluation gives answer to what effect an institution setting has in the quality of education and care given to health care consumers. This includes the setting and the infrastructure used to provide training and care. Such facilities include characteristics of administrative organization, qualification and education of health care providers as well as equipment needed for practicum.

This involves quality of leadership, institutional philosophy, mission statement, vision, management structure, relationship with staff, financial management, staff development policy, public relations and publicity, equal opportunities policies as well as other quality assurance systems, such as maintenance of safety and risk management where practicums are carried out.

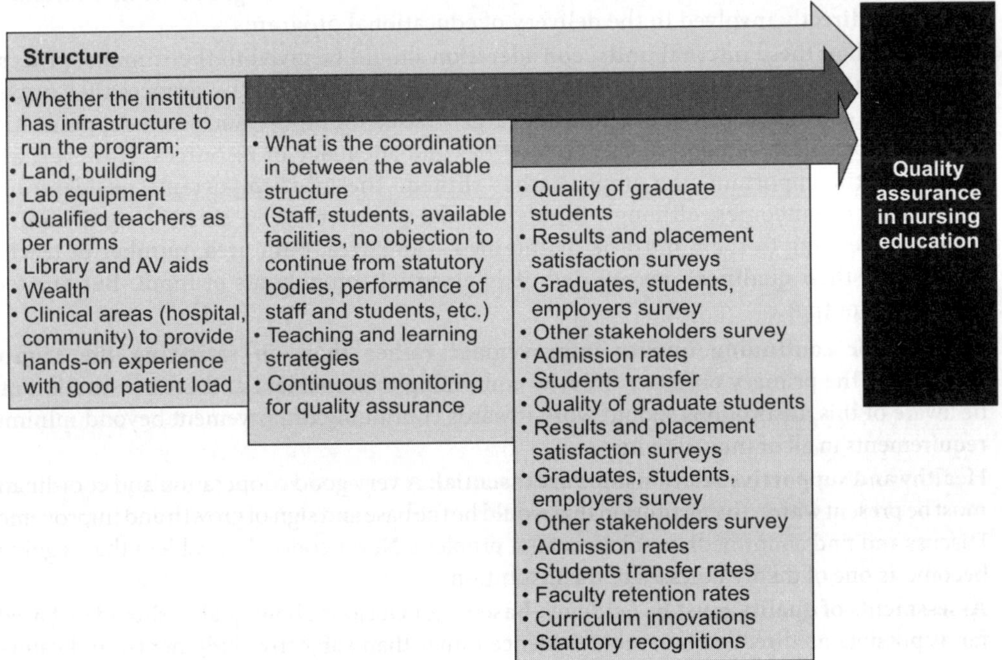

Fig. 26.1: Quality assurance in nursing education

Though the independent reviewers and external agencies are important to assure quality in educational institutions, the institution is fully responsible and accountable to provide quality education to its stakeholders.

Main Tenets of Quality Assurance in Nursing Education

- **Institution is responsible for assuring quality:** The institutions delivering program are responsible for the quality of those programs and for the quality of all of their facilities and activities. In most places, an 'institution' is the legal entity established with authority to grant academic awards.

  Though the external commission or quality agency can have an important role in assisting institutions to plan and introduce strategies for improvement and in evaluating and publicly reporting on what is achieved, this does not remove responsibility from the institution. An external authority can help, but it cannot deliver quality. It is solely the institution that has to take a role in maintaining the quality.

  The institution may decentralize some of its responsibilities or delegate authority to an internal unit, such as a college or department, this does not remove responsibility from the institution as a whole.

- **Quality not an isolated phenomenon:** Quality assurance relates to all functions and activities of the institution. Quality assurance processes in institutions should involve not only the educational programs, but also other matters, such as the facilities and equipment, staffing, relationships with the communities served by the institution and the administrative processes that link all these together. This means that a quality assurance system should involve individuals and academic and organizational units throughout an institution, not only those directly involved in the delivery of educational programs.

  Within each of these internal units, consideration should be given to their inputs, processes and outcomes, with an emphasis on the quality of the outcomes of the services they provide. In the past, considerations of quality were largely based on inputs, such as the qualifications of faculty, provision of equipment and facilities and adequacy of resources. However, while these are still important, the emphasis has shifted. The most important consideration is the quality of outcomes, although inputs and the processes used are still significant and standards relating to them must be maintained. Land area, built area, number of teaching faculty and their qualifications are definitely essential components of input. But our focus must be on output.

- **Support for continuing quality improvement rather than on satisfying the required standards:** The primary objective must be continuing improvement and each institution must be aware of this. Institutions should work towards continuing improvement beyond minimum requirements in all of their activities.

- **Healthy and supportive relationships are essential:** A very good cooperation and coordination must be present within the institution that would be the base and sign of growth and improvement. Discuss and find an immediate solution for a problem. Never conceal a problem that is going to become as one of the weaknesses of the institution.

- **Assessments of quality must be evidence-based:** Conclusions about quality should be based as far as possible on directly observable evidence rather than subjective judgments. Indicators of achievement should be identified in advance, related to valid benchmarks to establish appropriate standards of performance, and systematically reviewed.

- **Total institutional commitment to quality improvement should be achieved through effective leadership and widespread involvement:** A good educational institution should be a learning organization, in which all faculty and staff are involved in evaluating their performance and that of the units within which they work, and offer ideas and plan for improvement following that evaluation. There must be effective leadership and coordination at the level of the institution as a whole, but this leadership and coordination must be combined with wide participation in evaluation, planning and reporting. While effective leadership is essential at the most senior levels of the institution, it is also equally important in internal academic and administrative units.
- **Stakeholders are important:** The substantial involvement of stakeholders in planning and review processes and their regular feedback are necessary. Stakeholders include students and graduates, staff, employers, providers of funds, members of the communities served by the institution and any other groups with which the institution is involved.

  The eleven broad standards apply to both institutions and programs though there are differences in how they are applied for these different kinds of evaluation.

Various Sections of Quality Standards

Various higher educational institutions classify the required standards for assuring quality under specific sections with various substandards under each section. Following are the broader sections under which substandards are organized. Institutions must show great interest and concern in assuring quality in education.

- **A good leadership and program administration:** This must provide effective leadership and reflect an appropriate balance between accountability to senior management and the governing board of the institution within which the program is offered, and flexibility to meet the specific requirements of the program concerned. Planning processes must involve stakeholders (e.g. students, professional bodies, industry representatives, teaching staff). Some of the actions to support the quality assurance in program administration are:
  - Program administrators should have sufficient authority to ensure compliance within the program with formally established or agreed institutional or program policies and procedures.
  - Program administrators should provide leadership, and encourage and reward initiative on the part of teaching and other staff.
  - Program administrators should accept responsibility for the effectiveness of action taken within their area of responsibility regardless of whether that action is taken by them personally or by others responsible to them.
  - Regular feedback should be given on performance of teaching and other staff by the head of the department.
  - Delegations of responsibility should be formally specified in documents signed by the person delegating and the person given delegated authority, that describe clearly the limits of delegated responsibility and responsibility for reporting on decisions made.

Planning Processes

Planning must combine coordinated strategic planning with flexibility to adapt to results achieved and changing circumstances. Planning processes must be managed effectively to achieve the mission and goals of the program through cooperative action by the instructional team and, program and course reporting and decision-making.

To satisfy these requirements, some of the steps are:

- Planning should be strategic, incorporating priorities for development and appropriate sequencing of action to produce the most effective short-term and long-term results.
- Plans should take full and realistic account of aspects of the external environment affecting demand for graduates and the skills they require.
- Planning processes should provide for involvement of teaching and other staff, students and other stakeholders.
- Plans should be effectively communicated to all concerned with impacts and requirement for different constituencies made clear.
- Implementation of plans should be monitored with checks made against short-term and medium-term targets and outcomes evaluated.
- Planning should provide for regular reports on key performance indicators to senior management in the institution.
- Plans should be reviewed, adapted and modified, with corrective action taken as required in response to operational developments, formative evaluation, and changing circumstances.
- **Staff and faculty:** If there is no manpower (teachers), educational show cannot be run. This is one of the most important resources in nurse education training. The staff members must be appointed after a thorough process of evaluation of their qualification and past experiences at work. The institution must also ensure that an annual appraisal of each member of staff is performed for development and formative purposes. It is important also for the institution to provide staff development opportunities so as to maintain quality of service. Staff-student ratio should be such that it will encourage quality in the training of students. Administrative and support staff should be adequate to prevent work overload of academic staff.
  Teaching staff and library/support staff, qualification, motivation, morale, staff-student ratio, staff development opportunities and individual performance review when properly put in place ensures quality assurance of the nurses trained from an institution since these will equip them to deliver quality nursing care wherever they are to practice.

Integrity

- Teaching and other staff involved with the program must meet high ethical standards of honesty and integrity including avoidance of conflicts of interest and avoidance of plagiarism in their teaching, research, administrative and service functions.
- Teaching and other staff and students should comply with codes of practice relating to ethical conduct in research, teaching, performance evaluation and assessment, committee decision making and in the conduct of administrative and service activities.
- Declarations of pecuniary interest should be made whenever they exist and conflicts of interest should be avoided in all dealings by teaching and other staff.
- Advertising and promotional material should always be truthful, avoid any actual or implied misrepresentations or exaggerated claims, or negative comments about other programs or institutions.
- **Internal policies and regulations:** Policies and regulations function as a guide for the administrator. For every action in the institution, there need to be policies.
  Policies and regulations must be established that clearly define the major responsibilities and procedure for the administration of the program and for committees and teaching and other staff and students involved.

To satisfy this requirement, terms of reference and operating procedures associated with the program should be established for major committees and administrative positions.

Policies and regulations should be made available to staff and students and kept in locations that are readily accessible to all teaching and other staff and students who are affected by them, including new members of teaching and other staff, and members of committees.

Decisions made by committees on procedural and academic matters should be recorded and referred to as a guide in future-related decisions to ensure consistency.

Guidelines or regulations should be established for dealing with recurring procedural or academic issues.

All policies, regulations, terms of reference and statements of responsibility relating to the management and delivery of the program should be periodically reviewed and amended as required in the light of changing circumstances.

- **Management of program quality assurance:** Regular evaluations of quality must be undertaken within each course based on valid evidence and appropriate benchmarks, and plans for improvement made and implemented. Quality must be assessed by reference to evidence and include consideration of specific performance indicators and challenging external benchmarks. Teaching and other staff involved in the program must regularly evaluate their own performance and be committed to improving both their own performance and the quality of the program as a whole.

To satisfy this standard

- All teaching and other staff should participate in self-evaluations and cooperate with reporting and improvement processes in their sphere of activity.
- Innovation and creativity should be encouraged within a framework of clear policy guidelines and accountability processes.
- Mistakes and weaknesses should be recognized by those responsible and used as a basis for planning for improvement.
- Improvements in performance should be acknowledged and outstanding achievements recognized.
- Evaluation processes and planning for improvement should be integrated into normal administrative processes.

- **Teaching and Learning:** There are two types of teachers, like inborn and made teachers. It is easy for the inborn teachers to adopt and practice any kind of strict regulations related to quality but made teachers struggle and stress them. Teaching staff are major elements of the institutions that grab attention of the learners to seek admission in any given organization. Teaching staff must be appropriately qualified and experienced for their particular teaching responsibilities, use teaching strategies suitable for different kinds of learning outcomes and participate in activities to improve their teaching effectiveness. Teaching quality and the effectiveness of programs must be evaluated through student assessments and graduate and employer surveys with evidence from these sources used as a basis for plans for improvement.

Student Learning Outcomes

Intended student learning outcomes must be consistent with the National Qualifications Framework, and with generally accepted standards for the field of study concerned including requirements for any professions for which students are being prepared.

Some scales to the standards

- Relevant academic and professional advice should be considered when defining intended learning outcomes.
- Intended learning outcomes should be consistent with the National Qualifications Framework. It differs as per the national policy and requirements.
- Programs leading to professional qualifications should develop learning outcomes that meet requirements for professional practice in a given country in the fields concerned.
- Any special student attributes specified by the institution for its graduates, or in the program, should be incorporated as intended learning outcomes.
- Appropriate program evaluation mechanisms including graduating student surveys, employment outcome data, employer feedback and subsequent performance of graduates should be used to provide evidence about the appropriateness of intended learning outcomes and the extent to which they are achieved.

We need to check on the following aspects to meet the above:

- Program development processes
- Program specifications
- Course specifications
- Content and course delivery
- Evaluation and feedback.

Program Evaluation and Review Processes

Program is monitored regularly through appropriate evaluation mechanisms:

- Courses and programs should be evaluated and reported annually and reports should include information about the effectiveness of planned strategies and the extent to which intended learning outcomes are being achieved.
- When changes are made as a result of evaluations, details of those changes and the reasons for them should be retained in course and program portfolios.
- Quality indicators that include learning outcome measures should be established for all courses and the program.
- Records of student completion rates should be kept for all courses and for the program, and included among quality indicators.
- Reports on the program should be reviewed annually by senior administrators and quality committees.
- Systems should be established for central recording and analysis of course completion and program progression and completion rates and student course and program evaluations, with summaries and comparative data distributed automatically to departments, colleges, senior administrators and relevant committees at least once each year.
- If problems are found through program evaluations, appropriate and timely action should be taken to make improvements.
- In addition to annual evaluations, a comprehensive reassessment of the program should be conducted at least once every five years. Procedures for conducting these reassessments should be consistent with policies and procedures established for the institution.
- Program reviews, should involve experienced people from relevant industries and professions, and experienced teaching staff from other institutions.

- In program reviews, opinions about the program should be obtained from students and graduates through surveys and interviews, discussions with teaching staff, and other stakeholders, such as employers.

Student Assessment

- Student assessment processes must be appropriate for the intended learning outcomes
- Student assessment mechanisms should be appropriate for the different forms of learning sought
- Assessment practices should be clearly communicated to students at the beginning of courses
- Appropriate, valid and reliable mechanisms should be used
- Grading of students' tests, assignments and projects should be assisted by the use of matrices or other means to ensure that the planned range of domains of student learning outcomes are addressed
- Arrangements should be made within the institution for training of teaching staff in the theory and practice of student assessment
- Policies and procedures should include action to be taken to deal with situations where standards of student achievement are inadequate or inconsistently assessed
- Prompt feedback to students on their performance. Assessments of student work should be conducted fairly and objectively
- Criteria and processes for academic appeals should be made known to students and administered equitably.

Quality of Teaching

Teaching must be of high quality with appropriate strategies used for different categories of learning outcomes.

- Effective orientation and training programs should be provided within the institution for new, short-term and part-time teaching staff
- Teaching strategies should be appropriate for the different types of learning outcomes the program is intended to develop
- Strategies of teaching and assessment set out in program and course specifications should be followed by teaching staff with flexibility to respond to the needs of different groups of students
- Students should be fully informed about course requirements in advance through course descriptions that include knowledge and skills to be developed, work requirements and assessment processes
- The conduct of courses should be consistent with the outlines provided to students and with the course specifications
- Textbooks and reference material should be up-to-date and incorporate the latest developments in the field of study
- Textbooks and other required materials should be available in sufficient quantities before classes commence
- Attendance requirements in courses should be made clear to students and compliance with these requirements monitored and enforced
- Effective systems should be used for evaluation of courses and of teaching
- The effectiveness of different planned teaching strategies in achieving learning outcomes in different domains of learning should be regularly reviewed and adjustments should be made in response to evidence about their effectiveness

- Reports should be provided to program administrators on the delivery of each course and these should include details if any planned content could not be dealt with and any difficulties found in using planned strategies
- Appropriate adjustments should be made in plans for teaching if needed after consideration of course reports.

Support for Improvements in Quality of Teaching

The program administrators and teaching staff should support continuing improvement in quality of teaching.

- Training programs in teaching skills should be provided within the institution
- Training programs in teaching should include effective use of new and emerging technology
- Opportunities should be provided for additional professional development of teaching staff
- The extent to which teaching staff are involved in professional development to improve quality of teaching should be monitored
- Teaching staff should be encouraged to develop strategies for improvement of their own teaching. Formal recognition should be given to outstanding teaching, and encouragement given for innovation and creativity
- Strategies for improving quality of teaching should include improving the quality of learning materials and the teaching strategies incorporated in them.

Qualifications and Experience of Teaching Staff

Teaching staff should have appropriate qualifications and experience for the courses they teach. (For undergraduate and masters degree programs, this would normally require academic qualifications in their specific teaching area at least one level above that of the program in which they teach.)

If part-time teaching staff are appointed (for example, in a professional program, where current industry experience may be sought), there should be an appropriate mix of full-time and part-time teaching staff. (As a general guideline, at least 75% of faculty should be employed on a full-time basis.)

- All teaching staff should be involved on a continuing basis in scholarly activities that ensure they remain up-to-date with the latest developments in their field and can involve their students in learning that incorporates those developments.
- Full-time staff teaching postgraduate courses should be active in scholarship and research in the fields of study they teach.

Quality and Adequacy of Facilities and Equipment

Facilities and equipment must be of good quality with effective strategies used to evaluate their adequacy for the program, their quality and the services associated with them.

- Facilities should meet health and safety requirements.
- Quality assessment processes should include both feedback from principal users about the adequacy and quality of facilities, and mechanisms for considering and responding to their views.
- Standards of provision of teaching, laboratory and research facilities should be adequate for the program and should be benchmarked through comparisons with other comparable institutions.

(This includes such things as classroom space, laboratory facilities and equipment, access to computing facilities and associated software, private study facilities, and research equipment.)

- Adequate facilities should be provided for confidential consultations between teaching staff and students.
- Appropriate provision should be made for students and teaching and other staff with physical disabilities or other special needs.

Resources for Learning

There is a growing technology that is closely associated to education. Learning resource materials and associated services must be adequate for the requirements of the program and the courses offered within it and accessible when required for students in the program. Information about requirements must be made available by teaching staff in sufficient time for necessary provisions to be made for resources required, and staff and students must be involved in evaluations of what is provided. This means the adequacy of book stock and periodicals, opening hours, students support, information technology and media resources as well as secretarial and administrative support. The librarians and other staff members should be appointed as per the standards set by the national advisory boards. Library need to be providing current information in printed version or there need to be online provision for accessing the current information. Online data sources and adequate computer terminals to provided in match to the students numbers in the institution.

Steps to plan for and evaluate the learning resources

- Teaching staff responsible for the program and for courses within it should regularly provide advice on materials required to support teaching and learning
- Teaching staff and students should participate in user surveys dealing with adequacy of resources and services, extent of usage, and consistency with requirements for teaching and learning
- Data on the extent of usage of learning resources for the program should be used in evaluations of learning and teaching in the program
- In addition to participation in surveys, program administrators and teaching staff should have opportunities to provide input to evaluations of forward planning for provision of resources and services
- Teaching staff should provide regular advice on material that should be held in reserve in the library to ensure access to necessary materials and this advice should be responded to appropriately
- Library and resource centers and associated facilities and services should be available for sufficient extended hours to ensure access when required by users in the program
- Heavy-demand and required reading materials required for the program should be held in reserve collections
- Provision should be made for reliable and efficient access to online databases and research and journal material relevant to the program.

Help and support to library users

- Orientation and training programs should be provided for new students and other users to prepare them to access facilities and services
- Assistance should be available to help users in conducting researches and locating and using information

- A reference service should be provided through which in-depth questions can be answered by qualified librarians
- Electronic and/or other automated systems with search facilities should be available to assist in locating resources within the institution and in other collections
- Teaching staff and students in the program should be kept informed about library developments, such as acquisition of new materials, training programs, or changes in services or opening hours.

When these services are put in place, learning is often made easy and the quality of the trained nurses is shown in their area of practice.

Financial Planning and Management

Financial resources must be sufficient for the effective delivery of the program. Program requirements must be made known sufficiently far in advance to be considered in institutional budgeting. Budgetary processes should allow for long-term planning over at least a three-year period. Sufficient flexibility must be provided for effective management and responses to unexpected events and this flexibility must be combined with appropriate accountability and reporting mechanisms.

- Sufficient delegations of spending authority should be given to the program manager/head of department for effective program administration
- Any financial delegations should be clearly specified, and accompanied by appropriate accountability and reporting processes
- The program manager/head of department should be involved in the budget planning process, and be held accountable for expenditure within the approved budgets
- The accounting system should provide for accurate monitoring of expenditure and commitments against budgets with regular reports prepared throughout the year for the program/department.

Relationships with the Community

Commitment to service to the community by the department or program must be clearly specified, clear in its nature and scope, consistent with the community service policies of the institution and appropriate for the particular skills and knowledge of staff teaching in the program. The service commitment should be supported by policies to encourage involvement and regular reports prepared on activities that take place.

To meet the standards

- The service commitment of the program should be defined in a way that reflects the community or communities, within which the institution operates, and the skills and abilities of staff teaching in the program
- Contributions to the community by staff teaching in the program should be observed
- Community contributions should be included in promotion criteria and staff assessments
- Program initiatives in working with the community should be coordinated with responsible units in the institution to avoid duplication and possible confusion.

RESEARCH

The importance of research was established by Florence Nightingale in 1854, when during the Crimean war she found the military hospital and barracks to be overcrowded, filthy, rat- and flea-infected and lacking in food, drugs and essential medical supplies which she found led to the men dying from starvation, waterborne diseases and infection from wounds. This she achieved through systematically collecting, organizing and reporting data. Data analysis helped institute sanitary reforms and thus significantly reduced morbidity and mortality rates among the soldiers.

Today, nurses are actively generating, publishing and applying research in practice to improve client care and enhance nursing scientific knowledge base. The standards of clinical nursing practice published by American Nurses Association (ANA, 1998) include research as one of the standards of professional performance should be based on standards attained by students' degree classification.

Student Guidance and Counseling

Guidance and counseling by teachers and availability of school counseling services always encourage students to review their learning objectives and sort out other matters that may affect their learning negatively. Process evaluation in nursing also focuses on the manner in which the students use training given during theory and practicum. Process evaluation evaluates activities as they relate to standards in nursing profession and expectations of institution and health providers. Quinn (2001) opines that the management of nurse training evaluation can be collected through direct observations during teacher-student interactions, review towards quality in records, audit, checklist approach and the criteria-mapping approach. All these are employed to establish the student nurse's encounter protocol.

Outcome Evaluation

This involves evaluation of specific behavior/skills students exhibit during training and in the clinical setting. Outcome evaluation thus looks at the net changes that occur as a result of training (education) given (Johnson, Maas and Moorhead, 2000). The data of this can be collected from records kept by the school through questionnaire as well as nursing care services rendered to clients during practicum. Outcome evaluation can be referred to as summative evaluation, which is concerned with the product or results of the teaching learning process. It is the final or overall assessment of students' performance or achievement after a successful completion of unit study (Page, 1999).

Educational Institutions should get feedback about the course (each subject), students' experience in the institution and program performance from their existing students and graduating students. Some of the useful methods that would give a fine feedback to the institutions are:

- **Course Evaluation Survey:** All the courses (subjects) are to be evaluated. It is done at the end of the semester or year. The survey does not directly assess the quality of teaching by individual instructors. However the evaluation of the course is seen as a reasonable measure of the quality of teaching in a way that minimizes personal issues that could inhibit responses from students.
- **Student Experience Survey:** This is intended as a general survey that might be distributed to all students part way through their program—midway of the four-year program is recommended. The survey deals with the student's life at the institution including both major elements of the program in which they are enrolled and a number of general items relating to services and facilities.
- **Program Evaluation Survey:** This survey is intended for use at the time students have finished their program and are about to graduate. It is recommended that it be distributed shortly before final year classes are finished so their opinion of the total program at that stage can be assessed.

In addition to these, educational institutions should also analyze and measure some happenings of the program and conduct stakeholders' surveys to get the feedback about the institution and the different programs offered by the institution.

Measurements and Surveys

Some of the useful methods that would give a fine feedback to the institutions in this regard are:

Clear organization chart : This must indicate the levels of the position, reporting hierarchy and control. Dual reporting always causes problems. Team work under guidance of one boss (For example, Nursing Dean or Principal or Principal coordinator of the programme). Quality assurance team reports the head of the institution. Quality monitoring unit is always having the eye on the entire process of the educational programme.

Policies and procedures for any kind of work

Some examples are:

- Executive policies
- Staff conduct policies
- Students' code of conduct policy
- Admission policy
- Faculty, staff recruitment policy
- Policies for different committees (Examples: Curriculum committee, students' support services committee, disciplinary committee, program evaluation committee, examination committee, question paper vetting committee)
- Service rules and regulations policy
- Learning contract policy
- Workload—Faculty, teaching staff and students
- Students' appeal policy
- Attendance policy
- Assignment grading policy
- Limits of delegation policy
- To assure quality in educational institutions, the institutions must have clear-cut policies that would help us function without any delay.

The following are some of the figures which alert as well as give feedback.

The following are some of the examples:

- Students' dropout rates
- Students' sickness rates and reasons
- Students' transfer rates
- Students' pass rate in each course/subject
- Program completion within stipulated duration of the program
- Students' pass rates in each year
- Admission rates
- Staff-turnover rates
- Number of continuing education programs conducted
- Staff participation in educational activities—conferences, workshops, seminars, journal clubs, etc.
- Students' participation in educational activities
- Mentoring programs

- Continuing nursing education sessions
- Frequency in changing the leadership of the institution
- Parents' survey
- Graduates' destination survey
- Number of graduates going for higher education
- Survey on unemployed graduates
- Employers' satisfaction survey
- Good-practice survey among faculty and teaching staff.

Outcome Evaluation in Clinical Area

In the clinical area, outcome evaluation employs several methods to ensure and enhance quality.

These include using the following:

- **The tracer method:** This is a measure of both process and outcome of care. To use the tracer method, a nurse must be able to identify a volume of client with a particular characteristic resuming specific health care management. This method provides nurses with data to show the differences in outcome as a result of nursing care standards.
- **The sentinel method:** It is an outcome measure for examining specific instances of client care. It uses characteristics such as: the circumstances surrounding an event that require detailed examination, the review of morbidity and mortality as an index for action, health status indicator, such as changes in social, economic, political and environmental factors which may have effect on health outcomes are reviewed, as well as counting of unnecessary disease, disability and death.
- **Client satisfaction:** Nursing audit is the tool used to assess client satisfaction of care. Data collected from client is used to measure structure, process and outcome of caregivers. When deficiencies identified by the audit report are corrected, the benefits go to the consumers of nursing services (N & MCN, 2005).

Index